Modules for
Basic Nursing Skills Volume 2

Houghton Mifflin offers two other books for introductory nursing, which can be used either in conjunction with the present volume or independently.

Ellis/Nowlis: Nursing: A Human Needs Approach presents the theory and rationale that underlie nursing practice.

Ellis/Nowlis/Bentz: Modules for Basic Nursing Skills, Second Edition, Volume 1, contains the following skill topics: Assessment; Charting; Medical Asepsis; Basic Body Mechanics; Feeding Adult Patients; Bedmaking; Assisting with Elimination and Perineal Care; Hygiene; Basic Infant Care; Admission and Discharge; Intake and Output; Moving the Patient in Bed and Positioning; Applying Restraints; Range-of-Motion Exercises; Transfer; Ambulation; Postmortem Care; Collecting Specimens; Administering Enemas; Temperature, Pulse, and Respiration; Blood Pressure; Isolation Technique; Assisting with Examinations and Procedures; Applying Bandages and Binders; Applying Heat and Cold; and Cardiopulmonary Resuscitation.

Modules for Basic Nursing Skills   Volume 2

Second Edition

Janice Rider Ellis, R.N., M.N.
Elizabeth Ann Nowlis, R.N., M.N.
Patricia M. Bentz, R.N., M.S.N.
Shoreline Community College

Houghton Mifflin Company   Boston
Dallas   Geneva, Illinois   Hopewell, New Jersey
Palo Alto   London

Cover photo by Fredrik D. Bodin

Illustrations by Jeremy Elkin and Richard Spencer

Printed in the U.S.A.

Library of Congress Catalog Card Number: 79-89521

ISBN: 0-395-28655-7

Contents

List of Skills

The following skills are included in this volume. For easy reference, a module number and page number are provided for each skill.

To the Instructor

Modules for Basic Nursing Skills, Second Edition, is a two-volume text designed to teach beginning nursing students how to perform basic skills and procedures. It can be used in the clinical practice laboratory of an introductory nursing course or in any other suitable setting.

Skills are arranged in a progression from simple to complex throughout the two volumes, but each skill module is self-contained to permit instructors to omit or reorder skills according to the needs of their own programs. In the second edition, we have doubled the number of skills covered in the first edition and now present forty-eight modules in two volumes. Volume 1 contains the most basic skills and may be appropriate by itself for some courses enrolling LPN/LVN students, as well as for courses for nursing aides and nursing assistants. Volumes 1 and 2 together may be most useful in programs for RN students. Because programs vary considerably from state to state and from institution to institution, we have tried to make our second edition as adaptable as possible to many different programs by offering comprehensive coverage of nursing skills.

The format of the modules focuses on the student's practice and mastery of skills and procedures. It is designed for independent learning and self-instruction. Each module contains a main objective, a rationale, a list of prerequisites, specific learning objectives, a set of learning activities, a vocabulary list, a core of background and step-by-step instructions with carefully chosen photographs and illustrations, a performance checklist, and a quiz. These parts are described in detail in the next section entitled "To The Student." At the back of each volume of modules, we have given a glossary containing definitions of the words in the vocabulary lists and answer keys to the quizzes. The two volumes are three-hole punched with perforated pages, so students can tear out pages and hand them in or keep the modules in notebooks.

Modules for Basic Nursing Skills, Second Edition, Volumes 1 and 2 can be used in conjunction with the text by Ellis and Nowlis, *Nursing: A Human Needs Approach,* which treats the theory behind nursing practice. The two volumes of modules are designed to stand alone, however, and can be used by themselves in a course addressing nursing skills. *Modules for Basic Nursing Skills* can also be used in conjunction with any other text covering nursing theory or fundamentals.

We would like to thank the following individuals for their reviews of our manuscript at various stages and their many useful suggestions: the late Susan T. Reynolds, Bryn Mawr Hospital; Joan Long, University of North Carolina; Ramona Gonzales, College of Santa Fe; Betty Fallath, Community College of Baltimore; Teresa Gherkin, Montgomery County Community College; Martha Worthington, St. Petersburg Junior College; Marilee Creelan, Isabelle Firestone School of Nursing, Akron City Hospital; the late Dorothea T. Schmidt Penta, Middlesex Community College, Massachusetts; and Elizabeth Winning, R.N., Group Health Cooperative of Puget Sound, Seattle, Washington. We are especially grateful to our students and colleagues who have worked with the modules as they were originally written, through the changes made for the first published edition, and in planning for this revision. Their constant feedback has been essential to us.

To the Student

This set of modules is designed to enable you to learn the procedures basic to your role as a nurse. Each module has the following parts, unless they are not applicable to a particular skill:

Main Objective   A general statement of the basic skill that is taught in the module.

Rationale   The reason why you need to learn the skill.

Prerequisites   A list of specific skills or abilities needed to master the new skill. Also listed are other modules whose contents are necessary for an understanding of the skill.

Specific Learning Objectives   A table that breaks down the basic skill you are studying into specific subskills that you can test yourself on after completing the module.

Learning Activities   Activities designed to help you progress safely and gradually into carrying out the new skill. Practice, in whatever setting is available, is essential to skillful performance. Different students will need differing amounts of practice, depending on their manual dexterity and previous experience. Your school may provide audiovisual aids to use with the module. If so, view them after reading the module but before going on to actually practice the skill. Do not hesitate to contact your instructor if you encounter difficulties.

Vocabulary   A list of special terms used in the module. The glossary will give the definitions of most. Some terms will be best understood in the context of the module itself.

Module Core   Necessary background information and a step-by-step guide to performing the skill, including photographs and illustrations where necessary.

Performance Checklist   A brief guide both to use while you are practicing the skill and to judge your performance by.

Quiz   A brief review for self-testing.

Key   The answers at the back of the text allow you to score yourself.

Glossary   At the end of the volume, a glossary provides definitions for the key vocabulary terms.

There are, of course, many advanced nursing procedures not covered in the modules, but the skills that are included are basic to the educational preparation of the nurse.

As authors, we hope you will find gaining these essential skills to be a satisfying endeavor, and we wish you our best as you begin your studies.

Janice Rider Ellis
Elizabeth Ann Nowlis
Patricia M. Bentz

Module 27 Common Laboratory Tests

MAIN OBJECTIVE

To be able to perform with accuracy the common laboratory tests that are used in nursing practice.

RATIONALE

Laboratory tests remain an important part of establishing a diagnosis. In addition, laboratory tests indicate a patient's progress and can serve as the basis for planning therapy.

Modern technology has made many laboratory tests very simple to perform. Because no elaborate laboratory equipment or technical skills are needed, the tests are often performed on the unit. This makes the results immediately available.

Although not technically difficult, the tests must be done carefully and accurately. This places an additional burden on the nurse, who must know the purpose of the tests and the procedures to be followed. (Consult your medical-surgical textbook for information on why these tests are performed and the significance of the results of the tests.)

PREREQUISITES

Successful completion of the following modules:

VOLUME 1
Charting
Medical Asepsis
Collecting Specimens

SPECIFIC LEARNING OBJECTIVES

	Know Facts and Principles	Apply Facts and Principles	Demonstrate Ability	Evaluate Performance
1. Equipment	Name equipment used to test or measure in each procedure	Given a situation, select correct equipment for specific test	In the clinical setting, select equipment to perform test on patient's specimen	Evaluate with instructor
2. Specific gravity	Define specific gravity. Know normal range for specific gravity of urine.	When measuring specific gravity of urine in the practice setting, determine if finding is normal	In the clinical setting, correctly measure specific gravity of patient's urine	Evaluate with instructor
3. pH	Define pH. Know normal range for pH of urine.	When measuring pH of urine in the practice setting, determine if finding is normal	In the clinical setting, correctly measure pH of urine of patient	Evaluate accuracy with instructor
4. Using tablets and strips to test urine, blood, and feces	Identify various methods for testing or measuring substances in urine, blood, and feces	In the practice setting, successfully carry out the various tests on urine, blood, and feces	In the clinical setting, correctly carry out available test procedures on urine, blood, and feces, under supervision of instructor	Evaluate own performance using Performance Checklist
5. Recording	State how results of each procedure should be recorded	Given a specific situation, demonstrate accurate recording of results	In the clinical setting, accurately record results on chart	Evaluate recording with instructor

LEARNING ACTIVITIES

1. Review the Specific Learning Objectives.
2. Look up the module vocabulary terms in the glossary.
3. Read through the module.
4. In the practice setting:
   a. Inspect the urinometer, culture tubes, and various tablets and strips used in performing tests.
   b. Read the various accompanying instructional inserts.
   c. For practice, using a urine specimen obtained from yourself or a partner, test for specific gravity, blood, glucose, and ketone bodies using the methods available.
   d. Take home a tongue blade and folder to collect a smear of feces. Bring the folder to the practice laboratory and complete the procedure for checking your own fecal sample for occult blood.
   e. Using culture equipment (it need not be sterile), culture your partner's throat. Complete the procedure as if the specimen were being sent to the laboratory. Discard the culture.
5. In the clinical setting:
   a. With your instructor's supervision, perform any of the following activities using the method of your facility:
      (1) Measuring specific gravity of urine
      (2) Testing for glucose in the urine
      (3) Measuring the glucose level of the blood
      (4) Testing for ketone bodies in the urine
      (5) Testing for blood in the urine, stool, or gastric secretions
      (6) Obtaining cultures of feces, urine, or body fluids

VOCABULARY

acetone
acid
alkaline
ampule
bilirubin
caustic
displacement
exudate
feces
glucose
guaiac
hydrometer
ketone body
litmus paper
meniscus
occult
pH
protein
reagent
urinometer

COMMON LABORATORY TESTS

In this module, we will discuss the following tests: specific gravity of urine, pH of urine, urine glucose and ketone bodies, and occult blood in the urine and feces. (See Figure 27.1.) We will also look at how cultures are obtained. All the names of the tablets and strips described are brand names.

Equipment

The equipment for performing tests on bodily excretions is usually kept in the utility room. Those patients who require frequent testing of one type or another may have their own equipment kept in the bathroom. The equipment for cultures is usually kept with other sterile supplies.

You should know where, in your facility, to obtain new items or to restock the equipment used to perform tests. Reagent tablets, strips, and litmus paper usually come from the pharmacy; glass urinometers and culture tubes, as well as Culturettes, are often ordered from the central supply department.

But facilities do vary, so be familiar with the arrangement in yours.

Tablets, strips, and litmus paper can be kept indefinitely, so long as they are not unnecessarily exposed to bright light or moisture. Keep the brown glass bottles and the boxes used for these items tightly capped or closed. Keep all directions, packet inserts, and color charts with the appropriate products, so that errors do not occur.

Specific Gravity of Urine

Specific gravity is a measurement of the concentration of urine. Overhydration, or any disease that affects the body's ability to concentrate particles in the urine, leads to a low specific gravity figure. Conversely, dehydration, or any condition that increases water reabsorption, results in a high specific-gravity figure. The numbers used to delineate the normal range vary slightly, depending on the facility in which you practice or the text that you consult. Generally, the normal specific gravity range for urine is approximately 1.010 to 1.030 G/ml (grams per milliliter).

Reagent	Type	Specimen	Measures or Tests
Clinitest	Tablet	Urine	Glucose
Clinistix	Strip	Urine	Glucose
Diastix	Strip	Urine	Glucose
Testape	Tape	Urine	Glucose
Dextrostix	Strip	Blood	Glucose
Acetest	Tablet	Urine	Ketone bodies
Ketostix	Strip	Urine	Ketone bodies
Ketodiastix	Strip	Urine	Glucose, ketone bodies
Uristix	Strip	Urine	Glucose, ketone bodies
Combistix	Strip	Urine	Glucose, ketone bodies, pH
Labstix	Strip	Urine	Glucose, ketone bodies, pH, protein, blood
Bili-Labstix	Strip	Urine	Glucose, ketone bodies, pH, protein, blood, bilirubin
Hemastix	Strip	Urine	Blood
Hematest	Tablet	Feces	Blood
Hemoccult slide	Envelope	Feces	Blood

FIGURE 27.1   AVAILABLE TESTING PRODUCTS

EQUIPMENT

Specific gravity is measured with a *urinometer*—a device that measures the concentration of the urine by the simple principle of displacement. The particles that are in the urine displace or push the bulb of the urinometer upward. The specific gravity is read as the number at the meniscus of the urine. Because a heavy concentration of particles in the urine pushes the bulb higher, you will find a higher number at the meniscus as the specific gravity increases. (See Figure 27.2.)

MEASURING SPECIFIC GRAVITY

1. Collect at least 20 ml urine. The urine must be collected in a clean container so that extraneous particles do not alter the true concentration of the urine.
2. Obtain a urinometer (urine hydrometer).
3. Pour at least 20 ml of urine into the urinometer so that the base of the bulb floats and does not touch the bottom.
4. Twist the stem of the bulb slightly so that the bulb floats freely and is not "hung up" on the side of the container.
5. Elevate the urinometer to eye level, or place it on a firm surface and stoop to read it.
6. Read the lower meniscus. If the meniscus falls directly between two lines, always read to the next higher.
7. Record the number on paper; you will include it later in the patient's chart. (Often nurses attempt to remember readings of various procedures in an effort to save time, only to have to repeat the procedure later when their recall is not accurate. It is better to record numbers when you first obtain them.)
8. Dispose of the specimen and clean the equipment with soap and water.
9. Wash your hands.
10. Record data on the patient's chart.

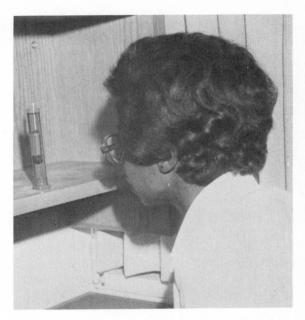

FIGURE 27.2 URINOMETER (urine hydrometer)
Courtesy Lawrence Cherkas. Urinometer courtesy of Francis Freas Glassworks

pH of Urine

Students of chemistry will remember that pH is a measurement of the concentration of hydrogen ions. These values are given on a scale from 1 to 14. The value 7 is neutral; lower is acid, and higher is base (alkaline). The normal pH range of urine is between 6 and 7, or slightly acid. Using litmus paper, you report in general terms (acid or alkaline).

EQUIPMENT

Blue litmus paper that turns red on contact with acid and remains blue in the presence of a base is most commonly used. A red litmus paper that remains red in the presence of acid and turns blue when in contact with a base may also be used. Whichever litmus paper is used, remember that *blue* (with a *B*) is always *base* (with a *B*) to avoid confusion.

MEASURING THE pH OF URINE

1. Obtain the urine specimen.
2. Obtain the litmus paper.
3. Dip the litmus paper into the urine.

4. Tap the paper on the side of the container to remove excess urine.
5. Read as acid for red (pink) and alkaline for blue. (This is a general test for pH. If a more definitive test is needed, with a quantitative number for pH, send a urine specimen to the laboratory, where a reactive agent will be used to test it.)
6. Discard the specimen and the litmus paper.
7. Wash your hands.
8. Record the reading as "acid" or "alkaline" on the patient's record.

Urine Glucose

Glucose in the urine is most often caused by high blood glucose levels. Thus, urine glucose measurement is a simple indirect method of identifying blood glucose level. However, in patients with kidney disease or in patients taking certain drugs, urine glucose may not be a reliable indicator of blood glucose level. For these persons, direct laboratory measurement of blood glucose may be needed. Often, both blood and urine glucose measurements are made, so that the physician can deter-

mine whether the urine glucose does accurately reflect blood glucose.

If you identify anything that will interfere with the accuracy of a urine glucose measurement, consult the physician.

EQUIPMENT

Many different commercial products are available to test for glucose in the urine. Among the most common are Clinistix, Clinitest, Dextrostix, Diastix, and Testape. Each has advantages and disadvantages. One problem is that false readings on each product can be caused by a variety of different drugs. Compare the literature regarding each product with the list of drugs the patient is taking, so that you can choose the correct product for the test. (See Figure 27.3.) Most facilities routinely keep at least two products available.

Each product uses a color scale to reflect differences in glucose content. The color scale is based on the reactions of the chemicals used in that product. Therefore, the color scales are *not* interchangeable.

Traditionally, products that tested for glucose in the urine had a scale that reported

Drug	Clinitest	Testape	Acetest
Aldomet	False positive		
Ascorbic acid (large doses)	False positive	False negative	
Benemid	False positive		
Cancer metabolites		False negative	
Cephalosporins (Keflex, Keflin, Loridine)	False positive		
Chloral hydrate (large doses)	False positive		
Chloromycetin	False positive		
INH (isoniazid)	False positive		
Levodopa (L-dopa)	False positive	False negative	False positive
Paraldehyde			False positive
Pyridium		False positive or negative	
Skelaxin	False positive		
Sulfonamides	False positive		
Tetracyclines	False positive		

FIGURE 27.3   DRUG INTERFERENCE WITH URINE TESTING

results as *negative, trace, one plus* (+ or 1+) *two plus* (++ or 2+), *three plus* (+++ or 3+), and so forth. Each of these represents a specific percentage of glucose. As new products have come on the market, their scales have also been set up with pluses. However, the pluses in one product *do not* correspond to the same percentage of glucose as do the pluses in another product. For example, Clinitest (5-drop method) 2+ equals .75 percent glucose, while Testape 2+ equals .25 percent glucose.

Because therapy (drugs, diet, and the like) is often prescribed on the basis of glucose in the urine, the potential for confusion can be dangerous. Therefore, some facilities recommend that all glucose readings be reported as percentages. This would help eliminate one source of error. You must follow the policy in your facility, however. If pluses are used as a basis for prescribing therapy, it is your responsibility to clarify with the physician what product is to be used as the basis for the prescription. Be sure to consult further if you find you must use a different product than that agreed on because of drug interference.

Once a product has been chosen, use it consistently for that patient. Because there are minor differences in each product, you will have a more reliable and consistent record if you use the same product.

SPECIMEN COLLECTION

The timing of the collection of a urine specimen to test for glucose is critical. Urine that has accumulated in the bladder reflects conditions in the body at the time the urine was formed. Thus, the first specimen in the morning contains urine secreted throughout the night. It is impossible to know whether glucose in that specimen was secreted at midnight, 2:00 a.m., or 6:00 a.m.

Therefore, use a second-voided, or double-voided, specimen. Have the patient void. (In some facilities this first specimen is saved just in case a further specimen is not obtained.) Wait thirty minutes, and ask the patient to void again. Use this second specimen for the test. Because only 1 or 2 ml of urine are needed for the test, most patients have no difficulty voiding this amount. And, by using this method, you know you are testing freshly secreted urine.

If the patient cannot void again, test the first urine specimen. A negative reading can be recorded, since no glucose was secreted at any time since the last voiding. If, however, any glucose at all is present, you must test a second specimen.

GENERAL PROCEDURE

1. Collect 1 to 2 ml urine in a clean container. Use a second-voided specimen.
2. Obtain the correct product for that patient for testing the urine for glucose.
3. Review the directions on the product.
4. Place the correct color scale where it is clearly visible.
5. Proceed with steps a or b, depending on the type of product you are using.
   a. Clinitest:
      One of the first simple tests that were devised to test for urine glucose was the Clinitest. It has two advantages: first, it is easy to use; second, except for the test interference with drugs, it is relatively precise. There are, however, several disadvantages. First, the tablets are poisonous, which could be a concern if the patient must carry out the test at home, with small children around. Second, the tablets are caustic when moist and can burn fingers. Third, the tablets deteriorate on exposure to moisture. Fourth, the method requires the use of test tubes and droppers, and takes relatively more time than do other methods. And, finally, many drugs can cause false readings with the product.

      There are two methods for using Clinitest: the 5-drop method is the most common; the 2-drop method is used to detect more exact percentages when high levels of glucose are found

in the urine. Each has its own color scale. Follow these directions for the 5-drop method:

(1) Obtain a clean glass test tube, a test tube holder, a dropper, and tablets.

(2) Place the test tube in the holder. If necessary, you can hold the test tube carefully at the top edge. Remember that the part of the test tube in contact with the solution will become hot enough to burn.

(3) Using the dropper, place 5 drops of urine in the test tube. (Save the remainder of the specimen in case it is necessary to repeat the test.)

(4) Rinse the dropper.

(5) Using the same dropper, place 10 drops of water in the test tube.

(6) Using a dry hand or a container top, place 1 Clinitest tablet in the test tube.

(7) *Watch the tube carefully.* If, while you are watching, the color bubbles through orange and turns dark, this is called *pass-through.* Pass-through indicates a high percentage of glucose in the urine, so the 5-drop method will not be accurate. You should report this and usually, go on to do a 2-drop test. If the color does not turn dark, *when the bubbling stops,* begin timing for 15 seconds.

(8) After 15 seconds have elapsed, shake the tube gently and compare the color of the solution with the color chart.

For the 2-drop method, follow the 5-drop directions, using *2* drops of urine and *10* drops of water. Be sure to use the appropriate color chart for the method.

b. Reagent strip tests (Clinistix, Diastix, Testape):

These tests use a clinical reagent im-pregnated in paper strips. The results of the reagent strip tests are less often altered by drugs and therefore are often recommended. The method of use for each is the same, although the timing and color charts are specific to the individual product.

(1) Remove a reagent strip from the container. Do not touch the area of the strip where the reagent is present.

(2) Dip the strip into the urine, tapping on the container to remove excess urine. For an in-continent patient or an infant, press the reagent strip onto the wet linen or wet diaper.

(3) Begin timing according to direc-tions.

(4) At end of the specified time period, compare the color on the strip with the correct color chart.

6. Record the results immediately on a piece of paper, for later transfer to the patient's chart.

7. Discard the urine and the strip, if used. Thoroughly rinse any equipment used and store.

8. Wash your hands.

9. Record the urine glucose results on the patient's chart. A flow sheet is often used to keep a tabular account of urine glucose. It usually is marked "Neg.," "1+," "2+," or "3+," as appropriate. If a table is not used, write a brief narrative note indicating the test results. For example:

9/10/80, 6:30 a.m. Urine specimen neg. for glucose.   J. Smith, RN

Blood Glucose

In some facilities, nurses perform finger and heel sticks for blood and check for blood glucose using a reagent strip. If this is a nursing responsibility in your facility, you should ask for direction and supervision to learn to do the "stick" correctly, Again, follow the directions on the package care-fully in using the reagent strip.

Ketone Bodies in Urine

Sometimes this test is called a test for *acetone.* Acetone is one of several ketones (ketone bodies) that can be produced in the body. All ketone bodies are significant, and the tests used do indicate all ketone bodies, not only to acetone.

Ketone bodies are a product of incomplete fat metabolism. They are present in urine only when fat is being broken down rapidly and incompletely. This can occur with rigid dieting or with uncontrolled diabetes. Most commonly, the urine is tested for ketone bodies in the diabetic patient to identify lack of control. Test the urine for ketones at the same time that you test it for glucose.

EQUIPMENT

Both tablets and reagent strips are available to test for ketones. The reagent strips are quicker and require less equipment.

PROCEDURE

1. Collect a fresh urine specimen. If ketones are present in the urine, they will increase as the urine stands at room temperature. Therefore, old urine gives an incorrect result.
2. Obtain the correct product and the directions for its use.
3. Review the directions.
4. Place the color chart where it is clearly visible.
5. Proceed with steps a or b, depending on the product you are using.
   a. Acetest tablets:
      (1) Place 1 tablet on a piece of filter paper or a paper towel.
      (2) Using a dropper, place 1 drop of urine on the tablet.
      (3) Begin timing.
      (4) Wait 15 seconds.
      (5) Compare the color of the tablet with the color chart.
   b. Reagent strips (Diastix, Ketostix, Uristix):
      (1) Remove the strip from the bottle, being careful not to touch

the area that is impregnated with the reagent.
      (2) Dip the strip into the urine.
      (3) Tap the strip on the edge of the container to remove excess urine.
      (4) Begin timing.
      (5) Time for 60 seconds.
      (6) Compare the strip to appropriate color chart.
6. Record the results (negative, positive, strongly positive) on paper immediately.
7. Discard the urine and the specimen, and clean any equipment used.
8. Wash your hands.
9. Transfer the information to the patient's chart. Frequently glucose and ketones are recorded together. The glucose result is given first, and then the ketone result. For example:

   Neg./Neg.
   1+/Neg.
   2+/Pos.

Blood in the Urine

Urine should be free of blood. Grossly bloody urine can result from disease conditions, trauma, or the menstrual flow. But, blood can be present in urine without being visible as such. The urine could have only a cloudy or hazy appearance. This is called *occult,* or hidden, blood.

Hemastix reagent strips are used to test for occult blood. Use them as you would other reagent strips. After 30 seconds, read the strip against the color chart.

Strip Combination Tests for Urine

There are now available reagent strips that test for several substances at the same time. These strips have a small area of reagent for each test being done. Although multiple strips are convenient, they do create opportunities for error. For example:

1. Confusing which area on the strip contains the reagent for which substance
2. Incorrectly timing the different areas

3. Comparing the color of the area on the strip with the wrong color chart

When you use multiple reagent strips, be especially careful about these three points.

Blood in Feces

Often, blood is not so visible in feces as it is in other body tissues and fluids. The undigested portions of oral iron preparations give the stool a black appearance that either can be mistaken for blood or can mask the presence of occult blood. Also, patients who have eaten rare red meat in the three days before the test may test positive for occult blood, which is why some physicians place patients on a red-meat-free diet for three days before the test.

GENERAL PROCEDURE

There are several methods of testing for occult blood, but we can draw the following guidelines:

1. Obtain a stool specimen. Use a tongue blade to place a small amount of stool in a container.
2. Wash your hands.
3. Obtain the test product.
4. Review the directions for that product.
5. Proceed with step a, b, or c, depending on the product you are using.
   a. Hematest:
      (1) Smear a thin layer of fecal material on the filter paper provided. This can be done with a tongue depressor.
      (2) Place a Hematest tablet in the center of the specimen.
      (3) Place 1 drop of water on the tablet.
      (4) Wait 10 seconds for the water to penetrate the tablet.
      (5) Add a second drop of water to thoroughly saturate the tablet and specimen; the water should run down the side of the tablet.
      (6) Wait an additional 20 seconds.
      (7) Observe the paper for the presence of a blue color. If blue is present, read positive for occult blood.
   b. Hemoccult slide:
      The Hemoccult slide is a small cardboard envelope. It was originally designed for the visiting nurse or patient at home to mail in a specimen for testing. (The envelope would be enclosed in a mailing envelope.) Because of its convenience, the Hemoccult slide is now widely used on nursing units.

      The envelope, with specimen enclosed (steps 1 and 2, below) can be sent to the laboratory for the actual test. The procedure below is for processing on the unit.
      (1) Open the envelope flap.
      (2) With an applicator, apply a thin smear of fecal material over the inside circle.
      (3) Drop the reagent solution onto the fecal smear.
      (4) Watch for a blue color to appear on the filter paper. Blue indicates the presence of occult blood, or a positive test.
   c. Guaiac:
      Guaiac is a gum resin that was once widely used for testing occult blood in feces. Newer agents are now used, but the term has stayed with us. Often a physician will write an order to "guaiac all stools." Rather than directing you to use the specific reagent guaiac, the physician is asking that the specimen be tested for occult blood. A few laboratories and facilities still use a guaiac solution, but most have changed to the more convenient strip or tablet method. If guaiac test is used, the solutions must be refrigerated because they deteriorate rapidly at room temperature.
      (1) Smear feces on filter paper or a paper towel.
      (2) Drop reagents onto the smear, following the order in the directions.

(3) Watch for a blue color. Again, blue represents the presence of occult blood or a positive test.

6. Record your results immediately on a slip of paper.
7. Dispose of specimen and any equipment used.
8. Wash your hands.
9. Transfer your information to the patient's chart.

Cultures

Cultures can be obtained from almost any body surface or orifice using a wet or dry method. Usually, cultures are made of fluids (secretions, exudates). All cultures should be sent to the laboratory promptly.

OBTAINING WET CULTURES

Wet cultures are often done using a Culturette. This is a plastic sealed tube that contains a transport medium (fluid) in the bottom of the tube, which is separated by an ampule from a cotton swab in the midportion. Following directions, crush the tube after the culture has been taken, breaking the ampule. This releases the transport medium, which saturates the swab. The purpose of the transport medium is to prevent drying and to maintain the bacterial concentration.

1. Remove the tube from its package.
2. Remove the swab stick from the tube. To prevent contamination with microorganisms, do not touch the end of the swab against your fingers or any objects.
3. Collect the specimen to be cultured on the cotton end of swab. Saturate the cotton.
4. Insert the swab in the tube and recap.
5. Note on the package, in the places designated, the patient's name, hospital number, and physician; the date; the time; and any antibiotics the patient is taking.
6. With the cap end down, crush the ampule at midpoint, releasing the transport medium.

7. Push the cap so that the swab moves down, making contact with the medium.
8. Send the package to the laboratory immediately. Any bacterial content can change in number or character if left standing.

OBTAINING DRY CULTURES

When a dry culture is ordered, use a sterile test tube and swab. Send the culture to the laboratory immediately.

URINE CULTURES

A clean catch specimen, as described in Module 18, Collecting Specimens, page 278, is usually sufficient for testing purposes. Use a sterile container. Although there is always a chance of infection when a patient is catheterized, occasionally the physician will order a catheterized specimen for culture. Because urine is normally sterile, this is the most accurate test for content or for pathogens.

PERFORMANCE CHECKLIST

	Unsatisfactory	Needs more practice	Satisfactory	Comments
Specific gravity of urine				
1. Collect 20 ml urine.				
2. Obtain urinometer.				
3. Pour 20 ml urine into urinometer.				
4. Twist stem of bulb so bulb floats freely.				
5. Elevate to eye level.				
6. Read lower meniscus.				
7. Dispose of specimen and clean equipment.				
8. Wash your hands.				
9. Record on patient's chart.				
pH of urine				
1. Obtain urine specimen.				
2. Obtain litmus paper.				
3. Dip litmus paper into urine.				
4. Tap paper on side of container to remove excess urine.				
5. Read acid for red or pink, alkaline for blue.				
6. Discard specimen and litmus paper.				
7. Wash your hands.				
8. Record reading (acid or alkaline) on patient's chart.				
Urine glucose				
1. Collect 1 to 2 ml urine.				
2. Obtain correct product for testing.				
3. Review directions.				
4. Place correct color scale where it is clearly visible.				

5. Proceed with steps a or b.
  a. Clinitest (5-drop method):
    (1) Obtain clean glass test tube, test tube holder, dropper, and tablets.				

(2) Place test tube in holder.				
(3) Using dropper, place 5 drops of urine in test tube.				
(4) Rinse dropper.				
(5) Using dropper, place 10 drops of water in test tube.				

	Unsatisfactory	Needs more practice	Satisfactory	Comments
(6) Using dry hand or container top, place 1 Clinitest tablet in test tube.				
(7) When bubbling action stops, wait 15 seconds. If pass-through occurs, repeat test using 2-drop method.[1]				
(8) Shake tube gently and compare color of solution with color chart.				
b. Reagent strip tests (Clinistix, Diastix, Testape): (1) Remove reagent strip from container.				
(2) Dip strip into urine and tap on side of container to remove excess.				
(3) Begin timing according to directions.				
(4) At end of time period, compare with correct color chart.				
6. Record results immediately on paper.				
7. Discard specimen and strip. Clean equipment.				
8. Wash your hands.				
9. Record test results on patient's chart.				
Ketone bodies in urine				
1. Collect fresh urine specimen.				
2. Obtain correct product and directions for use.				
3. Read directions.				
4. Place color chart where it is clearly visible.				
5. Proceed with step a or b. a. Acetest tablets: (1) Place 1 tablet on filter paper or paper towel.				
(2) Using dropper, place 1 drop of urine on tablet.				
(3) Begin timing.				
(4) Wait 15 seconds.				
(5) Compare color of tablet with color chart.				

[1] For 2-drop method, use 2 drops of urine and 10 drops of water. Change to appropriate color chart.

	Unsatisfactory	Needs more practice	Satisfactory	Comments
b. Reagent strips (Diastix, Ketostix, Uristix): (1) Remove strip from bottle.				
(2) Dip strip into urine.				
(3) Tap on edge of container to remove excess urine.				
(4) Begin timing.				
(5) Time for 60 seconds.				
(6) Compare to appropriate color chart.				
6. Record results immediately on paper.				
7. Discard urine and strip, and clean equipment.				
8. Wash your hands.				
9. Transfer information to patient's chart.				
Blood in urine (using Hemastix)				
1. Use the checklist for ketone bodies. For step 5, do the following: a. Dip strip into urine.				
b. Tap against side to remove excess urine.				
c. Wait 30 seconds.				
d. Read against color chart.				
Blood in feces				
1. Obtain stool specimen.				
2. Wash your hands.				
3. Obtain test product.				
4. Review directions for product.				
5. Proceed with step a, b, or c. a. Hematest: (1) Smear thin layer of fecal material on filter paper.				
(2) Place Hematest tablet in center of specimen.				
(3) Place 1 drop of water on tablet.				
(4) Wait 10 seconds for water to penetrate.				
(5) Add second drop of water to saturate tablet.				

	Unsatisfactory	Needs more practice	Satisfactory	Comments
(6) Wait 20 seconds.				
(7) Read (blue is positive for occult blood).				
b. Hemoccult slide: (1) Open envelope flap.				
(2) Apply thin smear of fecal material over inside circle.				
(3) Drop reagent solution onto fecal smear.				
(4) Read (blue is positive for occult blood).				
c. Guaiac: (1) Smear feces on filter paper or paper towel.				
(2) Drop reagents onto smear in order.				
(3) Read (blue is positive for occult blood).				
6. Record your results immediately on paper.				
7. Dispose of equipment and specimen.				
8. Wash your hands.				
9. Transfer information to patient's chart.				
Obtaining wet cultures (using Culturette)				
1. Remove tube from package.				
2. Remove swab stick from tube.				
3. Collect specimen on end of swab.				
4. Insert swab in tube and recap.				
5. Note on label patient's name, hospital number, and physician; date; time; and any antibiotics patient is taking.				
6. With cap end down, crush ampule at midpoint, releasing transport medium.				
7. Push cap so that swab makes contact with medium.				
8. Send to laboratory immediately.				
Obtaining dry cultures				
Follow directions for wet culture, steps 1–5, using sterile culture tube and swab. Send to laboratory immediately.				

Obtaining urine cultures	Unsatisfactory	Needs more practice	Satisfactory	Comments
Send 3 to 5 ml urine in sterile container to laboratory, obtained either by clean-catch or catheterization, according to physician's orders. (See Module 18, Collecting Specimens, and Module 39, Catheterization.)				

QUIZ

Short-Answer Questions

1. What instrument is used to measure specific gravity? _____

2. Define *specific gravity*. _____

3. Define *pH*. _____

4. Why is a reagent strip generally recommended for measuring the glucose content of urine? _____

5. What measure would be more accurate in reporting the glucose content of urine than pluses? _____

6. What method could you use to test for urine glucose on a diaper or the the bedding of an incontinent patient? _____

7. What factor can lead to inaccuracy when testing for blood in feces?

   _____

8. Why should all cultures be sent to the laboratory immediately?

   _____

Multiple-Choice Questions

_____ 9. Normal specific gravity is

   a. 1.000.
   b. 1.020.
   c. 1.300.
   d. 2.010.

_____ 10. Normal pH of urine is

   a. moderately alkaline.
   b. slightly alkaline.
   c. moderately acid.
   d. slightly acid.

_____ 11. Blue litmus paper means the urine is

   a. acid.
   b. alkaline.

Module 28 Gastric Intubation

MAIN OBJECTIVE

To be able to insert nasogastric tubes, for the purpose of feeding, instilling medications, irrigating the stomach, or initiating gastric suction.

RATIONALE

As a rule, food and fluids are withheld from patients for six to eight hours before they undergo major surgery, in order to empty the stomach. If intake were not restricted, vomiting with aspiration could occur during surgery. However, nausea and general discomfort can still occur following surgery. To prevent this, physicians may order a nasogastric tube, which is inserted through the nares and into the stomach. When suction is applied to the tube, gastric secretions and any accumulated gas are removed, leaving the post-op patient more comfortable.

A nasogastric tube also can be used to instill prescribed medications or to feed patients who are unable to swallow a sufficient diet for one reason or another. Feeding the patient in this manner is called *gastric gavage*.

A nasogastric tube is also used when a patient has ingested toxic substances. The stomach is emptied and washed. The term for this procedure is *lavage*.

Today, surgical procedures are performed on many persons who at one time would have been considered poor surgical risks. Depending on the procedure involved, many surgeons order a nasogastric tube inserted for these patients before surgery, to remove gastric secretions and gas and thereby to decrease distention. Distention is not only uncomfortable; it can place undue tension on an abdominal suture line. Because many of these patients cannot take food orally after surgery, long-term tube feeding in convalescence is frequently necessary. Also, physical and muscular debilitation caused by stroke or other conditions can make tube feeding necessary for at least a period of time.

Although the use of the nasogastric tube is a routine procedure in most facilities today, it can be frightening and unfamiliar to patients. It is the nurse's responsibility to help patients overcome their anxieties about this procedure.

PREREQUISITES

Successful completion of the following
modules:

VOLUME 1
Assessment
Charting
Medical Asepsis
Hygiene
Intake and Output

SPECIFIC LEARNING OBJECTIVES

	Know Facts and Principles	Apply Facts and Principles	Demonstrate Ability	Evaluate Performance
1. *Types and uses of tubes*	Identify characteristics of nasogastric tubes	Know when to ice tubes and how to lubricate	Ice tube if needed. Lubricate tube correctly.	Evaluate own performance with instructor
2. *Equipment*	Recognize types of equipment needed and whether it should be clean or sterile		Select appropriate equipment and assemble tray	Evaluate own performance with instructor
3. *Psychological support*	Know importance of preparing patient for procedure. Explain how to ascertain correct distance to insert tube.	Identify psychological problems of given patient	In the clinical area, explain procedure and elicit cooperation from patient	Review interaction with instructor
4. *Inserting tube*	Describe placement of tube in pharynx and esophagus		Under supervision, insert nasogastric tube	
5. *Placing tube properly*	List three methods for determining proper placement	Determine which method is most reliable	Use a reliable method to determine correct placement. Do not proceed until sure.	Evaluate using Performance Checklist
6. *Attaching suction equipment*	Know types of suction equipment used in facility	Take safety factors into account in planning	Attach suction equipment only after testing	Have procedure checked by staff nurse or instructor
7. *Carrying out irrigation*	State purposes of gastric irrigation	Select proper solution and equipment	Instill solution slowly and aspirate with care	Evaluate own performance with instructor
8. *Recording*	List essential data for recording procedure and know important observations to be made	Adapt data for recording to specific patient situation	Make routine data entries as well as specific observations for given patient	Have instructor review entries

LEARNING ACTIVITIES

1. Review the Specific Learning Objectives.
2. Read the section on the effects of immobility (in the chapter on activity and rest) in Ellis and Nowlis, *Nursing: A Human Needs Approach,* or comparable material in another textbook.
3. Look up the module vocabulary terms in the glossary.
4. Review the anatomy of the upper GI tract.
5. Read through the module.
6. In the practice setting:
   a. Inspect the various nasogastric tubes available. Note the differences in size and lumen.
   b. After carefully reading over the procedure and the Performance Checklist, report to the laboratory at your appointed time and insert a nasogastric tube into a mannequin.
   c. Give instructions and explanations to the mannequin as if it were a real patient.
7. In the clinical setting:
   a. Observe the insertion of a nasogastric tube by either your instructor or a staff nurse. Were the steps followed precisely? What was the patient's response?
   b. Familiarize yourself with the kind of nasogastric suction used in your facility. If the patient in step a, above, is to have suction applied, observe how this is done.
   c. Observe the procedure for a patient who requires gastric irrigation.
   d. When you feel you are ready, and with your instructor's supervision, perform the following activities in the clinical area:
      (1) Insert a nasogastric tube.
      (2) If ordered, attach it to suction.
      (3) If ordered, irrigate the tube.
   e. After performing each procedure, again review the Performance Checklist and evaluate your skills.
   f. Consult your instructor regarding any problems you encounter.

VOCABULARY

asepto syringe
aspirate
dyspnea
gag reflex
gavage
intubation
lavage
Levin tube
lumen
nasogastric tube
sternum
trachea

GASTRIC INTUBATION

The nasogastric tube, which is sometimes called a *Levin tube,* comes in several sizes. Generally, choose a tube with a larger lumen if the suctioned secretions contain blood or other substances that could occlude the tube. Most standard-sized tubes are stocked by all facilities; small tubes for children and infants are also available.

Nasogastric tubes are available in either rubber or plastic. A rubber tube must be thoroughly chilled before intubation, to make the tube more rigid and easier to pass. Plastic tubes, the more common of the two types, should be kept dry in a folded towel.

Procedure

1. Check the orders regarding the patient's name, room number, and type of procedure.
2. Wash your hands.
3. Assemble the equipment. On a clean tray (this is not a sterile procedure), place the proper-sized nasogastric tube.
   a. Chill a rubber tube for 15 to 20 minutes in a basin of ice chips.
   b. Keep a plastic tube dry in a folded towel.
   In addition to the tube, you will need a water-soluble lubricant, an emesis basin, tape, tissues, a towel, a glass, a straw, and a large syringe with an adapter or an asepto syringe.
4. Check the patient's name tag.
5. Explain the procedure to the patient and your reasons for doing it. Because the patient is apt to be anxious, do not explain the procedure too far in advance. Tell the patient that the procedure will not be painful but may be a little uncomfortable. Explain how he or she can help. For example, relaxation is important; ask the patient to breathe deeply, explaining as you proceed. Your confidence will also help the patient to relax.
6. Place the patient in high-Fowler's position if possible.
7. Place a clean towel on the patient's chest.
8. Give the patient a glass of cool water and a straw. Explain that, as he or she sips the water and swallows, you will advance the tube.
9. Standing to the patient's right, if you are right-handed, measure the distance of the portion of tube to be inserted by extending it from the tip of the patient's nose to the earlobe and then to the lower end of the sternum. Mark the tube with a piece of tape.
10. With a water-soluble lubricant, lubricate this portion of the tube, so as not to damage the nasopharyngeal mucosa when you insert it. Do not use an oily lubricant—if aspirated, it could cause lipoidal pneumonia.
11. Flex the patient's head forward slightly, grasp the tube with your right hand about 3 inches from the end, and gently insert it into the nostril, guiding it straight back along the floor of the nose.
12. Have a basin in the patient's lap and tissues handy. As the patient sips water and swallows, gently but steadily advance the tube. There may be some temporary gagging, caused by the gag reflex, but this should subside as the tube is progressed. If any coughing persists or dyspnea occurs, remove the tube immediately because you may have entered the trachea by accident.
13. Secure the tube to the bridge of the nose with a cross tape, to ensure that it remains in position while you check its placement. (See Figure 28.1.)
14. Check to be sure that the end of the tube is in the stomach. There are several methods for doing this, some of which are more reliable than others.
    a. Hold the free end of the tube to your ear, listening for crackling sounds, or place the free end of the tube in a glass of water and observe whether bubbling occurs. The absence of either crackling sounds or bubbling only proves that the tube

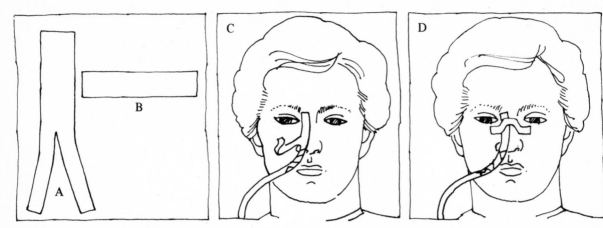

FIGURE 28.1   SECURING THE NASOGASTRIC TUBE   *A:* Tape torn lengthwise for several inches, to be placed lengthwise on nose with tails hanging beyond end of nose; *B:* second tape, to be placed crosswise over bridge of nose to secure tape A; *C:* tape A in place, one tail wrapped around tube in a spiral; *D:* second tail of tape A wrapped around tube, spiraling in opposite direction; tape B has been placed across bridge of nose, securing tape A.

is not in the lungs; however, it may be curled in the pharynx or not yet low enough to be in the stomach. Therefore, this is not the most reliable method of checking placement.

b. By placing a stethoscope over the gastric region and introducing a small amount of air into the open end of the tube with a syringe, you can clearly hear the crackle of air exiting from the tube in the stomach. This method is quite reliable.

c. If the tube is in the stomach, attaching a syringe to the free end of the tube and aspirating will return gastric secretions that are constantly in the stomach and can be easily identified. Once you have ascertained the tube's position, return the aspirated secretions to the stomach with the syringe. Gastric secretions contain electrolytes that are important to maintain the body's chemical balance.

   Note: If you think the tube is entering the trachea, ask the patient to hum. If the tube is even partially in the trachea, the patient, although able to talk, will *not* be able to hum.

15. To prevent air from entering the stomach, which could cause distention, plug the free end of the tube at all times, except when checking position, tube feeding, or irrigating.

16. To irrigate the tube:
   a. Slowly instill 10 to 20 ml solution, usually water or normal saline, with a syringe.
   b. Gently aspirate. If any bleeding is apparent, stop the aspiration and report your observations to the physician. Use sterile technique if the patient has had gastrointestinal surgery. Also, in this event, carefully measure all gastric secretions which must be considered output. (See Module 38, Irrigations.)

17. To suction:
   a. Turn the equipment on *before* you attach it to the patient's nasogastric tube. Place your finger over the suction tube opening, to determine whether the suction is malfunctioning or is too strong. Always use a low setting for suction.
   b. Attach the suction to the patient's nasogastric tube, using an adapter.
   c. Check equipment regularly, observe

drainage, and record amount and characteristics.

18. Secure the tube to the patient's nose using tape. Place a vertical strip down the bridge of the nose. Cut the lower end of the tape into two "tails" and wrap them around the tube (Figure 28.1). This method is comfortable for the patient and prevents abrasion to the side of the nostril. Fasten the length of tube to the patient's gown with a rubber band and safety pin, so that the patient can move freely in bed without pulling and dislodging the tube.

19. Make the patient comfortable.

20. Wash your hands.

21. Record the procedure and your observations.

22. Any patient with a nasogastric tube in place needs frequent oral and nasal care. This is because the tube irritates the nostrils and the back of the throat, producing a drying condition. Also, the mouth becomes particularly dry because the patient is mouth-breathing and is neither eating nor taking fluids.

Intubation of the Unconscious Patient

An unconscious patient often requires a nasogastric tube to relieve gastric distention or for feeding the patient.

Observe all of the principles described in the procedure above, with the following important adaptations:

1. Position the patient in low- to mid-Fowler's, again, with the head flexed forward slightly.

2. The main danger is the possible insertion of the tube through the bronchus into the lung. The unconscious patient may have lost both gag and cough reflexes, so you may not accurately know the position of the tube because the patient will not cough if the tube is misplaced. A simple but effective way to avoid this problem is to insert an oropharyngeal airway into the patient's mouth. The distal end of the airway acts

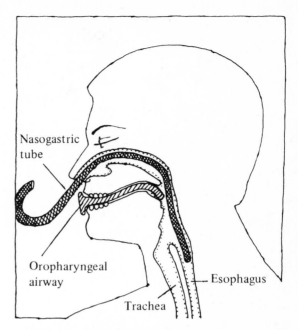

FIGURE 28.2   NASOGASTRIC INTUBATION OF AN UNCONSCIOUS PATIENT   The oropharyngeal airway prevents the nasogastric tube from coiling forward, so the tube passes easily into the esophagus.

as a guide, moving the tube smoothly down into the esophagus (see Figure 28.2). Even if you have used an airway, carefully check the placement. Once you are sure the location is correct, remove the airway.

PERFORMANCE CHECKLIST

	Unsatisfactory	Needs more practice	Satisfactory	Comments
1. Check orders				
2. Wash your hands.				
3. Assemble equipment, chilling tube if necessary.				
4. Check patient's name band.				
5. Explain procedure and its purpose to patient. Tell patient how he or she might help.				
6. Position patient in high-Fowler's, with head slightly flexed.				
7. Put clean towel on patient's chest.				
8. Give patient water to sip.				
9. Measure distance of tube to be inserted and mark with tape.				
10. Lubricate portion to be inserted.				
11. Introduce tube through nostril, guiding gently but steadily.				
12. Observe for gagging, coughing, or dyspnea.				
13. Temporarily tape tube to bridge of nose.				
14. Using reliable method, check for proper position.				
15. To irrigate tube: a. Slowly introduce 10 to 20 ml solution.				
b. Aspirate gently, observing return.				
16. To suction: a. Check equipment for proper functioning *before* attaching to nasogastric tube.				
b. Use the adapter to attach suction.				
c. Check equipment regularly; observe drainage and record amount.				
17. Secure tube to patient's nose, and fasten to gown.				
18. Help patient to comfortable position.				
19. Wash your hands.				
20. Record procedure and observations.				
21. Administer frequent oral and nasal care.				

QUIZ

Short-Answer Questions

1. List three reasons why a nasogastric tube would be inserted.

    a. _____

    b. _____

    c. _____

2. Why is the nasogastric tube lubricated? _____

Multiple-Choice Questions

_____ 3. To determine the proper distance to insert the nasogastric tube, measure

    a. from the tip of the earlobe to the cricoid.
    b. from the nose to the umbilicus.
    c. from the tip of the nose to the earlobe, and then to the lower sternum.
    d. from the tip of the earlobe to the nose, and then to the umbilicus.

_____ 4. When passing the tube, have the patient's head

    a. in extension.
    b. in flexion.
    c. turned to one side.

_____ 5. The nasogastric tube is passed more easily if the patient is

    a. in low-Fowler's position.
    b. flat in bed.
    c. in high-Fowler's position.
    d. positioned on the left side.

_____ 6. To check the position of the tube, which of the following methods is *least* reliable?

    a. Place the free end of the tube in a glass of water and watch for possible bubbling.
    b. Introduce a small amount of air into the tube and listen with a stethoscope over the gastric region for the entrance of air into the stomach.
    c. Aspirate the gastric contents gently with a syringe.

_____ 7. If fresh bleeding is observed when irrigating a nasogastric tube, you should

    a. complete the irrigation and report it to the physician.
    b. irrigate more slowly.
    c. use a larger amount of solution.
    d. stop the aspiration and report it to the physician.

_____ 8. A primary safety factor to remember when applying suction to a patient's nasogastric tube is to

   a. always turn the equipment on to the *low* position.
   b. test the functioning of the equipment *before* attaching it to the patient's tube.
   c. *be sure* the seals on the collection bottle are tight.
   d. *never* use extension cords.

Module 29 Tube Feeding

MAIN OBJECTIVE

To administer tube feeding, using the appropriate formula and water in proper amounts and observing safety precautions.

RATIONALE

The purpose of tube feeding is to enhance the nutritional status of patients who are unable to take food normally. For example, unconscious patients need nutrients supplied for them until they regain consciousness. Tube-feeding formulas can supply them with a well-balanced and complete diet (except for fiber or roughage). It is one of the nurse's primary functions to carefully and efficiently provide feedings via nasogastric tube until patients can eat unaided.

PREREQUISITES

Successful completion of the following modules

VOLUME 1
Assessment
Charting
Medical Asepsis
Intake and Output

VOLUME 2
Gastric Intubation (optional)

SPECIFIC LEARNING OBJECTIVES

	Know Facts and Principles	Apply Facts and Principles	Demonstrate Ability	Evaluate Performance
1. *Formulas*	Know components of various basic formulas and proper temperature for administration	State relationship of formula chosen to needs of patient	In clinical situation, choose formula ordered	
2. *Equipment*	List items needed to carry out tube feeding	Select or adapt equipment to complete tray	Use equipment in safe efficient manner	Using Performance Checklist, review type and completeness of equipment with instructor
3. *Safety*	Name methods for checking placement of tube	Decide which are the more reliable methods	Use reliable methods correctly in practice	Evaluate own performance using Performance Checklist
4. *Psychological support*	Verbalize importance of presenting a *meal* rather than treatment to patient	Adapt equipment to improve patient's psychological response	Maintain attitude that allows patient dignity	
5. *Carrying out tube feeding*	Outline correct procedure and reasons for various steps	Identify modifications needed for individual patients	Carry out tube feeding using proper technique	Evaluate own performance using Performance Checklist
6. *Recording*	State format and items to be recorded, including pertinent observations	Investigate recording used in specific facility	Record procedure using proper format and including pertinent observations	Evaluate own performance using Performance Checklist

LEARNING ACTIVITIES

1. Review the Specific Learning Objectives.
2. Read the chapter on nutrition in Ellis and Nowlis, *Nursing: A Human Needs Approach,* or a comparable chapter in another textbook.
3. Look up the module vocabulary terms in the glossary.
4. Read through the module.
5. Review the anatomy of the gastrointestinal and respiratory tracts.
6. In the practice setting:
   a. If tube feeding equipment is available, arrange for time to become familiar with the equipment you will need to carry out the procedure.
   b. If a mannequin is available, simulate the procedure using different types of equipment.
   c. Evaluate your performance with a partner or your instructor.
7. In the clinical setting:
   a. Observe the administration of a tube feeding. Was the procedure properly followed?
   b. When you are ready, perform a tube feeding with your instructor's supervision.
   c. Review your performance with your instructor.
   d. Record the procedure and your observations.
   e. Share your recording with your instructor.

VOCABULARY

asepto syringe
aspiration
burette
comatose
distention
gastric gavage
gastrostomy
Levin tube
lumen
nasal mucosa
nasogastric tube
patent
semi-Fowler's position

TUBE FEEDING

Types of Gastric Tubes

Tube feeding, sometimes called *gastric gavage,* is usually done by introducing the feeding or formula through a tube. The tube most commonly used is a nasogastric tube, which is passed through the nose, down the esophagus, and into the stomach. Tubes come in three general sizes: adult, pediatric (for small children), and infant.

In adults and children, the tube is passed and remains in place for individual or continuous feedings. The clean tube should be inserted into the other nostril when it is (1) no longer patent, (2) irritating the nasal mucosa, or (3) possibly harboring microorganisms. Because there are not clearly defined times, the decision to change the tube rests with the nurse.

For infants who must be fed by a nasogastric tube, you may introduce the tube each time through the mouth, administer the formula, and remove the tube.

Occasionally, you will care for a patient who is being fed through a tube that has been placed surgically through the abdominal wall directly into the stomach. This surgical procedure is called a *gastrostomy.* The tube used has a much larger lumen than the nasogastric tube and is usually secured under a light dressing. The feeding procedure is the same. Although it will appear that the end of the tube must be in the stomach, make sure each time by aspirating a portion of the gastric contents.

Formulas for Tube Feeding

Many types of formulas are used for tube feeding, some offering a more balanced diet than others. More often in long-term facilities than in hospitals, a "house" formula is available, which consists primarily of eggs, milk, corn syrup, salt, a blenderized vegetable, and water. This formula yields approximately 1 calorie per milliliter. After it has been established that a patient can tolerate this formula without vomiting or diarrhea (diarrhea is a common occurrence), pureed

meat and cereal as well as fruit juice are sometimes added to it.

Also, a variety of tube-feeding preparations can be purchased commercially. Many of these preparations provide the basic nutrients through a process that liquefies food, including meat products. Most are available in cans, although prefilled bottles, ready to be administered, are now available as well. (See Figure 29.3.)

Oral medications too can be given with tube feeding. Ideally, medications should be in liquid form, to pass through the tube easily. However, tablets and capsules can be administered. Tablets should be finely crushed, and capsules should be opened and the contents mixed with water and added to the formula. It is best to give medication at the beginning of a feeding, so that if, for any reason, the full amount of formula is not given, the medication will have been administered.

Preparation

Some patients are fed by tube because they are in a state of coma; others may be alert but suffering from paralysis or pathology of the mouth, pharynx, or esophagus. Whether the patient is comatose or alert, regardless of his or her problem, the feeding procedure should be carried out carefully, always maintaining the patient's dignity.

Do not hurry or force the feeding; this can cause distention and discomfort. In fact, if the patient is alert, you will find that the time for feeding is excellent for communication and assessment.

Use clean technique when you administer a tube feeding, and remember that this feeding is actually the patient's *meal.* Although the formula and additional water used are ordered by the physician and you measure them in a container, they can be poured into attractive glasses and served on a colorful tray.

Warm the formula; although it has been shown that cold formula is as easily digested as warm formula, it can be unpleasant to the patient or cause chilling.

Procedure

1. Check the order regarding the patient's name, type of formula and amount of water to be given, time, and any oral medications.
2. Wash your hands.
3. Warm the formula to room temperature.
4. Prepare the tray. Use the method of administration and appropriate equipment for your facility. (See step 8, below.)
5. Explain to the patient what you are going to do.
6. Place the patient in semi-Fowler's position.
7. Test the placement of the tube. Because the tube may have become dislodged in the interval between feedings, it is important that you check for position and patency *each* time before feeding. Three methods are described in Module 28, in the procedure for gastric intubation, step 14, page 23. It is best to use the most reliable method; that is, aspirating the gastric contents. This is both a positive determination as well as a check for digestion of the previous feeding. If the aspirated contents contain formula that appears noncurded, or much like the fresh formula, the feeding may be omitted or decreased in amount. In some hospitals, if more than 50 ml undigested formula contents is aspirated, the next feeding is withheld and the aspirated material is reinstilled through the tube. Again, remember that gastric contents of any amount should always be returned to the stomach, so as not to disturb the chemical balance.
8. Depending on the equipment used in your facility, administer a small amount of water first (to ensure that the tube is patent), any medications ordered, and the formula. Follow with the remainder of the water, which rinses the tube of formula.
   a. Burette method:
      In most facilities where a burette is used, it is used more than once.

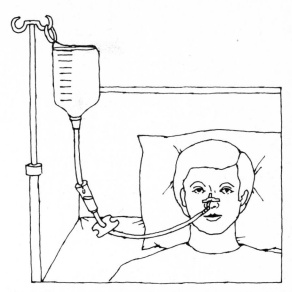

FIGURE 29.1   BURETTE METHOD OF TUBE FEEDING

Therefore, it must be kept thoroughly cleaned between feedings, so that microorganisms are not harbored in the bag. The burette consists of a square-shaped plastic bag with markings calibrated in milliliters. Attached to the bag is a drip chamber and tubing (Figure 29.1).
(1) Hold the top of the bag open as you instill a portion of the water ordered.
(2) Open the stopcock until the water has displaced the air left in the tube.
(3) Attach the tube to the patient's nasogastric tube, and allow the water to enter.
(4) Clamp before air enters from the bag.
(5) Pour the formula into the bag and regulate the drip using the stopcock.
(6) Before the formula runs completely down the tube, introduce the remainder of the water.
(7) Close the stopcock and detach the burette tubing from the nasogastric tube.
(8) Clean thoroughly.

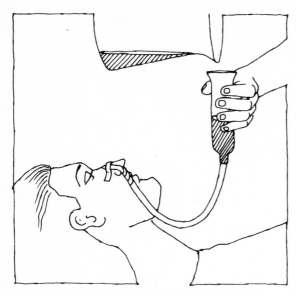

FIGURE 29.2   ASEPTO-SYRINGE METHOD OF TUBE FEEDING

b. Asepto-syringe method:
When you use this method, hold the syringe manually, and fill and refill in the same sequence used with the burette method. Again, do not allow the water or formula to fall below the narrowing at the bottom of the syringe, to prevent the entrance of air through the nasogastric tube. (See Figure 29.2.)

c. Prefilled tube-feeding set:
These sets are available commercially and consist of premeasured formula in a minibottle with a drip chamber and tubing.

(1) Remove the sealed screw cap and screw in its place the cap with the drip chamber and tubing.

(2) Hang the bottle on an intravenous pole.

(3) Introduce a small amount of water at this time with an asepto syringe, to ensure that the nasogastric tube is patent.

(4) Start the flow from the mini-bottle to fill the tubing with formula instead of air, so that air is not introduced into the stomach.

(5) When the formula has filled the tubing, attach the set to the patient's nasogastric tube and begin the feeding.

(6) Follow with water, using the asepto syringe. (See Figure 29.3.)
If this equipment is not available, a sterile, empty IV bottle and tubing can be successfully adapted for use.

Note: All three methods use gravity flow to move the formula through the tube. If the flow slows down or stops, gentle pressure with the asepto bulb or "milking" the tubing may help. If the patient gags during the feeding, stop the procedure.

9. After the feeding, clamp the tube tightly or plug it.

10. Reposition the patient in low- or semi-Fowler's position. If the patient is comatose, his or her head should be turned to one side, to prevent aspiration into the lungs if vomiting occurs.

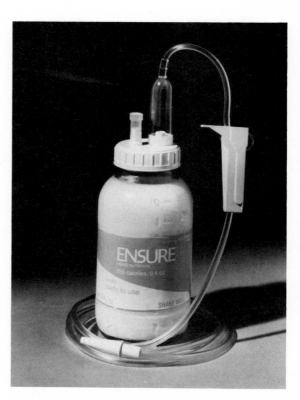

FIGURE 29.3   PREFILLED TUBE-FEEDING SET
Courtesy Ross Laboratories, Columbus, Ohio

11. Wash your hands.
12. Record on the medication sheet or progress notes. Your notes should include date, time, type and amount of formula, amount of water, and the patient's response. Most patients being fed by tube are on intake—output, so a proper entry should be made after each feeding.
13. Check the patient in approximately 30 minutes, to determine retention and tolerance.

PERFORMANCE CHECKLIST

	Unsatisfactory	Needs more practice	Satisfactory	Comments
1. Check order.				
2. Wash your hands.				
3. Warm formula to room temperature.				
4. Prepare tray.				
5. Explain procedure to patient.				
6. Position patient in semi-Fowler's position.				
7. Test for placement of tube by aspirating gastric contents.				
8. Using a burette, asepto syringe, or prefilled set, administer small amount of water, medications ordered, feeding, and then remainder of water.				
9. Tightly clamp or replug tube.				
10. Reposition patient. Turn head of comatose patient to side.				
11. Wash your hands.				
12. Record procedure and pertinent observations.				
13. Check patient in 30 minutes for tolerance and retention.				

QUIZ

Multiple-Choice Questions

_____ 1. Each milliliter of house formula yields approximately

   a. 1 calorie.
   b. 5 calories.
   c. 10 calories.

_____ 2. For administration, the formula should be

   a. hot.
   b. cold.
   c. at room temperature.

_____ 3. To prevent gastric distention you should
   a. feed the patient only every four hours.
   b. allow as little air as possible to enter the tube.
   c. rinse the tube well with water after the feeding.

_____ 4. The head of a comatose patient should be turned to the side after feeding in order to prevent

   a. vomiting.
   b. aspiration.
   c. distention.
   d. indigestion.

_____ 5. The patient should be checked approximately 30 minutes after feeding for

   a. vomiting.
   b. drowsiness.
   c. anorexia.

_____ 6. If the tubing does not appear to be in the stomach when you check it, you should

   a. give the feeding slowly.
   b. remove the tube immediately.
   c. not give the feeding.

_____ 7. If the patient begins to gag while you are tube feeding, you should

   a. stop the feeding for a time.
   b. continue with the feeding as planned.
   c. give additional feeding.
   d. give medication for nausea.

Module 30 Ostomy Care

MAIN OBJECTIVE

To care for patients with an "ostomy," using correct technique while maintaining cleanliness and an environment conducive to patients' dignity and self-respect.

RATIONALE

More advanced surgical techniques have led to increasing numbers of patients with surgical diversions of fecal- and urinary-elimination pathways. Comprehensive care requires that the nurse understand the different types of diversions and the reasons for them. Cleanliness, skin care, and odor control are other concerns. Because a surgical diversion is a profound change in body structure and function, the nurse must also provide supportive care, helping patients to make the necessary psychosocial adjustments.

PREREQUISITES

1. Successful completion of the following modules:

   VOLUME 1
   Assessment
   Charting
   Medical Asepsis
   Hygiene
   Administering Enemas

2. A review of the anatomy and physiology of the gastrointestinal and urinary systems

SPECIFIC LEARNING OBJECTIVES

	Know Facts and Principles	Apply Facts and Principles	Demonstrate Ability	Evaluate Performance
1. *Types of ostomies*	Differentiate between various types of ostomies	Explain why skin care is different for different ostomies based on effect of urine and feces on skin	Correctly identify type of drainage to be expected when assigned patient with ostomy	Verify identification with instructor
2. *Appliances*	Describe various appliances available	Given a patient situation, choose suitable appliance		
3. *Changing a colostomy-ileostomy bag*	List steps in procedure for changing colostomy bag	Given a patient situation, decide whether bag should be changed	Change colostomy or ileostomy bag correctly	Check bag for security, leaks, and cleanliness. Evaluate own performance using Performance Checklist.
4. *Colostomy dressing*	List steps in procedure for changing colostomy dressing. State rationale for forming base of gauze around stoma.		Change colostomy dressing correctly	Check patient for cleanliness and comfort. Evaluate own performance using Performance Checklist.
5. *Colostomy irrigation*	Describe two types of irrigation, based on purpose. List equipment needed for both types of irrigation. State fluid volume used for each type of irrigation. State distance to insert catheter into stoma.	Given a patient situation, identify appropriate type of irrigation	Irrigate colostomy using correct technique according to type of procedure	Evaluate effectiveness of irrigation by checking for fecal and fluid return. Evaluate own performance using Performance Checklist.

6. *Changing a urinary-drainage appliance*	State rationale for exceptional attention to cleanliness. Describe process for removing old appliance. Discuss steps in applying urinary drainage appliance.	Change urinary drainage appliance correctly	Evaluate by checking appliance for leaks. Evaluate own performance using Performance Checklist.
7. *Charting*	State pertinent information to be charted regarding ostomy care	Chart appropriate information regarding ostomy care	Evaluate own charting by reviewing for completeness and consulting with instructor

LEARNING ACTIVITIES

1. Review the Specific Learning Objectives.
2. Look up the module vocabulary terms in the glossary.
3. Read through the module.
4. In the practice setting:
   a. Examine the various types of appliances available.
   b. Read the instructions on any appliances and adhesives available.
   c. Examine colostomy irrigation equipment.
   d. Using a simulated ostomy on a mannequin:
      (1) Change the ostomy dressing using the Performance Checklist as a guide.
      (2) Change the ostomy bag using the Performance Checklist as a guide.
      (3) Set up a colostomy irrigation using the equipment available. Do a mock irrigation if possible, using the Performance Checklist as a guide.
      (4) When you believe you have mastered these skills, ask your instructor to check your performance.

VOCABULARY

adhesive
appliance
cecostomy
colostomy
double-barreled colostomy
ileoconduit (ileobladder, ileoloop)
ileostomy
karaya
ostomate
ostomy
sigmoidostomy
stoma
ureterostomy

OSTOMY CARE

Ostomies usually drain either urine or fecal material; only rarely does the same ostomy drain both. Urinary-diversion ostomies and bowel-diversion ostomies, although similar in appearance and certain appliances used, differ in one important element: urine drains from the sterile ureters, and any opening into the urinary system offers a pathway for infection directly to the kidneys. Also, the liquid nature and chemical composition of urine make it more irritating to the skin and more difficult to contain than fecal material.

Bowel Diversions

Bowel-diversion ostomies drain fecal material. The consistency of the material depends on the portion of the bowel that remains and the length of time the ostomy has been in place.

An *ileostomy* empties from the end of the small intestine. Therefore, the contents are liquid, drain constantly, and contain some digestive enzymes that break down the skin. Odor is not usually a major problem.

A *cecostomy* empties from the first part of the large intestine. Digestive enzymes are not usually present, but the stool is still quite liquid. A person with this type of ostomy, as well as the person with the ileostomy, must wear a drainage bag constantly. These two types of ostomies are not irrigated.

A *colostomy* can be located anywhere along the entire length of the large intestine. The further along the bowel it is located, the more solid the stool, because the large intestine reabsorbs water. Also, the larger the portion of intestine that remains, the less frequent the bowel movements, because there is space for fecal material to accumulate.

A *sigmoidostomy* empties from the sigmoid colon, and stools appear normal in consistency. A person with this type of ostomy is most regular, and may not have to wear an appliance at all times.

The longer a bowel-diversion ostomy has been in place, the more normal the consistency of the stool, because other portions of the intestine increase water reabsorption to compensate for the lost area. Still, drainage from the ileostomy and cecostomy remains relatively liquid.

The surgeon determines the location of the ostomy. The location can be optional, leaving the surgeon free to select the site on the abdomen that will allow for a well-fitting appliance. Site selection can be limited, however, by the extent of surgery that must be performed. Thus, some ostomies are in locations that are more difficult to fit with a tight-sealing appliance. (See Figure 30.1.)

Urinary Diversions

A *ureterostomy* is an opening of a ureter directly onto the abdominal surface. Ureterostomies can be right, left, or bilateral, in which case each ureterostomy is covered by a separate appliance. They are very small— about as large as a pencil—and drain urine continuously.

To simplify the actual diversion, a more elaborate surgical procedure may be performed. This procedure is called *ileoloop, ileobladder,* or *ileoconduit.* (The prefix can also be written "ileal.") This requires that a section of the ileum (small intestine) be cut out of the rest of the intestine, and then that the intestinal ends be reattached. Both ureters are then attached to this separate segment of the ileum, draining into it. One end of this segment of ileum is closed, and the other is opened onto the abdomen as a stoma. (See Figure 30.2.) This stoma is the size of an ileostomy (about 1½ inches in diameter) and drains urine continuously. The advantage of this type of urinary diversion is having one stoma that is larger and more easily fitted with an appliance. There is also less chance of ascending kidney infection because the mucous membrane of the intestinal segment serves as a barrier to microorganisms.

A newer technique—sometimes called a continent ilealconduit—is in limited use. In

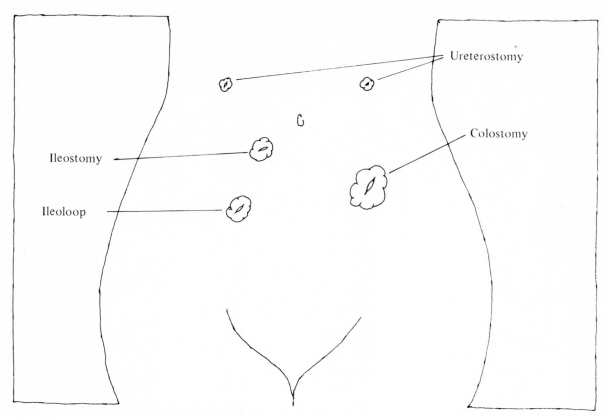

FIGURE 30.1   COMMON LOCATIONS OF OSTOMIES

this technique, the ileoloop is folded back on itself inside the peritoneum. The muscles of the ileoloop then create a pseudosphincter, causing the urine to be retained in the ileoloop until a drainage catheter is inserted. This stops the continuous drainage of urine.

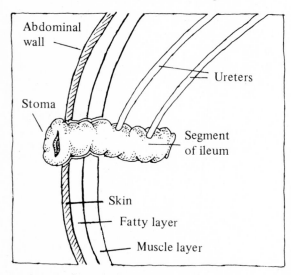

FIGURE 30.2   ILEOLOOP

Ostomy Appliances

Several companies make ostomy appliances, and no one type is best for all patients. An enterostomal therapist is the best resource person to consult when selecting an appropriate appliance. When no therapist is available, a salesperson at the surgical supply store may be helpful in explaining the various types of appliances. For convenience, many facilities carry only one brand, but the patient should be made aware of all available options, so that he or she can make a personal choice for long-term care. Ostomy appliances can also be ordered at most pharmacies.

A temporary appliance may be used in the hospital. This is a disposable bag that has a peel-off adhesive square. To use, cut a hole in the square to the size of the stoma. Allow only the mucous membrane of the stoma to project through the hole. (The mucus protects the membrane from irritation.) The skin surrounding the stoma can be irritated easily if urine or stool drains across it. After the hole is cut, peel off the covering from the adhesive and apply the bag to the skin. Each time the bag is full, it may be removed and replaced. Some temporary bags can be opened and drained from the bottom, so they don't need to be replaced as frequently. Removing and reapplying adhesive bags can irritate the skin.

Permanent appliances usually have a solid ring faceplate that fits around the stoma. These come in a variety of sizes, and the size needed may change over time. The bag is fastened to the faceplate. The faceplate is held in place by an adhesive, either a karaya gum ring, solid-type adhesive (such as Stomadhesive), or a liquid adhesive. A belt is usually attached to the ring. The belt is designed to support the weight of the bag as it fills, preventing it from pulling the adhesive loose and causing leakage. Not all patients wear a belt. Usually, the bag has a closure at the bottom, so it can be drained. The closure clip may be reusable even if the bag is disposable. (See Figure 30.3.)

Persons with a well-controlled colostomy

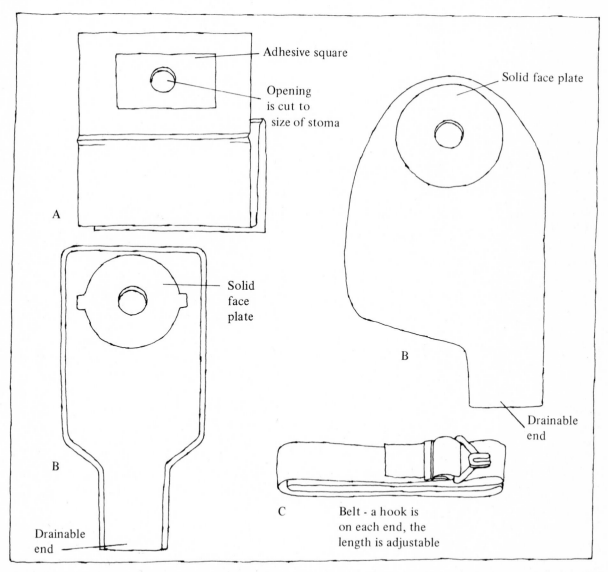

FIGURE 30.3 DRAINAGE BAGS FOR COLOSTOMY *A:* Temporary bag; *B:* permanent bags; *C:* belt with hook on each end, length adjustable.

may wear only a flat dressing over the stoma except when irrigating the colostomy. This is done only after good control has been positively established.

The appliances used for urinary-drainage ostomies are very similar to those already described. (See Figure 30.4.) Special adhesives are used that cannot be broken down by urine. Also, urinary appliances always can be drained from the bottom. They are usually replaced every three to five days, or when they begin to leak.

Changing a Colostomy-Ileostomy Bag

1. Wash your hands.
2. Check the patient's care plan to ascertain whether a protective substance is being applied to the skin and whether special procedures are being used.
3. Screen the patient.
4. Check the appliance in use. Note the type of bag, the method of sealing the bag, and the condition of the skin. Also check to see what equipment is at the bedside.
5. Explain to the patient what you plan to do.
6. Obtain all the equipment you will need. (Some items may be at the patient's bedside.)
   a. Cleansing supplies. You will need tissues for wiping away stool, warm water, a mild soap, a washcloth, and a towel. In some facilities, clean rags that can be thrown away are used for cleaning.

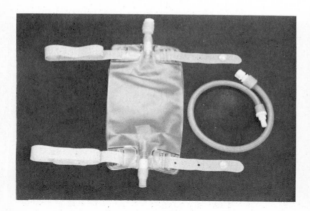
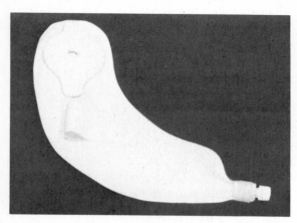
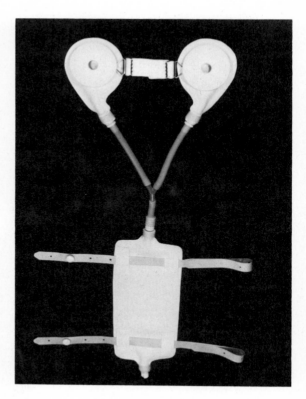

FIGURE 30.4   SEVERAL URINARY-DRAINAGE APPLIANCES
Courtesy Mason Laboratories, Inc., Horsham, PA

b. A clean bag of the type currently being used.

c. A seal or adhesive to prevent leakage. (This may be attached to the bag.)

d. A clean belt. The belt is used to support the weight of the appliance so that it does not loosen the seal as the bag fills. Temporary appliances may not have a belt. Belts are not disposable. The patient usually has two; one to be worn while the other is washed and dried. The belt being worn can be used again if it is clean.

e. A receptacle for the soiled bag. A bedpan can be used initially. For both aseptic and aesthetic reasons, place the soiled bag in a paper bag or wrap it in newspaper or paper towels for disposal. This keeps the linen clean and helps to contain odor.

f. A protective spray. The skin around the stoma may be protected by applying a coat of tincture of benzoin. Although a spray can is convenient to use, a liquid can be applied with an applicator or a gauze square.

g. Clean rubber (rectal) gloves.

7. To remove the old bag:

a. Unfasten the belt.

b. Check the method of adhesion. You may have to use an adhesive solvent to remove certain types of adhesive. Follow the directions carefully. A karaya gum seal will simply peel off.

c. Peel the bag gently away from the skin, being careful not to irritate or damage the skin.

d. Place the bag in a bedpan as it is removed. If a reusable clip is on the bottom of the bag, twist or fold the top of the bag to retain stool and carefully remove the clip. The bedpan will keep stool from getting on the patient and the linen. If the stool is very liquid, you may have to carry the bag to a toilet where you can empty it when you remove the clip.

e. Measure liquid stool for intake and output records.

Rubber gloves can be worn to handle the soiled bag. However, at home the patient will not wear gloves to care for the colostomy, and it can be helpful to the patient to see that others are able to care for a colostomy without gloves.

8. Using warm water and a mild soap, clean the skin around the stoma carefully. As you clean, inspect the skin for redness or irritation.

9. Cover the stoma with a tissue to prevent the stool from leaking onto the clean skin. Change this tissue as necessary.

10. Dry the skin around the stoma carefully, patting gently. Do not rub. Rubbing tends to irritate the skin.

11. Apply the protective material if needed. Use only a very thin coating.

12. Allow the skin to dry thoroughly. A lamp can be placed 18 to 24 inches from the area to dry it more quickly. *Do not* place the lamp too close or leave it for too long a time. A burn would be tragic.

13. Remove the tissue and apply the bag, using the adhesive as directed. For a karaya gum ring, either soften it slightly under the lamp before applying or run hot water over the bag before removing the cover on the karaya. Other adhesive materials must be cut to fit over the stoma, and still others are painted on the skin.

14. "Bunch" the bag over the stoma to provide room for the stool.

15. Place a deodorant solution in the bag to prevent odor, if wanted. Commercial solutions are available, but you can substitute a few drops of vanilla extract, which is less expensive. Aspirin is not recommended for odor control because of potential stoma irritation.

16. To relieve the accumulation of gas in the bag, prick a pinhole near the top of the bag. This does allow odor to escape also, and you will have to decide which is more of a problem. Sometimes a hole is made to allow accumulated gas to escape while the patient is in the bath-

room. Then a piece of tape is used to
cover the hole when the patient is
around others.

17. Fasten the closure clip on the bottom of
the bag if necessary.
18. Fasten the clean belt in place, adjusting
as necessary for comfort and fit.
19. Discard or clean the bag.
    a. If the soiled bag is disposable, empty
    the stool into a toilet or flush sink
    and place the bag in the trash in the
    utility room. Do not leave it in a
    wastebasket in the patient's room be-
    cause it creates odor.
    b. If the bag is reusable, empty the stool
    and wash the bag with a mild deter-
    gent and water. Then, rinse and dry.
    An odor prevention material can be
    used in the rinse. If odor is a problem
    and no special rinse is available, a
    weak vinegar solution or Cepacol
    mouthwash often stops odor. Fill the
    bag with the solution and let it stand
    for 15 to 30 minutes; then, empty,
    rinse, and dry.
20. Wash the soiled belt in mild soap and
warm water. Rinse and hang to dry.
Usually, this is hung in the patient's
room so that it is not lost.
21. Wash your hands thoroughly. If odor
clings, use a weak vinegar solution or
toothpaste, which when used as a hand
soap also removes odor.
22. Make the patient comfortable.
23. Chart the bag change. Also note your
observations of the stool and of the
skin around the stoma.

Colostomy Dressing

A new colostomy is sometimes covered
with a dressing instead of an appliance
because a new incision may make it inap-
propriate to adhere an appliance in place.
Because it is difficult to control fecal drainage with a dressing, a shift to an appliance is
usually made as soon as possible. This is a
clean, not a sterile, procedure.

1. Wash your hands.
2. Gather equipment.
    a. Cleansing supplies
    b. 4 X 4–inch gauze squares or fluffs
    (unfolded gauze)
    c. Large absorbent pads
    d. Tape
    e. Clean gloves
    f. Paper bag or newspaper
3. Drape and screen the patient.
4. Using gloves, remove the soiled dressing,
place it in the papers or the bag, and
cover (to help contain odor).
5. Carefully clean the area as described in
Changing a Colostomy-Ileostomy Bag,
step 8, page 47.
6. Remove soiled gloves.
7. Use unfolded 4 X 4s or fluffs to form a
circular base dressing around the stoma.
(See Figure 30.5.) This keeps the stoma
unobstructed and helps protect the skin.
8. Use the larger dressings over the top,
placing more of them in the direction of
the flow.
9. Tape the dressings in place. Montgomery
tapes may be used so repeated application and removal of tape is not necessary.
10. Dispose of the soiled dressings in the
utility room, not in the patient's room.
11. Wash your hands.
12. Chart the amount, color, and consistency
of the drainage, the skin condition, and

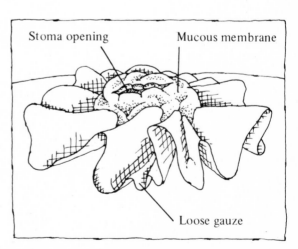

Stoma opening   Mucous membrane

Loose gauze

FIGURE 30.5   THE COLOSTOMY DRESSING
BASE

the procedure. Also note the patient's response to the colostomy and his or her emotional status.

Irrigating a Colostomy

The physician determines whether a colostomy should be irrigated. Not all colostomies need to be irrigated for effective functioning, although irrigation may be done if constipation develops. For some persons, a colostomy does not function well without irrigation. When performed daily, a regular routine should be established to facilitate cleanliness and odor control, and to prevent embarrassing emptying of the bowel at inconvenient times and places. To this end, set up a regular time, accommodating to the patient's personal schedule, for irrigation. Select a time when the patient will be more relaxed and able to pay careful attention to detail. The patient's privacy is also important. Often, you will be teaching the procedure to the patient. The more the irrigation in the hospital can be made to resemble the way it will be done at home, the easier the patient's transition.

Two general types of irrigation are currently in use. The physician may decide the type of irrigation, or your facility may have a policy regarding the type to be used.

The first is the *large-volume, enema-type irrigation.* The purpose of this type of irrigation is to wash out the bowel contents. Some patients using this method may have to irrigate only every two or three days. Its disadvantages include the retention of fluid and later dribbling, excessive distention of the colon, electrolyte depletion, and the amount of time needed for the procedure. Also, some patients increase the volume of the irrigation beyond what is ordered or insert the tubing a long distance into the colon, both of which can cause damage to the colon.

The second type is the *small-volume, bulb syringe method.* Its purpose is to stimulate the bowel to do its own emptying. Because the tip on the syringe is so short, it is impossible for the patient to insert it too far

and cause bowel damage. A disadvantage of the method is that it may not empty the bowel adequately, allowing stool to be excreted later. Also, the hard bulb may be too stiff for weak or arthritic elderly persons to squeeze. In this case, the enema-type equipment is used for a smaller-volume irrigation. The small-volume irrigation usually must be done daily.

Both methods are described below.

1. Explain the procedure and its purpose to the patient.
2. Wash your hands.
3. Obtain the necessary equipment.
   a. For either method:
      (1) Bath blanket or large towel
      (2) Lubricant
      (3) Clean rubber gloves
      (4) Paper bag for soiled bag or dressings
      (5) Clean colostomy bag or dressings
      (6) Irrigation sleeve, or bag
      (7) A bedpan and two disposable pads (if the patient must remain in bed)
   b. Large-volume method (Figure 30.6):
      (1) Irrigating bag with 1,000 ml warm tap water or other solution

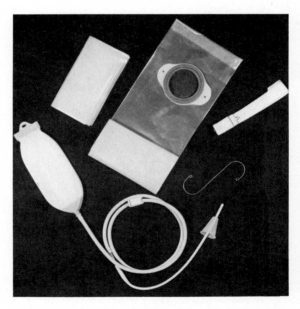

FIGURE 30.6   EQUIPMENT FOR A LARGE-VOLUME IRRIGATION
Courtesy Mason Laboratories, Inc., Horsham, PA

as ordered. This bag is usually equipped with a flow regulator and a number 28 rubber catheter. A cone can be substituted for the catheter. An advantage of the cone is that it cannot be inserted too far.

(2) An IV pole. (This is not necessary when there is a hook where the irrigation is to be given.)

(3) A rubber nipple to prevent backflow. (This fits over the catheter. It is not necessary if a cone tip is on the tubing.)

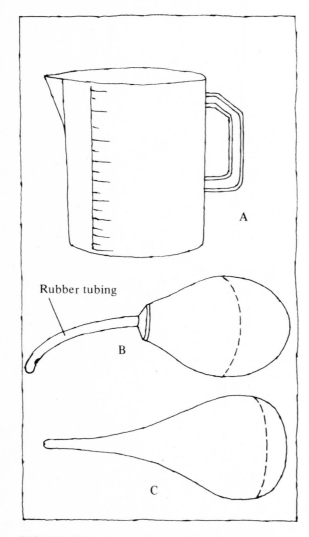

Rubber tubing

FIGURE 30.7   BULB SYRINGE COLOSTOMY IRRIGATING EQUIPMENT   *A:* Measuring container; *B:* 8-ounce rubber bulb; *C:* large-size ear syringe

c. Bulb syringe method (See Figure 30.7):

(1) An 8-ounce bulb syringe with a Number 28 rubber catheter attached. A large-sized ear syringe without a catheter can be substituted.

(2) A container filled with 750 ml warm tap water.

4. Provide for the patient's privacy, either by closing the bed curtains (if done at bedside) or by taking the patient to the bathroom.

5. Remove the soiled bag.

6. Put the irrigating bag or sleeve on the patient, over the colostomy.

7. Position and drape the patient.

a. In the bathroom, the patient sits on the toilet or commode. Place the end of the irrigating bag between the legs, so that it can drain directly into the toilet. Drape a towel or bath blanket over the patient's lap for warmth and modesty. (See Figure 30.8.)

b. In bed, position the patient on his or her side. You will use two disposable pads and a bedpan. Place the bedpan on a protective pad on the bed. Then place the end of the irrigating sleeve in the bedpan. (See Figure 30.9.) Use the other disposable pad to cover the bedpan as the colostomy empties. This helps to contain odor. Sometimes a patient who cannot sit on a commode but can sit in bed is placed in a high-Fowler's position. The bedpan is then placed beside the patient's hips.

8. Irrigate the colostomy.

a. Large-volume method:

(1) Hang the irrigating container on the IV pole with the fluid level approximately 12 to 18 inches above the stoma. This positions the bottom of the container at the patient's shoulder.

(2) Expel all air from the tubing.

(3) Place the nipple over the end of the catheter, approximately 3 to 5 inches from the end, or attach the cone to the tubing.

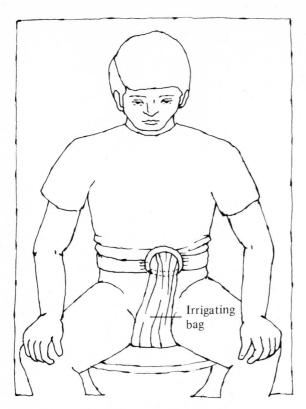

FIGURE 30.8   PATIENT SITTING ON A COM-
MODE FOR IRRIGATION OF A COLOSTOMY
A lap drape has been omitted to make the position
of the drainage bag clear.

(4) Lubricate the tip of the catheter
or the cone.
(5) Put on a rubber glove and lubricate your little finger.
(6) Gently dilate the stoma by putting your lubricated finger
through the open top of the

irrigation bag (or the hole provided in the bag) into the opening. Check for the direction of
the lumen. If the colostomy is
double-barreled (has two stomas),
you will be irrigating the proximal loop.
(7) Gently thread the catheter
through the opening in the irrigation bag on into the stoma. Insert only 3 to 5 inches. If you
meet an obstruction, do not
force the catheter. Rotate it
gently, allowing a small amount
of fluid to flow in. This often
opens the lumen. If you cannot
insert it, seek help. It is possible
to perforate a bowel or to
severely traumatize the mucosa
by forceful pushing. The cone
tip fits into the stoma only a
short distance.
(8) Press the nipple or cone firmly
against the stoma to occlude the
opening around the catheter. If a
nipple or cone is not available,
press with the fingers to close
the stoma around the catheter.
(9) Open the tubing and allow all of
the fluid to flow into the bowel.
If cramping occurs, stop the
flow and wait, as you would with
a conventional enema.
(10) When all the fluid is in, remove
the catheter or cone, and allow
the bowel contents to empty.

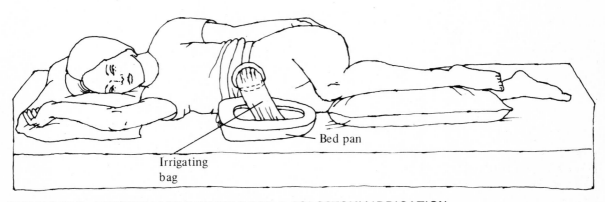

FIGURE 30.9   PATIENT LYING ON SIDE FOR A COLOSTOMY IRRIGATION

b. Bulb syringe (small-volume) method:
   (1) Fill the syringe with water. Be sure to turn the opening up and expel all air.
   (2) Dilate the stoma with your lubricated and gloved little finger.
   (3) Gently insert the catheter of the syringe 3 to 5 inches into the stoma.
   (4) Gently squeeze the bulb, instilling all of the water, as you press around the stoma to prevent backflow. Do not allow the bulb to reinflate while in the stoma. There may be some return after the catheter is withdrawn.
   (5) Refill the syringe two more times, for a total of three syringes full (720 ml) of fluid. Do not give more than this amount even if some fluid returned between instillations.

9. Have the patient sit for approximately 15 minutes to allow the bowel to empty. By gently massaging the abdomen, you can encourage emptying.
10. Clean off the bottom of the irrigating sleeve, fold it up, and fasten it closed.
11. Wait 30 more minutes to allow the colostomy to complete emptying. During this time the patient can move around, shave, bathe, and so on.
12. Drain the irrigating sleeve again and remove it.
13. Put a clean regular bag or dressing in place.
14. Clean all the equipment, dry it, and put it away for future use.
15. Wash your hands.
16. Chart the irrigation. Include the amount of fluid used and returned, a description of return, and the patient's reaction.

PROBLEMS

1. *The fluid does not return* Consider the fluid as intake, and notify the physician. *Do not* use additional irrigating fluid. Watch the patient carefully for later fluid return.

2. *No stool returns* If the bulb syringe method is used, you can repeat the procedure immediately, wait a few hours and repeat, or wait 24 hours and then repeat. This depends on the physician's decision and your facility's procedure. Repeating the procedure immediately can excessively fatigue the patient. The large-volume irrigation is not usually repeated without specific consultation with the physician because of electrolyte depletion.

3. *The fluid flows out as fast as you put it in* This will not allow for adequate emptying of the bowel. Stop the irrigation and devise a better way to occlude the stoma opening before you begin again.

4. *A patient with an old colostomy says that he or she uses a lot more fluid than you are planning to use* Some patients increase fluid on their own at home and have been known to instill 4,000 to 5,000 ml, and to take two hours for an irrigation. Explain to the patient the rationale for the procedure as you are going to do it. Then consult with your team leader or head nurse. You may have to increase the amount of fluid to obtain any results. Also, inform the physician of the patient's current practice.

5. *The patient states that he or she always inserts the catheter 8 or 10 inches* Explain the rationale for the short distance and do not insert the catheter any farther. One of the advantages of the bulb syringe (or cone) is that the patient cannot insert the device too far because it is so short.

Changing a Urinary-Drainage Appliance

You must pay particular attention to cleanliness whenever you work with a urinary diversion because of the potential for urinary-tract infection.

1. Wash your hands.
2. Gather the necessary equipment:

a. Adhesive solvent
b. Cotton-tipped applicators
c. Cleansing materials
d. Tissues
e. Clean bag
f. Adhesive
g. Paper sack for the soiled bag
h. Protective spray for skin, if ordered
i. Stoma guidestrip if available. This is a dissolvable paper material especially made for this purpose.

3. Position the patient on his or her back and drape.
4. Dip the applicators in the adhesive solvent.
5. Starting at one corner, roll the applicator against the edge, loosening the adhesive.
6. Continue pulling from the one corner while you roll the applicator against the point where the adhesive meets the skin. Do not try to pull the appliance off until the solvent has loosened the adhesive or you may damage the skin.
7. Carefully clean the skin with clear warm water. Rinse thoroughly and pat dry.
8. Fold a tissue over the stoma to absorb urine. Change as necessary to keep the skin dry.

9. Put the protective spray on the skin if ordered.
10. Put adhesive on the appliance face.
11. When the adhesive has dried as much as the directions indicate, remove the tissue from the stoma.
12. Curl the stoma guidestrip onto the stoma opening. This will help you place the appliance correctly over the stoma. (See Figure 30.10.)
13. Center the appliance carefully over the stoma, using the guidestrip for placement.
14. Press the appliance firmly into place. The guidestrip will drop into the appliance and dissolve.
15. Hook the belt into place.
16. Clean the used appliance according to your facility's procedure.
17. Wash your hands.
18. Chart the appliance change, including your assessment of the skin and the patient's reaction.

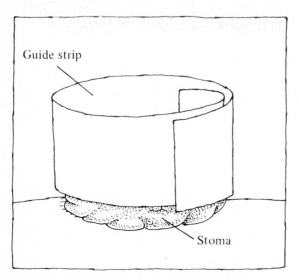

Guide strip

Stoma

FIGURE 30.10 STOMA GUIDESTRIP BEING POSITIONED

PERFORMANCE CHECKLIST

Changing a colostomy-ileostomy bag	Unsatisfactory	Needs more practice	Satisfactory	Comments
1. Wash your hands.				
2. Check care plan.				
3. Provide for patient's privacy.				
4. Check appliance in use and equipment available at bedside.				
5. Explain procedure to patient.				
6. Obtain equipment: a. Cleansing supplies				
b. Clean bag				
c. Seal or adhesive				
d. Clean belt				
e. Paper bag, paper towels, or newspaper				
f. Protective spray (tincture of benzoin)				
g. Clean rubber gloves				
7. Remove old bag, and place on paper or in paper bag. Save closure clip if necessary.				
8. Clean around stoma.				
9. Cover stoma with tissue.				
10. Dry area thoroughly.				
11. Apply protective material if needed.				
12. Allow to dry thoroughly.				
13. Remove tissue from stoma and, following directions for adhesive, apply bag.				
14. "Bunch" bag.				
15. Add deodorant solution if wanted.				
16. Prick hole in bag if wanted.				
17. Fasten closure clip at bottom of bag.				
18. Fasten clean belt in place.				
19. Dispose of soiled bag: discard disposable bag; empty and clean reusable bag.				
20. Wash soiled belt for future use.				
21. Wash your hands.				
22. Make patient comfortable.				
23. Chart.				

Colostomy dressing	Unsatisfactory	Needs more practice	Satisfactory	Comments
1. Wash your hands.				
2. Gather equipment.				
3. Drape and screen patient.				
4. Using gloves, remove soiled dressing and place in bag or paper.				
5. Clean area.				
6. Remove soiled gloves.				
7. Form circular gauze base.				
8. Place large dressings over top, putting more in direction of flow.				
9. Tape dressing in place.				
10. Dispose of soiled dressings.				
11. Wash your hands.				
12. Chart.				
Irrigating a colostomy				
1. Explain procedure to patient.				
2. Wash your hands.				
3. Obtain necessary equipment.				
4. Provide for patient's privacy.				
5. Remove soiled bag.				
6. Put irrigating sleeve on patient.				
7. Position and drape patient.				
8. Irrigate colostomy. a. Large-volume method: (1) Hang container.				
(2) Expel air from tubing.				
(3) Place cone or nipple.				
(4) Lubricate tip of catheter.				
(5) Lubricate gloved finger.				
(6) Dilate stoma.				
(7) Thread catheter in 3 to 5 inches or insert cone.				
(8) Occlude stoma opening.				

	Unsatisfactory	Needs more practice	Satisfactory	Comments
(9) Allow fluid to run in.				
(10) Remove catheter.				
b. Small-volume method: (1) Fill bulb syringe.				
(2) Dilate stoma with lubricated gloved finger.				
(3) Insert catheter of syringe 3 to 5 inches.				
(4) Squeeze bulb, instilling all water, while pressing around stoma to prevent backflow.				
(5) Refill syringe and repeat twice.				
9. Have patient sit for 15 minutes.				
10. Clean bottom of irrigating sleeve and close.				
11. Wait 30 minutes.				
12. Drain irrigating sleeve again and remove it.				
13. Put on clean bag or dressing.				
14. Clean equipment.				
15. Wash your hands.				
16. Chart.				
Changing a urinary-drainage appliance				
1. Wash your hands.				
2. Gather equipment.				
3. Position patient and drape.				
4. Dip applicators in adhesive solvent.				
5. Start removing at one corner.				
6. Continue removing by rolling applicator against adhesive.				
7. Clean skin and dry.				
8. Cover stoma with tissue.				
9. Put protective spray (if ordered) on skin.				
10. Put adhesive on appliance face.				
11. When adhesive is dry, remove tissue.				
12. Place stoma guidestrip.				

	Unsatisfactory	Needs more practice	Satisfactory	Comments
13. Place appliance, centering over stoma.				
14. Press appliance in place.				
15. Hook belt on appliance.				
16. Clean used appliance.				
17. Wash your hands.				
18. Chart.				

QUIZ

Short-Answer Questions

1. What is an ileostomy? _____

2. What special problems does a patient with an ileostomy have?

   _____

3. How is an ileoloop different from an ileostomy? _____

   _____

4. List two reasons why a base of gauze is placed around the stoma.

   a. _____

   b. _____

5. What is the best position for the patient having a colostomy irrigation?

   _____

6. How many milliliters of fluid are used for a large-volume colostomy irrigation? _____

7. How many milliliters of fluid are used for a bulb syringe (small-volume) irrigation? _____

8. How far is the catheter inserted for a colostomy irrigation? _____

9. How long should the patient remain on the toilet after the irrigation fluid is instilled? _____

10. After the initial draining, how long should the irrigation bag be left in place before putting on the regular appliance or dressing? _____

11. Why is special attention to cleanliness necessary when changing a urinary-drainage appliance? _____

Module 31 Administering Oxygen

MAIN OBJECTIVE

To administer oxygen to patients, using the equipment appropriate in a safe and effective manner.

RATIONALE

Emergency patients, post-op patients, and the increasing number of patients with heart or lung disease often require the administration of oxygen. As much skill and knowledge are required to administer oxygen as are needed in the administration of medication. There are certain hazards inherent in the use of oxygen, and thus the nurse must be familiar with the equipment and skilled in its utilization.

PREREQUISITES

Successful completion of the following modules:

VOLUME 1
Assessment
Charting
Medical Asepsis
Hygiene
Temperature, Pulse, and Respiration

SPECIFIC LEARNING OBJECTIVES

	Know Facts and Principles	Apply Facts and Principles	Demonstrate Ability	Evaluate Performance
1. Patients who need oxygen	List general conditions that necessitate oxygen administration	Give rationale for oxygen administration when assigned a patient		
2. Methods of administration	Name four methods of oxygen administration	Describe appropriate situation for use of each method. Determine methods used in a given facility.		
3. Psychological support	Know impact of fear and anxiety on breathing	Assess for level of anxiety in patient	Reassure and make adequate explanations to patient	Evaluate patient's emotional status in terms of relaxation and decreased anxiety
4. Administering oxygen	State hazards of oxygen	Prepare room properly to prevent fire	Implement oxygen administration with emphasis on patient's comfort and safety	Evaluate own performance using Performance Checklist
5. Recording	Know essential information to be recorded	Use proper format and know responses patient may have to administration	Record data and patient's responses	Review own performance with instructor

LEARNING ACTIVITIES

1. Review the Specific Learning Objectives.
2. Read the section on respiration in Ellis and Nowlis, *Nursing: A Human Needs Approach,* or comparable material in another textbook.
3. Look up the module vocabulary terms in the glossary.
4. Read through the module.
5. In the practice setting, if oxygen equipment is available:
   a. Inspect and handle the equipment.
   b. Practice applying a mask and a nasal cannula on a partner.
   c. Have your partner apply the mask and nasal cannula on you.
6. In the clinical setting:
   a. Become familiar with the oxygen equipment used in your clinical facility.
   b. By talking to a patient who is receiving oxygen, ascertain what he or she has been told regarding the procedure.
   c. Review the types of patients who are receiving oxygen.
   d. On a specific patient, observe the administration of oxygen. Were all safety precautions observed?
   e. Under supervision, plan and initiate oxygen therapy as ordered on a patient.
   f. Chart the procedure properly, and share your notes with your instructor.

VOCABULARY

anoxia
cannula
catheter
claustrophobia
combustion
dyspnea
explosive
flowmeter
humidifier
hypoxemia
hypoxia
liter
lumen
prongs
uvula

ADMINISTERING OXYGEN

Oxygen is essential to life, and an optimum level of oxygen must be maintained to sustain mental functioning. Approximately one fifth, or 20 percent, of the air we normally breathe is oxygen.

In persons who have problems of the respiratory tract or systemic conditions that affect respiration, the exchange of oxygen in the lungs is often compromised, leading to a state of hypoxia. Trauma or injury (hemorrhage) can also interfere with the process of oxygenating the blood (hypoxemia). In such cases, administering additional oxygen to increase its concentration in the blood is essential.

Psychological Problems for the Patient

The administration of oxygen, although a commonplace procedure, can make patients anxious, which invariably leads to difficulty in breathing. You will find that many patients perceive the administration of oxygen as a lifesaving measure, or as an indication that they are seriously ill. This is not always the case. Others find a mask or tent oppressive and experience feelings of claustrophobia during the process. By explaining the procedure (in simple terms) to the patient and the patient's family, as well as by maintaining a calm attitude, you can help to allay many unnecessary fears. For this reason, even semicomatose patients should be given explanations.

Safety

There are inherent dangers in administering oxygen. Although oxygen itself is not explosive, it supports combustion. This means that extremely rapid burning takes place in the presence of a high oxygen concentration, almost as if the oxygen itself were explosive. Thus, it is essential that you take precautionary steps to prevent sparks or fire in an environment where oxygen is being used. Some precautions follow.

1. Display a No Smoking sign prominently on the patient's door, which cautions all persons in the room, including the patient, not to smoke.
2. Inspect all electrical equipment in the immediate vicinity of the patient for frayed cords and defective plugs that could cause sparks.
3. Do not allow the patient to use an electric razor.
4. Avoid the use of woolen blankets because they produce static electricity, which is another cause of sparks.
5. Because of the enclosed high concentration of oxygen, take special precautions with patients in oxygen tents to further avoid sparks and possible fire. Do not comb hair or allow call bells to be operated in a closed tent.

Oxygen can be stored in several ways. Most facilities have a piped-in system with outlets on the wall by the bedside; a special flowmeter is available that attaches to the wall outlet. This oxygen comes from a large holding tank, which is usually located separate from the facility. When oxygen is not piped in, facilities use a tank (usually painted green) that holds oxygen at more than 2,000 pounds pressure per square inch. Because of the extreme pressure, these tanks should be handled with great care. Large tanks are chained to a stand.

For outpatients who need intermittent therapy, there are smaller, portable tanks of liquid oxygen that can be wheeled by the patient or strapped to the body for use. Oxygen in this form is safe because of its low pressure.

Regardless of the method or appliance used, oxygen should always be turned on and checked *before* you administer it directly to a patient. All oxygen is under pressure, and gauges and flowmeters do malfunction, so *each time* oxygen is to be started on a patient, check all equipment first.

The physician usually writes an order for oxygen, which includes the date and time, the method of administration, and the num-

ber of liters per minute that are to be delivered. If at any time you assess that a
patient is in a state of anoxia (lacking oxygen) you can start oxygen without a doctor's
order, notifying the physician later. This
decision requires skilled nursing judgment,
however. Frequently a physician will order
oxygen p.r.n. (as needed), so that the nurse
can start or discontinue its administration
according to the patient's needs.

Equipment

A *flowmeter* is a device that is attached to
the oxygen outlet to regulate the amount
and pressure of oxygen delivered. (See
Figure 31.1.) Flowmeters are usually of
two types: mercury ball and gauge. They
both register the number of liters delivered
per minute.

An additional gauge is used with tank
oxygen. The gauge attaches directly to the
tank and registers the amount of oxygen in
it. When the tank is almost empty, the

needle points to a red area, warning that the
tank will need replacing shortly.

Below the flowmeter may be a *humidifier
bottle,* which moistens the flow of dry
oxygen. Currently, opinion differs as to
whether a humidifer should be used. Those
advocating its use feel that moistening the
flowing oxygen decreases the drying effect
on the oronasal mucosa. Those opposed
argue that the danger of infection from
microorganisms harbored in the bottle
outweighs any advantages. A partial answer
to this position is to fill the container with
sterile water. Studies may soon give us
guidelines, but, for the time being, follow
the policy of your facility.

Methods of Administration

OXYGEN TENTS

Tents (Figure 31.2) are seldom used now,
except for pediatric patients, because of
several disadvantages. Most tents are constructed of a transparent plastic canopy
that is suspended from a frame with an
electric cooling unit and an oxygen gauge
on the back. The bottom of the tent must
be secured in folds of linen and under the
mattress to prevent leakage. Some patients

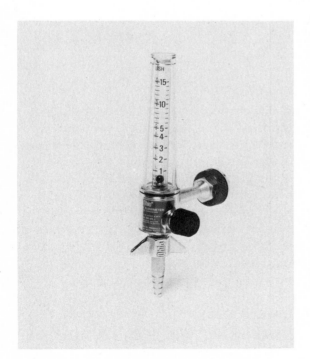

FIGURE 31.1   OXYGEN FLOWMETER
*Courtesy Ohio Medical Products, Division of
Airco, Inc.*

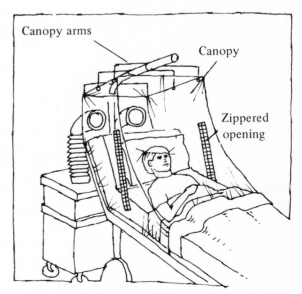

FIGURE 31.2   OXYGEN TENT

experience an unpleasant, closed-in feeling when they are in an oxygen tent; and they cannot move about in bed freely without disturbing the tucked edges. Tents also require much more oxygen to maintain the desired concentration and are, therefore, costly to operate. Furthermore, it is difficult to maintain a comfortable temperature for a patient in the tent. Another disadvantage is that tents are difficult to clean, although disposable canopies are now available. However, tents do provide relative comfort for a small child who finds a face device unpleasant.

NASAL CATHETERS

Nasal catheters—plastic or rubber catheters with a small lumen (Figure 31.3)—are also used infrequently because they can irritate a patient's nostrils and are unpleasant to have inserted.

1. To measure for insertion, hold the tip of the catheter from the tip of the patient's nose to the earlobe, and mark the length with tape.
2. Apply a water-soluble lubricant to the catheter for easy passage. The lubricant must be water soluble so that it is not hazardous if a small amount accidentally enters the lungs.

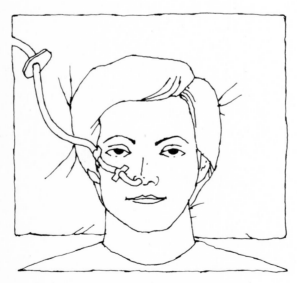

FIGURE 31.3   NASAL CATHETER

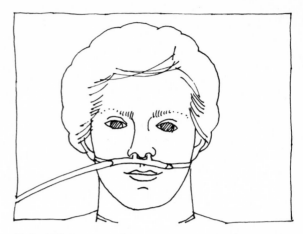

FIGURE 31.4   NASAL CANNULA

3. Then, direct the catheter into the nostril and guide it backward along the floor of the nose.
4. Check the position by inspecting the back of the throat. The tip of the catheter should be visible at a position near the uvula.
5. Turn on the oxygen and adjust to the proper flow rate *before* you attach the adapter to the patient's catheter.
6. Change the nasal catheter every 48 hours.

NASAL CANNULAS

This is the most common method of administering oxygen, because it is easy to apply and comfortable for the patient. (See Figure 31.4.) The administration of 3 liters per minute by a cannula is a sufficient amount of oxygen for most patients. Although patients often mouthbreathe and it appears that they are not receiving the oxygen, it has been found that the oxygen flows downward over the mouth because it is heavier than air and is, in fact, breathed in.

OXYGEN MASKS

Mask oxygen (Figure 31.5) is the method of choice in emergency situations or at times when patients need a relatively high concentration of oxygen promptly.

1. Prepare the patient. The application of a mask can be frightening.

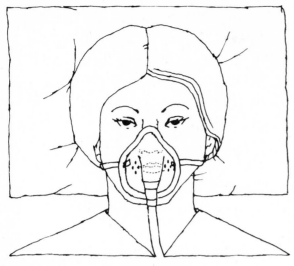

FIGURE 31.5   OXYGEN MASK

2. Attach the mask to the oxygen source tube.
3. Regulate the flow. More than 3 liters per minute may be needed initially until the patient becomes acclimated to the mask and breathes more regularly.
4. Securely fit the mask against the face to prevent leaks.
5. Make sure the patient is comfortable.

Oronasal Care

Oxygen dries the mucous membranes. It is good nursing practice to administer frequent oral and nasal care to any patient who requires oxygen.

PERFORMANCE CHECKLIST

General procedure	Unsatisfactory	Needs more practice	Satisfactory	Comments
1. Explain procedure to patient and elicit patient's cooperation (if possible).				
2. Wash your hands.				
3. Obtain equipment.				
4. Place No Smoking sign on door of patient's room.				
5. Check all electrical equipment and outlets.				
6. Attach flowmeter and filled humidifer (if used) to tank or wall outlet.				
7. Check equipment for proper functioning.				
8. Follow directions for equipment to be used. (See checklists below.)				
9. Wash your hands.				
10. Chart procedure, numbers of liters of oxygen delivered, method, and patient's response.				
11. Evaluate patient's tolerance of procedure, administering appropriate oronasal care for dryness.				
Oxygen tents				
1. Place tent, untucked, over patient, with controls to side or head of bed.				
2. Plug into electrical outlet.				
3. Set temperature at approximately 70° F.				
4. Attach oxygen flowmeter to outlet.				
5. Flood tent. (Set flow between 10 and 12 liters per minute until tent holds sufficient concentration of oxygen.)				
6. Secure back and sides of tent under mattress.				
7. Using edges of bedding in tuck-fold manner, secure bottom edges of front side for tight fit.				
8. Readjust flow to desired level.				
9. As you work, continually reassure patient.				

	Unsatisfactory	Needs more practice	Satisfactory	Comments
Nasal catheters				
1. Measure from tip of nose to earlobe, and mark.				
2. Lubricate with water-soluble lubricant.				
3. Insert gently along floor of nostril to marking.				
4. Check position.				
5. Attach to preadjusted oxygen supply.				
6. Change every 48 hours.				
Nasal cannulas				
Fit cannula to patient's nostrils, adjusting head strap comfortably. (Some patients prefer loose loop over ears and tightening plastic ring under chin.)				
Oxygen masks				
1. Attach mask outlet to oxygen supply tubing.				
2. Regulate flow.				
3. Snugly fit mask to patient's face.				
4. Check patient's comfort.				

QUIZ

Short-Answer Question

1. List four methods to deliver oxygen.

   a. _____

   b. _____

   c. _____

   d. _____

Multiple-Choice Questions

_____ 2. Oxygen is potentially dangerous because it

   a. burns rapidly.   c. supports combustion.
   b. is explosive.   d. combines with nitrogen.

_____ 3. Regardless of the method used, it is important to test and regulate oxygen flow before applying to the patient because

   a. it is easier to observe the flow rates.
   b. it guards the patient from the danger of a malfunction.
   c. it guards the patient from an explosion.
   d. it limits the amount of oxygen intake.

_____ 4. Oxygen flow (liters per minute)

   a. should never exceed 3 liters/min.
   b. should remain under 8 liters/min.
   c. should be changed every eight hours.
   d. is determined by the delivery method and the physician's order.

_____ 5. In an emergency situation, the method most frequently used would be the

   a. mask.   c. nasal catheter.
   b. tent.   d. nasal cannula.

_____ 6. The least advantageous method, which is used infrequently, is the

   a. mask.   c. nasal catheter.
   b. tent.   d. nasal cannula.

_____ 7. Frequent oral and nasal care should be given to the patient receiving oxygen *primarily* because

   a. of the patient's high anxiety level.
   b. oxygen is drying to mucous membranes.
   c. oxygen is irritating to the skin.
   d. secretions are increased.

_____ 8. Patients who receive oxygen therapy need explanations and reassurance because (1) the patient or family may think the patient is seriously ill when this is not so; (2) it may bring on a feeling of claustrophobia; (3) the patient has had no previous experience with it; (4) some oxygen appliances are uncomfortable to wear.

    a. 1 only   **c.** 1, 2, and 4 only
    b. 2 and 3 only   **d.** All of the above

Module 32 Inspection, Palpation, Auscultation, and Percussion

MAIN OBJECTIVE

To achieve beginning skills in inspection, palpation, auscultation, and percussion, and thereby to enhance assessment and nursing care.

RATIONALE

The nurse is expected to perform various aspects of the basic physical exam on a daily basis when caring for hospitalized patients. The observations of the nurse, augmented by skills in inspection, palpation, auscultation, and percussion, give the nurse a better data base for nursing care and give the physician valuable input into the diagnosis and treatment of patients.

The development of the skills presented in this module require frequent practice. The module is not meant to provide you with the detail and depth necessary to do a complete physical examination; it is planned to give you the beginning skills that will enable you to make a more complete nursing assessment.

PREREQUISITES

Successful completion of the following modules:

VOLUME 1
Assessment
Charting
Temperature, Pulse, and Respiration
Blood Pressure

73

SPECIFIC LEARNING OBJECTIVES

	Know Facts and Principles	Apply Facts and Principles	Demonstrate Ability	Evaluate Performance
1. Inspection	Define inspection. List six areas to be included in inspection.		Include color, odor, size, shape, symmetry, and movement appropriately when performing inspection	Evaluate own performance with instructor
a. Pupils	List three aspects of pupils to include in inspection. Explain pupillary reaction to light. Explain accommodation.		Inspect pupils of patient for size, shape, and equality. Check pupillary reaction to light and accommodation.	Evaluate with instructor using Performance Checklist
b. Neck veins	State position in which neck veins are normally collapsed. Describe how to estimate venous pressure without special equipment. State normal venous pressure values in centimeters.	Place patient in position in which neck veins are normally collapsed. Given specific values, state whether venous pressure is within normal limits	Identify jugular veins of neck and assess. Estimate venous pressure of patient with distended neck veins	Evaluate with instructor using Performance Checklist
2. Palpation	Define palpation. List four areas or conditions that can be identified using palpation.	Given patient situations, choose parameters to be measured by palpation	Using palpation, identify softness, rigidity, temperature, position, and size appropriately	Evaluate own performance with instructor

a. Edema	State two items of information to be included in explanation to patient prior to palpation	Given a patient situation, state what should appropriately be included in explanation to patient	In the clinical setting, give appropriate explanation to patient before palpating	Evaluate with instructor using Performance Checklist
	State four areas of body where dependent edema might be found	Given a patient situation, state where dependent edema might be found	In the clinical setting, evaluate patient for presence of dependent edema.	Evaluate with instructor using Performance Checklist
	Define *periorbital edema* and *prettibial edema*		In the clinical setting, evaluate patient for presence of periorbital edema.	
b. Ascites	Define *ascites*	State one problem patient might have as result of ascites	In the clinical setting, test for presence of fluid wave	Evaluate own performance with instructor
	State how to differentiate between obesity and ascites			

	Know Facts and Principles	Apply Facts and Principles	Demonstrate Ability	Evaluate Performance
c. *Breasts*	List five parameters to be observed in inspecting breasts of male or female patients. Describe characteristics of breast tissue in younger female, older female, and menstruating female. Describe how to palpate breast.	Given a patient situation, describe what characteristics of breast tissue might be present	Include size, symmetry, skin color, vascularity, and skin retraction when inspecting breasts of male or female patient. In the clinical setting, palpate breasts of male or female patient.	Evaluate own performance with instructor. Evaluate with instructor using Performance Checklist.
d. *Abdomen and liver*	List four observations to be made when inspecting abdomen. List three parameters that may be demonstrated when palpating abdomen. Describe procedure for palpation of liver.		Include bulges, bruises, scars, and symmetry when inspecting abdomen of patient. Palpate abdomen moving systematically and gently. In the clinical setting, palpate for liver of patient.	Evaluate own performance with instructor. Evaluate with instructor using Performance Checklist.
e. *Digital exam of rectum*	List signs and symptoms of fecal impaction. Describe procedure for digital exam of rectum.		In the clinical setting, perform digital exam	Evaluate with instructor using Performance Checklist

3. *Auscultation*	Define *auscultation*. State two ways in which nurse can help control environmental noise level.	Given a patient situation, state what might be done to control noise level	Take steps to control noise level before attempting auscultation	Evaluate with instructor using Performance Checklist
a. *Heart*	List three areas commonly auscultated. List three aspects of heartbeat to be evaluated with use of auscultation. Describe where first and second heart sounds are usually most easily heard.		Accurately discern rate, rhythm, and intensity of heartbeat of assigned patient. Listen for first and second heart sounds in correct locations.	Evaluate with instructor using Performance Checklist
b. *Bowel sounds*	List situations in which bowel sounds may be diminished. List situations in which bowel sounds may be increased. State why auscultation of abdomen should be carried out prior to palpation and percussion.	Given a patient situation, predict whether bowel sounds will be diminished or increased	In the clinical setting, listen for bowel sounds in a systematic fashion	Evaluate with instructor using Performance Checklist

	Know Facts and Principles	Apply Facts and Principles	Demonstrate Ability	Evaluate Performance
c. *Lungs*	List situations in which breath sounds may be absent or decreased. State type of conditions that might cause breath sounds to be increased. Define *adventitious sounds.*	Given a patient situation, predict whether breath sounds will be decreased or increased	In the clinical setting, identify adventitious sounds on auscultation of lungs	Evaluate with instructor using Performance Checklist
4. Percussion *a. Chest* *b. Abdomen*	Define *percussion.* Describe percussion procedure. Define *resonance, tympany, dullness,* and *flatness.* State where and in what situation(s) each sound might be heard.	Given a patient situation, state what sound might be heard on percussion	In the clinical setting, demonstrate percussion of chest and abdomen	Evaluate with instructor using Performance Checklist
5. Charting	State observations that should be included in record with regard to inspection, palpation, auscultation, and percussion	Given a patient situation, chart appropriate items accurately	In the clinical setting, chart findings of inspection, palpation, auscultation, and percussion completely and accurately	Evaluate with instructor using Performance Checklist

LEARNING ACTIVITIES

1. Review the Specific Learning Objectives.
2. Read the section on observation (in the chapter on the nursing process) in Ellis and Nowlis, *Nursing: A Human Needs Approach,* or comparable material in another textbook.
3. Look up the module vocabulary terms in the glossary.
4. Read through the module.
5. In the practice setting, with a partner and under supervision:
   a. Test the reaction of your partner's pupils to light and accommodation, using the Performance Checklist as a guide. Chart your observations.
   b. Identify the jugular veins of your partner bilaterally, while he or she is lying supine. Gradually elevate the head of the bed to a 45-degree angle. Note when the jugular veins collapse. Is your partner's venous pressure within normal limits?
   c. Assess your partner for edema of the ankles. If any is present, rate it on a scale of 1+ to 4+. Is periorbital edema present?
   d. Inspect and palpate your partner's breasts. Practice communicating as you would with a patient.
   e. Observe and palpate the four quadrants of the abdomen.
   f. Palpate for the liver.
   g. Practice the digital exam for fecal impaction on a mannequin. Have your partner evaluate your performance, including communication, using the Performance Checklist.
   h. Using the diaphragm of the stethoscope:
      (1) Practice listening to your own cardiac rate and rhythm.
      (2) Identify first and second heart sounds using the carotid pulse as a guide.
      (3) Repeat steps (1) and (2) using your partner as a patient.
   i. Listen to all four quadrants of your partner's abdomen for bowel sounds.
   j. Systematically listen to your partner's lungs, both anteriorly and posteriorly. Then, listen to your partner's lungs in the supine and side-lying positions. If you hear rales, ask your partner to cough, and listen again to see if they have cleared.
   k. Practice percussion technique on a hard surface, such as a desk or table. Then, practice on your thigh to get used to percussing on a body surface. Using the procedure as a guide, practice percussing your partner for resonance, tympany, dullness, and flatness. Do systematic percussion of the chest and abdomen.
   l. Have your partner evaluate your technique using the various checklists. He or she should also evaluate your explanations and your regard for the "patient's" comfort and modesty.
   m. Change roles, and repeat steps a–l.
   n. When you are both satisfied with your performances, have your instructor evaluate you.
6. In the clinical setting:
   a. Practice inspection, palpation, auscultation, and percussion techniques as frequently as possible, with a staff nurse or your instructor to supervise, assist, and evaluate.
   b. Practice the above techniques independently, and compare your findings with those of the staff nurse responsible for the care of the patient.

VOCABULARY

accommodation
adventitious sounds
alveoli
apex
apical pulse
auscultation
base
bell
bronchi
constriction
dependent edema
diaphragm
diastole
dullness
edema
flatness
impaction
inspection
objective
palpation

percussion
periorbital edema
pretibial edema
rales
rebound tenderness
resonance
retraction
rhonchi
stethoscope
subjective
symmetry
symphysis pubis
systole
trachea
tympany
umbilicus
venous pressure
wheezes
xiphoid process

INSPECTION, PALPATION, AUSCULTATION, AND PERCUSSION

The four general processes included in a physical examination are difficult to separate totally from one another. Despite the overlapping of certain areas, we will attempt to discuss each of the processes as a single entity.

Inspection

Inspection is closely related to observation, but involves itself more specifically with physical, rather than social, information. Although primarily visual in nature, inspection includes the sense of smell as well.

You will want to work out your own system for the inspection process to avoid missing any area of information. You could use the body systems, a head-to-toe approach, or a combination of the two, but the emphasis should be on a *systematic* approach.

Whichever system you use, inspection should include color, odor, size, shape, symmetry, and movement (or lack of same). In each instance, you will be comparing what you see with what is "normal" for an individual of the patient's age group.

In the event that you observe something significant, you must elicit information about the finding. For example, what were the precipitating factors? How long has it existed in this state? Is there pain associated?

PUPILS

The nurse is frequently called on to observe the pupils and their reaction to light. Usually performed as a part of "neuro signs," this is often done when neurological disease is present or suspected.

1. Wash your hands.
2. Explain to the patient what you plan to do.
3. Inspect size, shape, and equality of pupils.

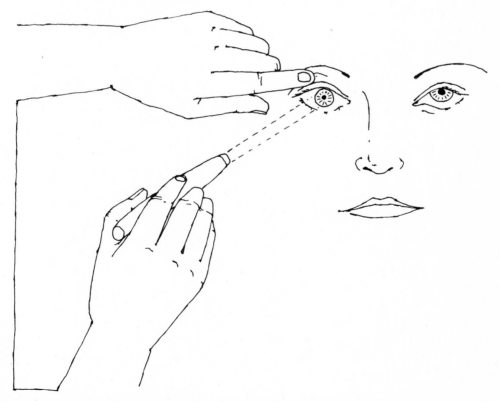

FIGURE 32.1   TESTING THE PUPILLARY REACTION TO LIGHT   The light source is brought in from the side.

4. Inspect the pupillary reaction to light.
   a. Holding the lid open with one hand, shine a light (a common flashlight is generally used) on one pupil at a time, bringing the light in from the side (Figure 32.1).
   b. Observe what happens to the pupil.
      (1) Does it constrict?
      (2) If it does constrict, does it do so rapidly or is it sluggish?
   c. Repeat step b on the opposite side.
      (1) Are the reactions the same?
5. Test the pupillary reaction to accommodation. (This is not routinely done in all settings.)
   a. Ask the patient to look at an object in the distance, and then at your fingers held 5 to 10 cm from the bridge of the patient's nose.
   b. Note the pupillary constriction (the pupils should constrict as they attempt to accommodate) and the convergence of the eyes.
6. Wash your hands.
7. Chart your observations. A variety of forms have been designed for pupillary observations (see Figure 32.2), and one of them may be in use in your clinical facility. Also, the abbreviations PERL (pupils equal and reactive to light) and PERLA (pupils equal and reactive to light and accommodation) are commonly used in charting pupillary observations.

NECK VEINS

You will often be called on to inspect the distention of the jugular veins for an estimation of venous pressure. When a person is standing or sitting in a position above 45 degrees, the jugular veins of the neck are normally collapsed. If these veins are distended in a position above 45 degrees, an abnormally high venous pressure is present.

1. Wash your hands.
2. Explain to the patient what you plan to do.
3. Have the patient lie flat on his or her back. Watch for dyspnea. (Patients with distended neck veins are often unable to lie flat without experiencing dyspnea.)
4. Identify the jugular veins bilaterally.
5. Gradually elevate the head of the bed to a 45-degree angle, watching to see when the jugular veins collapse.
6. If the jugular veins remain distended at 45 degrees, venous pressure may be estimated by measuring (in centimeters) the vertical distance from the right atrium level (midchest) to the upper level of distention. If this procedure is carried out frequently, mark the right atrial level on the patient's chest, to ensure consistent measurements. Venous pressure is considered normal between 4 and 10 cm.
7. Wash your hands.
8. Chart the estimated venous pressure.

Palpation

Palpation involves the sense of touch, and in most cases is used simultaneously with inspection. Using the palms, fingers, and tips of the fingers, the nurse can identify softness, rigidity, and temperature, as well as determine position and size. You have already used palpation to measure the rate and quality of the peripheral pulses.

Again, explanation is extremely important to obtain the cooperation of the patient as you palpate. Explain what is being done, why it is being done (if appropriate), and what the patient can do to make it easier for both of you.

EDEMA

Edema is the abnormal accumulation of fluid in the intercellular tissues of the body. Edema is often *dependent* in nature; that is, it occurs in dependent areas of the body (the hands, feet, ankles, and sacrum).

Periorbital edema (around the soft tissue of the eyes) is also relatively common. It may have diagnostic significance, or in women it may simply be related to cyclical hormonal changes. This type of edema is

VITAL SIGN RECORD

PUPIL SIZE AND REACTION			
0 - - 0	Equal	R	Reacts
. - - 0	Unequal	NR	Does not react
Example:	left smaller, no reaction		

O	R	.	NR

CONSCIOUSNESS
Normal
Responds verbally
Disoriented
Moves only to pain
Deeply comotose

MISCELLANEOUS
Medicines
Fluids
Treatments
Pain
Paralysis

DATE	HOUR	B.P.	P	R	TEMP	PUPILS		
						RIGHT	LEFT	

BALLARD COMMUNITY HOSPITAL

SEATTLE, WASHINGTON

VITAL SIGNS RECORD

FIGURE 32.2 A FORM FOR RECORDING PUPILLARY OBSERVATIONS
Courtesy Ballard Community Hospital, Seattle, Washington

usually soft and resilient, not pitting in nature.

To palpate for edema, use the fingertips of the index and middle fingers, pressing firmly over a bony area. (Figure 32.3) When you remove your fingers, observe the area for its appearance at that time, and continue to watch to see how long it takes for the depressed area to disappear. Edema is generally rated on a scale of 1+ to 4+. 1+ is a slight depression that disappears quickly; 4+ is a deep depression that disappears slowly. Because the scale is subjective, measurements of extremities are often used for more objective data, along with daily weights.

ASCITES

Ascites is a large accumulation of fluid in the peritoneal cavity, which can cause respira-

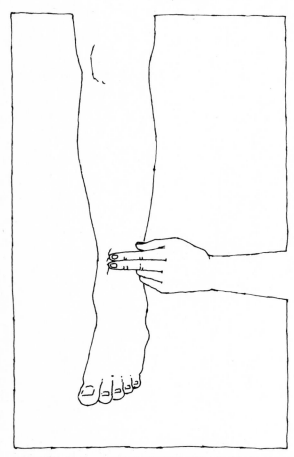

FIGURE 32.3   APPLY PRESSURE TO EVALU-
ATE PRETIBIAL EDEMA

tory distress because of the pressure of the fluid on the diaphragm. It is sometimes difficult to identify ascites, especially in an obese person. One way to differentiate between obesity and ascites is to test for a fluid wave, which indicates the presence of fluid in the peritoneal cavity.

1. Place the patient in the supine position.
2. Place the palm of your hand against the lateral abdominal wall.
3. With the other hand, tap the opposite wall of the abdomen.

If the impact of the tap is felt by the other hand, you have demonstrated the presence of a fluid wave.

Ongoing assessment of ascites usually includes a measurement of abdominal girth. Place the measuring tape around the patient at the point of widest girth. You can use a felt-tipped marker to mark the patient's abdomen in two places, so that measurement is consistently done at the same place and so that the tape is placed on an even plane around the patient.

BREASTS

The most common site of cancer in the female is the breast. The examination of the breasts in male patients is important, too. Although much less frequently than in females, cancer of the breast does occur in males. Again, the procedure is a combination of inspection and palpation.

1. Explain to the patient what you plan to do.
2. Screen the patient.
3. Wash your hands.
4. Ask the patient to disrobe to the waist and to be seated with hands in the lap.
5. Observe the nipples for color, discharge, and retraction ("dimpling").
6. Observe the breasts for size, symmetry, skin color, vascularity, and skin retraction.
7. Ask the patient to raise the hands above the head, and particularly observe for skin texture and/or dimpling.
8. Have the patient lie down.

9. Starting with the upper outer quadrant and moving systematically in one direction or the other, use the palmar aspect of your fingers to palpate each breast in turn. Palpate the breast by gently compressing the breast tissue against the chest wall. The consistency of breast tissue varies among females, primarily according to age: that of younger women is firm and elastic; that of older women is more stringy and nodular. In addition, be aware of the stage of the menstrual cycle of menstruating females because the breasts can be particularly sensitive at the time of menstruation.
10. Wash your hands.
11. Chart.

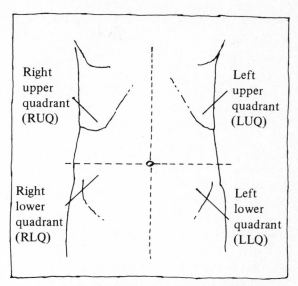

FIGURE 32.4   THE FOUR QUADRANTS OF THE ABDOMEN

ABDOMEN AND LIVER

Although the palpation of the abdomen can be a very sophisticated procedure, we include it here as a fairly simple endeavor. In a complete examination, first auscultate the abdomen, and then palpate and percuss. Palpation and percussion can change the bowel sounds.

Palpation of the liver is part of the overall procedure. The normal liver is not palpable. An enlarged nontender liver indicates chronic disease; an enlarged tender liver indicates acute disease.

1. Explain to the patient what you plan to do.
2. To make your examination systematic and to clarify your descriptions, mentally divide the abdomen into quadrants. The horizontal line extends across through the umbilicus; the vertical line extends downward from the xiphoid process to the symphysis pubis. The four quadrants are the *right upper quadrant* (RUQ), the *right lower quadrant* (RLQ), the *left lower quadrant* (LLQ), and the *left upper quadrant* (LUQ). (See Figure 32.4.)
3. Wash your hands in warm water. Cold hands will make the patient uncomfortable and may cause him or her to be tense.

4. Ask the patient to breathe through the mouth, to enhance relaxation.
5. Observe the abdomen. Note the condition of the skin, including any bulges, bruises, or scars, and observe for symmetry.
6. Use the palmar surfaces of your fingers to palpate.
7. Moving systematically, palpate gently for tone (softness versus rigidity), swelling, and tenderness.
8. Also assess for rebound tenderness, (pain that is elicited when you release your hand quickly after slow palpation). Rebound tenderness is a symptom of peritonitis.
9. Ask the patient to inhale.
10. Standing to the right of the patient, place your left hand under the rib cage and use the palmar surface of the fingers of your right hand to palpate just below the right costal margin. If the liver edge is palpable, it will descend below the right costal margin, and the number of centimeters it descends below the right costal margin should be noted.
11. Wash your hands.
12. Chart your findings.

DIGITAL EXAMINATION OF THE RECTUM

A digital examination of the rectum is usually performed when fecal impaction is suspected, and is usually based on the patient's complaint of long-term or abnormal constipation, or the leakage of watery stool in the absence of actual bowel movements.

1. Wash your hands.
2. Gather the necessary equipment:
   a. A clean rectal glove
   b. A lubricant
   c. A bedpan
3. Explain to the patient what you plan to do.
4. Assist the patient to the left lateral position, with the knees drawn up toward the abdomen. Other positions can be used, but this is usually the most comfortable for both patient and nurse.
5. Place a clean glove on the hand you will use to do the examination.
6. Lubricate the gloved index finger.
7. Spread the patient's buttocks apart with your other hand.
8. Ask the patient to bear down while you gently insert your index finger into the rectum.
9. Ask the patient to breathe in and out through the mouth (to enhance relaxation).
10. Move your examining finger in a circle. A hard mass that fills the rectum is probably a fecal impaction. You may be able to break it up and remove it with your gloved finger by bending the finger and gently removing small amounts at a time into the bedpan. (Sometimes oil-retention enemas are given to help soften the fecal mass and assist in its discharge.)
11. Remove the glove.
12. Wash your hands.
13. Chart your findings on the patient's record.

Auscultation

Auscultation refers to listening (usually with a stethoscope) to sounds produced by the body in order to differentiate normal from abnormal sounds. To perform auscultation, you must first be able to recognize the normal variation in sounds. Then gradually, through constant practice, you will begin to recognize deviations from normal. Only the sophisticated practitioner can evaluate the significance of the abnormal sounds.

Stethoscopes come equipped with a bell, a diaphragm, or preferably both. With this last type, you can switch from one to the other by turning the chestpiece or by flipping a lever. Low-pitched sounds are better heard with the bell placed lightly against the skin; high-pitched sounds are better heard with the diaphragm pressed firmly against the skin. Many nurses purchase their own stethoscopes to ensure quality and consistency.

An important aspect of auscultation is the control of the noise level in the environment. This is extremely important if you are to detect all sounds. In addition, instruct the patient not to talk during this aspect of the examination.

HEART

You can begin to recognize heart sounds by listening to your own heart and then to those of other students. Starting at the fifth left intercostal space near the sternum, listen all along over to the nipple line and laterally, until you find the position in which you can hear best.

In the clinical setting, if you have difficulty hearing the heart, have the supine patient roll partially over to the left, or have the sitting patient lean slightly forward. In either case, the sounds should be easier to hear because the heart has moved closer to the chest wall. Heart sounds that are very difficult to hear are termed *distant* and those easily heard termed *clear.* Heart sounds are often more difficult to hear in obese or barrel-chested patients.

Evaluate cardiac rate, rhythm, and intensity first. In some facilities, all patients who are receiving a digitalis preparation have an apical pulse taken prior to the administration of the digitalis, to ensure an accurate heart rate count. Note *regular* irregularities, as well as occasional missed or early beats (irregular irregularities). Abrupt changes in rate and/or rhythm should also be noted.

You should also be able to differentiate between the first and second heart sounds (S_1 and S_2). (This is more easily accomplished at normal and slow rates.) Heart sounds are created by the closing of valves in the heart. Systole occurs between the first and second sounds, and diastole between the second and first sounds. The first sound is more easily heard in the area of the fifth intercostal space near the nipple line (the apex); the second sound is more easily heard in the area of the second intercostal space immediately to the right of the sternum (the base). (See Figure 32.5.) The sounds over the apex are usually more easily heard with the bell of the stethoscope; the sounds over the base of the heart are usually more easily heard with the diaphragm. You should, however, feel free to experiment with both on any given patient to determine which gives you the best sound.

If you have difficulty distinguishing the sounds, identify the carotid pulse while you listen to the heart. The carotid pulse occurs simultaneously with the first heart sound.

There are often sounds (third and fourth) that are generally considered abnormal, as well as other sounds associated with cardiac pathology. These are beyond the scope of this text.

LUNGS

As you did with heart sounds, you can begin by listening to your own lungs, although it will probably be easier to listen to those of another student, or to a record of lung sounds if available. You should try to discern normal breath sounds and abnormal, or adventitious, sounds. Again, to attain any degree of skill, you must practice frequently.

Use the diaphragm of the stethoscope, pressed firmly against the skin, to auscultate the lungs. The patient should be in a sitting position if possible. If not, roll the patient from side to side, so that you can listen to all areas. If the patient is able to cooperate, ask that he or she breathe slowly in and out

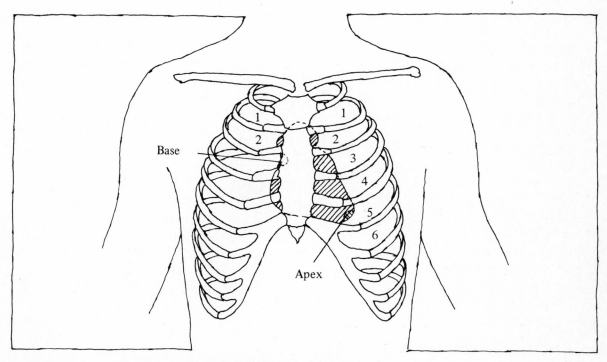

FIGURE 32.5   THE APEX AND THE BASE OF THE HEART

through an open mouth, when the stethoscope is placed on the back. Auscultation should be done both anteriorly and posteriorly in a systematic manner, comparing one side to the other. (See Figures 32.6 and 32.7.) Be sure to note the location of the lobes of the lungs in the figures. The lower lobes are heard only in a very small area on the anterior chest; conversely, the upper lobes are heard only in a small area of the posterior chest.

Breath sounds are the sounds created by the movement of air in the trachea, bronchi, and alveoli. Normally, the expiratory phase is twice as long as the inspiratory phase. On auscultation, however, you do not hear all of the expiratory phase, so that it will seem shorter than the inspiratory phase. In cases of bronchial obstruction, chronic lung disease, or shallow breathing (as might be seen in a patient with incisional pain after abdominal surgery), breath sounds may be absent or decreased. In a condition that causes consolidation of lung tissue, such as pneumonia, the breath sounds may be louder or increased.

There are many abnormal sounds, which you hear superimposed on the breath sounds. Among these are rales, rhonchi, wheezes, and friction rubs.

Rales   Rales result from air passing through moisture (due to secretions) in the respiratory passages. They are usually heard on inspiration. Fine rales have a crackling sound; coarse rales are similar in quality but louder. If you hear rales, ask the patient to cough and listen again. Often a patient who has been lying quietly has some rales in the bases that clear when he or she coughs.

Rhonchi   Rhonchi are caused by air passing through respiratory passages that have narrowed or been partially obstructed by secretions, edema, tumors, and the like. Rhonchi are usually low-pitched in quality and often alter in quality after the patient coughs.

Wheezes   Like rhonchi, wheezes are caused by air passing through partially obstructed respiratory passages, but they are higher pitched in quality because they originate in smaller passages. Wheezes have a whistle-type tone. Although they are more commonly

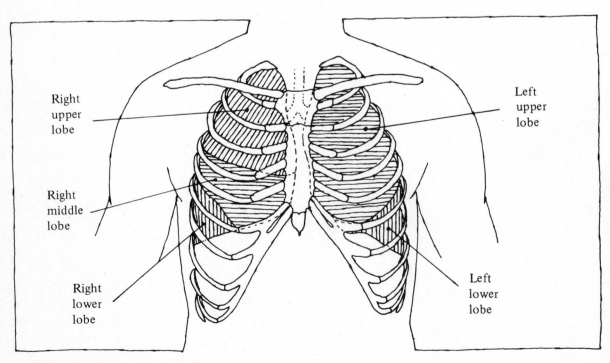

FIGURE 32.6   THE ANTERIOR CHEST

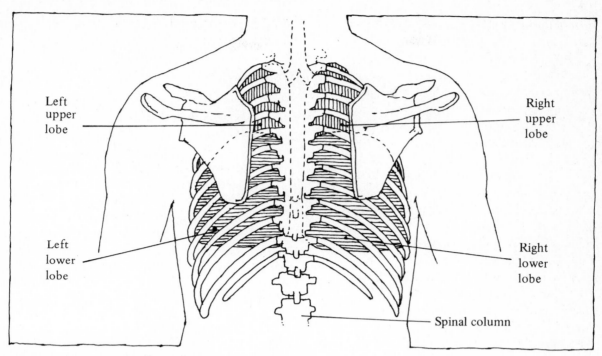

Left
upper
lobe

Right
upper
lobe

Left
lower
lobe

Right
lower
lobe

Spinal column

FIGURE 32.7   THE POSTERIOR CHEST

heard during expiration, rhonchi and wheezes can be heard during any phase of respiration.

Pleural Friction Rubs   Pleural friction rubs are caused by the rubbing together of inflamed and roughened pleural surfaces. The sound is rough and scratchy, somewhat like two pieces of sandpaper being rubbed together. Friction rubs are heard on both inspiration and expiration. If this sound correlates with the rate and rhythm of the heartbeat, and not the respirations, it is a pericardial friction rub.

BOWEL SOUNDS

Normal bowel sounds, which indicate normal peristaltic activity, occur every 5 to 15 seconds. The absence of sound or very soft sounds (commonly called *diminished bowel sounds*) indicate the inhibition of bowel mobility, as would occur in inflammatory processes or in the postoperative state. Increased bowel sounds (or *hyperactive bowel sounds*) occur with gastroenteritis or after a laxative has been taken. High-pitched rushing sounds may indicate a bowel obstruction.

To listen for bowel sounds, lightly place the diaphragm of the stethoscope on the abdomen. Auscultate all four quadrants in a systematic fashion. Start with the right lower quadrant because bowel sounds are often most pronounced (and more easily heard) there.

AUSCULTATION PROCEDURE

This procedure includes the auscultation of the three areas presented here: heart, bowels, and lungs.

1. Explain to the patient what you plan to do. Ask the patient not to speak while you are trying to listen.
2. Control the noise in the environment. For example, turn off the television and close the door.
3. Screen the patient.
4. Fan-fold the patient's gown or pajama top up to the shoulders.
5. Wash your hands.
6. To auscultate the heart:
   a. Place the patient in the supine position.

b. Fan-fold the bed linen down to the patient's waist.

c. Warm the diaphragm of the stethoscope in your hands.

d. Place it at the fifth left intercostal space near the sternum, and listen moving laterally until you can hear the heart sounds clearly.

e. Count the cardiac rate.

f. Evaluate the cardiac rhythm, noting any regular or irregular irregularities.

g. Listen for the first and second heart sounds, correlating the carotid pulse with the first heart sound.

7. To auscultate the bowels:

a. Fan-fold the patient's gown or pajama top down to cover the chest.

b. Fan-fold the bed linen down to the symphysis pubis.

c. Place the diaphragm of the stethoscope lightly against the skin of the right lower quadrant, moving systematically until you have listened to all four quadrants. If no sounds are heard, continue to listen in that quadrant for a minimum of two to five minutes.

8. To auscultate the lungs:

a. Assist the patient to a sitting position, if possible; if not, roll patient from side to side.

b. Ask the patient to breathe slowly in and out through an open mouth.

c. Using the diaphragm of the stethoscope, listen to the anterior chest, beginning with the apex on one side and comparing with the other side.

d. Then move to the posterior chest and listen, beginning with the upper lobes and moving to the lower.

e. If any rales or rhonchi are present, ask the patient to cough and listen again to see if they have cleared.

9. Replace the patient's gown.

10. Make the patient comfortable, repositioning the bed linen as he or she wants.

11. Return the environment to its previous state. Check to be sure the patient would like this done.

12. Wash your hands.

13. Chart your findings.

Percussion

Percussion involves striking a body surface to produce sounds that enable an experienced examiner to determine whether the underlying tissues are air-filled, fluid-filled, or solid. The examiner both *hears* (sounds change with the density of the tissue beneath) and *feels* the effects of percussion.

Because percussion penetrates only about 5 to 7 centimeters into the chest, it will not detect deep lesions.

SOUNDS

Resonance is the normal sound heard when the lung is percussed. You can elicit this sound by percussing the lung at the right anterior portion of the third interspace. The sound is low in pitch and not loud.

Tympany results from air trapped in an enclosed chamber. It is loud and high in frequency. You can hear this sound if you percuss over the stomach. It is especially marked after a carbonated beverage has been consumed.

Dullness occurs with the consolidation or increased density of lung tissue, as in the case of pneumonia. It is a short, high-pitched sound. You can elicit dullness by percussing over the diaphragm.

Flatness is a short, high-pitched sound completely without resonance or vibration. Fluid in the chest or abdomen can produce flatness. You can hear the sound by percussing over solid tissue, for example, your thigh.

METHOD

Although we can present the process here (the actual procedure appears in the Performance Checklist), along with the examples above of the kinds of sounds that can be elicited, you will have to practice on normal individuals to become familiar with normal sounds, in order to begin to be able to detect abnormal sounds.

1. Place the middle finger of your non-dominant hand firmly against the body surface to be percussed. Keep the palm and other fingers off the skin.
2. With the tip of the middle finger of your dominant hand, strike the base of the distal phalanx of the finger against the body surface, just behind the nail bed (Figure 32.8). Use a wrist action and make the blow brief. Remove the striking finger immediately to avoid attenuating the vibrations.
3. Systematically percuss the chest, comparing one side to the other.
4. Percuss each quadrant of the abdomen. Dullness may indicate the presence of fluid. Tympany in the left upper quadrant may indicate a gastric air bubble.

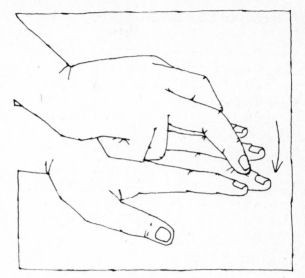

FIGURE 32.8   PERCUSSION

PERFORMANCE CHECKLIST

	Unsatisfactory	Needs more practice	Satisfactory	Comments
Inspecting the pupils				
1. Wash your hands.				
2. Explain procedure to patient.				
3. Inspect size, shape, and equality of pupils.				
4. Test reaction of pupils to light, one at a time.				
5. Test reaction of pupils to accommodation.				
6. Wash your hands.				
7. Chart.				
Inspecting the neck veins				
1. Wash your hands.				
2. Explain procedure to patient.				
3. Have patient lie flat on back.				
4. Identify jugular veins bilaterally.				
5. Gradually elevate head of bed to 45-degree angle.				
6. Measure vertical distance in centimeters from right atrium to upper level of distention.				
7. Wash your hands.				
8. Chart.				
Palpating the breasts				
1. Explain procedure to patient.				
2. Screen patient.				
3. Wash your hands.				
4. Have patient disrobe and be seated with hands in lap.				
5. Observe nipples for color, discharge, and dimpling.				
6. Observe breasts for size, symmetry, skin color, vascularity, and skin retraction.				
7. Have patient raise hands above head and observe for skin texture and dimpling.				
8. Have patient lie down.				
9. Palpate each breast systematically.				
10. Wash your hands.				
11. Chart.				

	Unsatisfactory	Needs more practice	Satisfactory	Comments
Palpating the abdomen and liver				
1. Explain procedure to patient.				
2. Mentally divide abdomen into quadrants.				
3. Wash your hands in warm water.				
4. Ask patient to mouth-breathe.				
5. Observe abdomen for skin condition and symmetry.				
6. Using palmar surfaces of your fingers, palpate patient's abdomen.				
7. Move systematically, palpating for tone, swelling, and tenderness.				
8. Assess for rebound tenderness.				
9. Ask patient to inhale.				
10. Palpate for liver.				
11. Wash your hands.				
12. Chart your findings.				
Examining the rectum for fecal impaction				
1. Wash your hands.				
2. Gather equipment.				
3. Explain procedure to patient.				
4. Position patient in left lateral position.				
5. Place glove on hand.				
6. Lubricate gloved index finger.				
7. Spread patient's buttocks.				
8. Gently insert finger into patient's rectum.				
9. Ask patient to mouth-breathe.				
10. Move examining finger in a circle, removing any fecal material found.				
11. Remove glove.				
12. Wash your hands.				
13. Chart your findings.				

Auscultating the heart, bowels, and lungs	Unsatisfactory	Needs more practice	Satisfactory	Comments
1. Explain procedure to patient.				
2. Control environmental noise.				
3. Screen patient.				
4. Raise patient's gown or pajama top to shoulders.				
5. Wash your hands.				
6. Heart: a. Place patient in supine position.				
b. Fan-fold bed linen to patient's waist.				
c. Warm diaphragm of stethoscope.				
d. Position diaphragm.				
e. Locate apical pulse and count rate.				
f. Evaluate rhythm.				
g. Listen for first and second heart sounds, correlating carotid pulse with first heart sound.				
7. Bowels: a. Fan-fold patient's gown or pajama top over chest.				
b. Fan-fold bed linen to patient's symphysis pubis.				
c. Systematically listen to all four quadrants of abdomen, beginning with right lower quadrant.				
8. Lungs: a. Assist patient to sitting position, or roll from side to side.				
b. Ask patient to mouth-breathe.				
c. Auscultate anterior chest.				
d. Auscultate posterior chest.				
e. If rales or rhonchi are present, have patient cough and listen again.				
9. Replace patient's gown.				
10. Assist patient to position of comfort.				
11. Readjust environment.				
12. Wash your hands.				
13. Chart.				

Percussing the chest and abdomen	Unsatisfactory	Needs more practice	Satisfactory	Comments
1. Explain procedure to patient.				
2. Screen patient.				
3. Remove patient's gown or pajama top.				
4. Fan-fold bed linen to patient's waist.				
5. Place patient in sitting position.				
6. Percuss patient's chest systematically.				
7. Have patient lie down.				
8. Percuss each quadrant of patient's abdomen.				
9. Replace patient's gown.				
10. Assist patient to position of comfort.				
11. Wash your hands.				
12. Chart.				

QUIZ

Short-Answer Questions

1. List five observations that should be included in inspection.

   a. _____

   b. _____

   c. _____

   d. _____

   e. _____

2. Before testing the pupillary reaction to light and accommodation, for what three things should the nurse inspect the pupils?

   a. _____

   b. _____

   c. _____

3. In what position are the jugular veins normally collapsed?

   _____

4. Between what values is venous pressure considered normal?

   _____

5. List three elements that the nurse should include in the explanation to the patient prior to palpation.

   a. _____

   b. _____

   c. _____

6. Where is periorbital edema found? _____

7. Why should the nurse be aware of the patient's stage in the menstrual cycle when palpating the breasts of a female? _____

8. When examining the abdomen, why should auscultation be done before palpation and percussion? _____

9. In what area is the first heart sound usually most easily heard?

   _____

10. Name one situation in which breath sounds might be absent or decreased.

   _____

Module 33 Respiratory Care Procedures

MAIN OBJECTIVE

To effectively assist patients with deep breathing, coughing, postural drainage, and percussion as necessary in their individual situations.

RATIONALE

Although most large hospitals have respiratory care departments that undertake technical respiratory care procedures, in many instances these procedures do become the responsibility of the nurse. Therefore, the nurse must be able to perform them competently. Even when the specific procedure is the responsibility of the respiratory care department, the nurse must remain responsible for total patient care. In addition, one of the nurse's regular responsibilities is to explain procedures to patients. In order to do this thoroughly, the nurse must understand the procedure.

Often these procedures must be taught to patients, so that the patients are able to carry them out independently. When this is true, the nurse must use the understanding of the process of patient teaching as well as the procedural information contained in this module.

PREREQUISITES

1. Successful completion of the following modules:

   VOLUME 1
   Assessment
   Charting
   Medical Asepsis
   Moving the Patient in Bed and
       Positioning

   VOLUME 2
   Inspection, Palpation, Auscultation,
       and Percussion

2. A review of the anatomy and physiology of the respiratory system, paying special attention to the physiology of the cough reflex.

SPECIFIC LEARNING OBJECTIVES

	Know Facts and Principles	Apply Facts and Principles	Demonstrate Ability	Evaluate Performance
1. *Deep breathing*	State reasons for deep breathing. Identify patient situations in which deep breathing is needed. Describe procedure for deep breathing. State purposes for blow bottles, incentive spirometer, and IPPB.	Given a patient situation, identify when deep breathing is needed	Assist patient to deep breathe effectively	Evaluate effectiveness of deep breathing by checking depth of patient's respiration (identifying extent of rise and fall of abdomen and chest as breath is taken)
2. *Coughing*	Define *cough*. State reasons for encouraging patient to cough. Identify patient situations in which coughing is needed. Describe procedure for effective coughing.	Given a patient situation, identify when coughing is needed	Assist patient to cough effectively	Evaluate effectiveness by checking for movement of secretions
3. *Postural drainage*	Define *postural drainage*. Identify patient situations in which postural drainage is often used. Describe positions used for postural drainage for all lung areas. Describe common problems of postural drainage.	Given a patient situation, identify which position for postural drainage would be most effective. Given a patient situation, identify problems occurring.	Assist patient in postural drainage. Recognize problems occurring during postural drainage and decide appropriate course of action related to problem.	Evaluate effectiveness of postural drainage by auscultation of lungs. Validate decision with instructor.

4. *Percussion and vibration*	State purpose of percussion and vibration. Describe procedure for percussion and vibration.	Identify situations where percussion and vibration might be helpful	Perform percussion and vibration correctly	Evaluate own performance using Performance Checklist. Evaluate by checking amount of secretions raised.
5. *Charting*	State information to be charted regarding respiratory care		Chart appropriate information when assisting with respiratory care	

LEARNING ACTIVITIES

1. Review the Specific Learning Objectives.
2. Read the material on respiration and the chapter on health teaching in Ellis and Nowlis, *Nursing: A Human Needs Approach,* or comparable chapters in another text.
3. Look up the module vocabulary terms in the glossary.
4. Read through the module.
5. Using the module directions as a guide:
   a. Practice deep breathing until you can do deep abdominal breathing easily.
   b. Practice coughing until you can create an effective cough.
   c. Practice postural drainage at home on your own bed.
      (1) Use pillows to position yourself in a moderately slanted position.
      (2) Try the jackknife position.
      (3) Consider the fatigue and discomfort caused by these positions.
6. In the practice setting:
   Obtain a partner. Each of you, in turn, will be the patient while your partner is the nurse. Practice each skill as though you were instructing a patient with no previous knowledge or skill. The person representing the patient should do *exactly* as told, not what he or she knows to be correct.
   a. Teach one another deep breathing.
   b. Evaluate one another using the Performance Checklist.
   c. Teach one another to cough effectively.
   d. Evaluate one another using the Performance Checklist.
   e. Assist one another in postural drainage.
   f. While the "patient" is in each position, use percussion and vibration over the area being drained.
   g. When you believe you can perform all skills correctly, ask your instructor to check your performance.

7. In the clinical area:
   a. Ask your instructor for an opportunity to observe respiratory care being given.
   b. Ask your instructor for opportunities to use these skills.

VOCABULARY

abdominal breathing
alveoli
atelectasis
auscultation
bronchiole
cough
diaphragm
expectorate
expiration
gatched bed
hyperventilation
hypoventilation
inspiration
intermittent
lobe
lung
mucous
mucus
nebulizer
percussion
postural hypotension
segment
sputum
Trendelenburg position
vibration

RESPIRATORY CARE PROCEDURES

Deep Breathing

All alveoli are not equally expanded during each breath taken. Normal respiration includes occasional deep breaths, which serve to fully expand all alveoli and encourage the movement of secretions. Whenever a person is bedridden or otherwise immobile, continuous shallow respirations are common. This tends to encourage the retention of secretions and the collapse of alveoli (atelectasis). Therefore, deep breathing is a planned part of the nursing care of every immobile patient, especially those who have had increased secretions (persons who have inhaled respiratory anesthetics or who have respiratory disease).

Deep breathing may be difficult and even painful for patients who have undergone abdominal or chest surgery. Therefore, you will have to exert greater effort and support when you assist these persons to deep-breathe.

1. Instruct the patient. Because the patient must carry out the procedure, he or she must understand what should be done and why it should be done. A person who understands and accepts the importance of deep breathing will be more likely to cooperate and participate in the exercise. As part of the instruction, you could demonstrate proper deep breathing for the patient. Remember to use the principles of health teaching as you plan for the patient's instruction.
2. Position the patient for maximum expansion of the lungs. To accomplish this, there should be no constriction of the chest. Having the patient sit up on the edge of the bed or in a chair is ideal. However, deep breathing can be done in any position necessitated by the patient's condition.
3. Relieve the patient's pain. A patient who has a surgical wound will feel pain when moving the muscles that have been cut in the surgery. You can minimize this pain by holding the incisional area firmly, decreasing movement. This is called *splinting.* You can spread your hands and hold them firmly over the incision, or the patient can hold the incision with his or her own hands, or a pillow can be held firmly over the incisional area to splint it. It also may be necessary to arrange for pain medication.
4. Have the patient inspire slowly. This allows for more comfortable alveolar expansion. (Slow movement usually creates less discomfort than does rapid movement.) Because normal expiration is twice as long as inspiration, it is helpful if you count slowly to 2 during inspiration.
5. Have the patient expire slowly while you count to 4. This preserves the normal inspiratory-expiratory ratio and encourages the maximum filling and emptying of the alveoli.
6. Watch the patient for chest and abdominal expansion. Maximum expansion of the lungs occurs when both abdomen and chest expand during inspiration. This is often called *abdominal breathing.* The expansion of the abdomen is caused by the diaphragm moving downward, displacing abdominal contents, to allow complete lung expansion. Observe the patient's breathing to see whether complete lung expansion occurs.
7. Correct the patient's breathing technique as necessary to encourage complete lung expansion.
8. Repeat the procedure, for a total of ten deep breaths.
9. Record on the patient's chart. Often there is a checklist on which deep breathing can simply be checked off. If not, make a brief narrative note indicating the time and the patient's performance (whether breaths were deep, how many were taken, and the patient's response).

MECHANISMS FOR ENCOURAGING DEEP BREATHING

Blow Bottles Blow bottles are usually 1-liter bottles. Each bottle has a cork with two tubings running through it, one of which connects the two bottles (Figure 33.1). One bottle is filled with fluid. In blowing into one bottle, the patient must exert enough expiratory force to push the fluid through the tube from one bottle to the other. These exercises encourage the development of the diaphragm and other expiratory muscles. Blow bottles are most commonly used for patients with chronic respiratory disease.

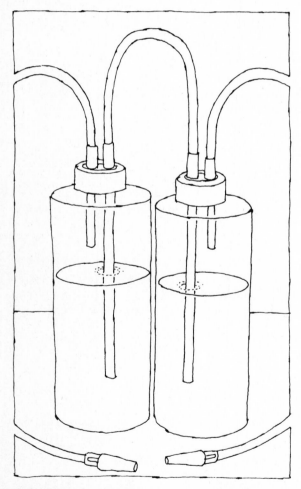

FIGURE 33.1 BLOW BOTTLES Blowing forcefully moves all of the water into one bottle. Then the water can be moved back by blowing on the other open tube.

Incentive Spirometers There are several models of incentive spirometers available, but all have been developed to encourage the patient to deep-breathe. The spirometer is set by the respiratory therapist so that a signal is activated when a prescribed inspiratory volume is achieved. The patient is instructed in deep breathing with particular emphasis on the long inspiratory effort. The patient expires normally, then places the mouthpiece in the mouth, and inspires only through the machine. If the inspiratory volume meets the preset amount, the signal is activated. Most incentive spirometers also have counters to indicate frequency of use.

The device is based on the learning theory that immediate objective feedback about performance increases motivation to learn and results in quicker learning. Set the achievement signal low at first, allowing the patient to master that level before moving higher. This also allows the patient to progress gradually. The devices are quite successful: many patients do far more deep breathing using them.

Some incentive spirometers function with expiratory effort, but the basic premise is the same: with maximum expiratory effort, maximum inspiration also will occur.

Intermittent Positive Pressure Breathing (IPPB) These devices use positive pressure to increase inspiration and to deliver nebulized moisture (with or without medication) deep into the lungs. Most often, IPPB is used for the patient with respiratory disease who needs to have a medication delivered to the lungs.

The actual procedure is specific to the brand of machine. The manufacturer provides a manual with directions for use.

Coughing

Coughing is always combined with deep breathing, although deep breathing may be done without coughing. Deep breathing fully expands the alveoli and enhances the normal respiratory function; coughing is used to raise respiratory secretions so that they do not plug the bronchioles (causing atelecta-sis) or provide a medium for bacterial growth. Also, large amounts of fluid in the lungs can create pneumonia. To prevent the accumulation of secretions, coughing may be encouraged even when a patient does not feel the need to cough.

1. Instruct the patient, explaining the reasons for coughing. Again, a patient who understands and accepts the reason for an activity will be more cooperative in performing that activity.

2. Place the patient in a sitting position if possible. This is usually the most effective position; however, other positions can be used depending on the needs of the patient.

3. Splint, as described in Deep Breathing, step 3, page 103, if necessary.

4. Have the patient deep-breathe, following steps 4 and 5 in Deep Breathing.

5. After the third deep breath, have the patient inspire and hold the air briefly.

6. Have the patient expire forcefully against the closed glottis, and then release the air abruptly while flexing forward. Exhaling against the closed glottis builds up pressure, which tends to create a force that raises secretions. Flexing forward causes abdominal pressure against the diaphragm, which further increases the force of the expired air, increasing the force sufficiently to carry secretions. (Use simpler language when explaining this to the patient. For example, instead of "Exhale against the closed glottis," say, "Hold your breath and then try to breath out when your throat is closed.")

7. Repeat for three deep coughs if possible, or repeat until mucus is expectorated. Do not prolong deep breathing and coughing, however, because this can cause hyperventilation. Watch for dizziness and the tingling of extremities, the most common symptoms of hyperventilation.

8. Check the lungs by auscultation.

9. Offer oral hygiene. Sputum often leaves a disagreeable taste in the mouth.

10. Chart the deep breathing and coughing, and the results of the coughing, if any. Also chart what you heard on auscultation.

11. Repeat deep breathing and coughing hourly, as needed to clear the lungs of secretions, or as ordered.

Postural Drainage

When large amounts of secretions are present in the lungs, it is sometimes impossible to raise all of them by deep breathing and coughing. Postural drainage—positioning the patient so that the force of gravity helps drain the lung secretions—may be necessary.

For most individuals, moderately slanted positions are successful in draining lungs. However, because of the branching structure of the lungs, it is necessary to use a wide variety of positions to adequately drain all of the segments of the lungs.

When postural drainage is used for a patient with chronic respiratory problems, but with no current acute difficulty, each position need be held for only 15 seconds to adequately drain the segments of the lung. In a person with an acute problem, however, it is usually recommended that five minutes be spent initially in each position. When it is determined in which position the majority of the secretions are raised, the time in some positions can be shortened and the times in other positions lengthened. Not all positions are necessary for every patient; only those positions that drain specific affected areas may be needed.

The positions in the procedure that follows are moderate. Although certain lung segments do not drain in these positions, if the entire sequence is used, most do.

1. Explain to the patient the purpose and method of postural drainage. Use the basic principles of health teaching as you plan the patient's instruction.

2. Obtain pillows and a sputum cup and

tissues for the patient to use for expectorated secretions.

3. Position the patient. Check the bed mechanism. Some beds can be "gatched" (raised in the middle) to provide the correct position for postural drainage. Some beds that cannot be gatched do have a foot section that can be lowered, in which case, you can position the patient with his or her head at the foot of the bed and use the foot drop to achieve the desired position. Some beds can be placed in a head-down (Trendelenburg) position. This position can be used for postural drainage, but having the feet raised may increase the patient's fatigue and is not necessary to the effectiveness of the procedure. If the bed cannot be positioned, you will need one large or two small pillows to place under the patient's hips to provide the correct position. You will also need another pillow to use to support the patient in the side-lying position.

4. Identify the specific segments of the lung to be drained. This may be part of the physician's order, or the areas with excessive secretions may be identified by the physician in the progress notes, or you may be able to identify the areas with excessive secretions through auscultation or by checking the chest x-ray report.

   Most often, the lower lobes are drained. It is assumed that most of the upper lobes will drain in normal daily activity, but this would not be true for a severely immobilized patient. The complete sequence is very tiring, and if necessary can be done with rest periods between positions. Pay special attention to elderly patients with heart disease who frequently experience difficulty with the procedure.

5. Drain the upper lobes.
   a. Have the patient sit upright if possible. (Sitting in a fairly straight chair is ideal.) You can also raise the head of the bed to its maximum height.
   b. Have the patient lean to the right

side for five minutes, to drain the left aspect of both upper lobes. Support the patient with pillows if necessary.
   c. Then have the patient lean to the left side for five minutes, to drain the upper right lobes. Again, support the patient with pillows if necessary.
   d. Have the patient lean forward at a 30- to 45-degree angle and stay in this position for five minutes. This drains the posterior segments of the upper lobes. Let the patient brace his or her elbows on the knees to maintain this position. Or, you can pad an overbed table and place it in front of the patient for him or her to lean on.
   e. Have the patient lean backward at a 30- to 45-degree angle for five minutes. This drains the anterior segments of the upper lobes. Help the patient maintain the position by having him or her lean back in bed with the headrest at the proper height.
   f. Have the patient lie on the abdomen, back, and both sides, while horizontal, to drain the remaining segments of the upper lobes.

6. Drain the lower lobes. Use pillows or adjust the bed so that the patient's head is 30 to 45 degrees down from the horizontal position. The 30-degree position is less tiring and creates fewer adverse circulatory effects than does the 45-degree angle.

   Remember that there are six positions. Each can be achieved if the patient starts out lying on one side and gradually turns like a rotisserie. Use the same sequence of positions each time to help you to remember them easily. To identify which segments of the lungs are drained with each position, refer to an anatomy text. The anatomical drawings outline the various lung segments. The patient should remain in each position for five minutes.
   a. Have the patient lie on the left side

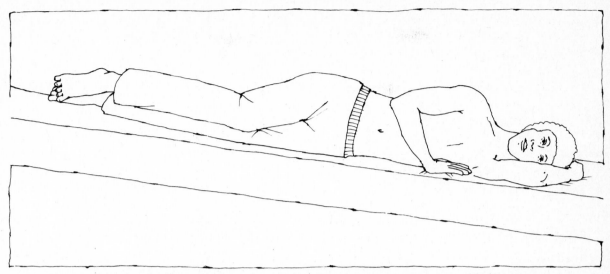

FIGURE 33.2 DRAINING THE LATERAL BASAL SEGMENT OF THE RIGHT LOWER LOBE

with the shoulders perpendicular to the bed. This drains the lateral basal segment of the right lower lobe (Figure 33.2). Use pillows to support the patient and place a small pillow under the head if essential to comfort.

b. Turn the patient halfway onto the back, so that the shoulders are at a 45-degree angle from the bed (Figure 33.3). This position drains the right middle lobe. Again, use pillows to support this position.

c. Turn the patient flat on the back (Figure 33.4). This position drains the anterior basal segments of the right and left lower lobes.

d. Turn the patient halfway to the right side, so that the shoulders are at a 45-degree angle to the bed (Figure 33.5). This position drains the lingula of the left lower lobe.

e. Turn the patient completely onto the right side, so that the shoulders are again at a 90-degree angle to the bed (Figure 33.6). This position drains

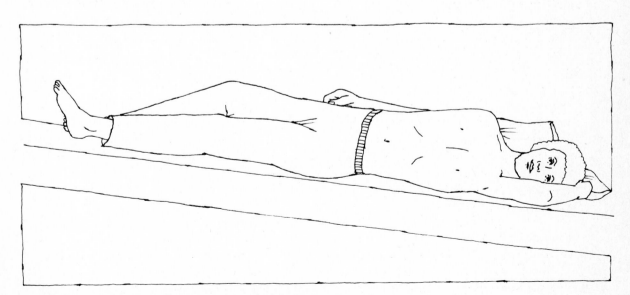

FIGURE 33.3 DRAINING THE RIGHT MIDDLE LOBE

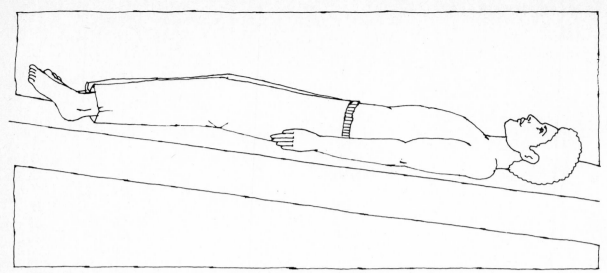

FIGURE 33.4   DRAINING THE ANTERIOR BASAL SEGMENTS OF BOTH LUNGS

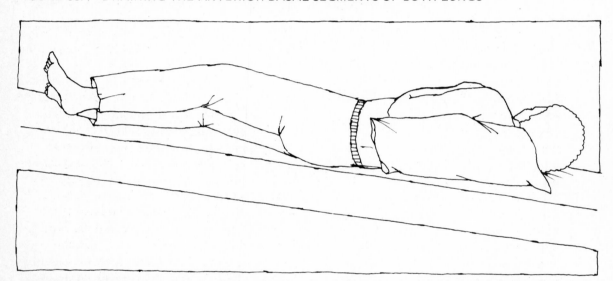

FIGURE 33.5   DRAINING THE LINGULA OF THE LEFT LOWER LOBE   Note the pillow for support.

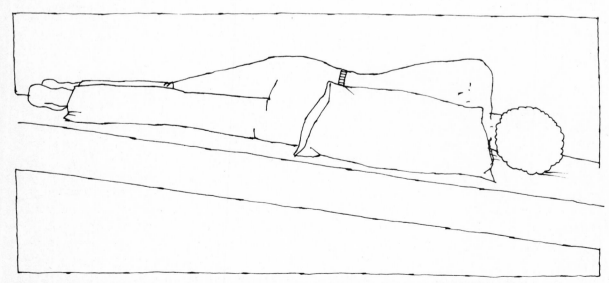

FIGURE 33.6   DRAINING THE LATERAL BASAL SEGMENTS OF THE LEFT LOWER LOBE

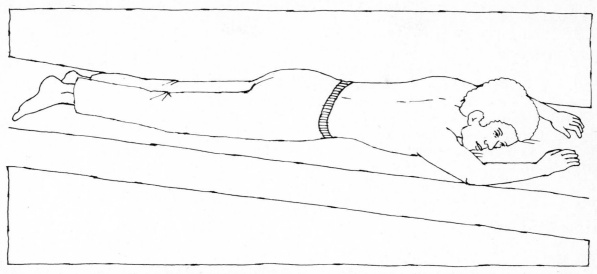

FIGURE 33.7   DRAINING THE POSTERIOR BASAL SEGMENTS OF THE LOWER LOBES   This position is used for coughing out secretions too.

the lateral basal segments of the left lower lobe.

   f. Have the patient turn onto the abdomen with the head turned to the side (Figure 33.7). This position drains the posterior basal segments of the lower lobes. This position is usually used last because secretions are often easier to cough out when the patient is on the abdomen.

7. Have the patient cough thoroughly (lying on the abdomen) to expel secretions.
8. Return the patient to a position of comfort.
9. Allow the patient to rest.
10. Chart.

PROBLEMS

Potential falling because of dizziness or fainting is a common concern when the patient is placed in postural drainage. This can occur while the patient is in the head-down position, but it is even more likely to occur when the patient is first returning to the normal position because of postural hypotension. By changing the positions slowly, you can help somewhat with this problem. In order to protect the patient, raise the side rails and make frequent observations during the procedure. Some patients cannot be left alone at all during the procedure, so use careful nursing judgment.

If a great many secretions are mobilized from the alveoli and small bronchioles at one time, a larger airway may be temporarily blocked, causing severe respiratory distress, anxiety, and fear. In fact, this experience can be so upsetting that the patient may resist future attempts at postural drainage. Explain what is happening and help the patient to cough out the secretions. Support the patient with your continued presence and reassurance.

Sometimes it is necessary to employ percussion (see below) to remove secretions. Also, suctioning may be required if the blockage is severe.

Percussion and Vibration

Perform percussion over areas that need to be drained. While the patient is in the postural-drainage position of choice, cup your hands and clap them over the chest wall. Do not strike hard enough to cause discomfort. By cupping your hands, you cause the percussive force to be transmitted through the forced air to the chest wall. The movement is then transmitted to deeper tissue, helping to loosen mucus.

Vibration is done for the same purpose

and is as effective as percussion if done correctly. Rather than clapping over the chest area, place your hands firmly against the chest wall and vibrate them back and forth rapidly. The vibration is transferred through the tissues and loosens mucus.

Mechanical vibrators also loosen secretions by transferring vibrations through the chest wall. Read the directions for the particular brand and model available (generally you place the vibrating head firmly against the chest wall over the area where secretions are retained).

PERFORMANCE CHECKLIST

	Unsatisfactory	Needs more practice	Satisfactory	Comments
Deep breathing				
1. Instruct patient, demonstrating if necessary.				
2. Position patient.				
3. Relieve pain or splint if necessary.				
4. Have patient inspire while counting slowly to 2.				
5. Have patient expire while counting slowly to 4.				
6. Observe patient for chest and abdominal expansion.				
7. Correct patient's technique as necessary.				
8. Repeat, for total of ten deep breaths.				
9. Chart.				
Coughing				
1. Instruct patient.				
2. Position patient.				
3. Relieve pain or splint if necessary.				
4. Have patient deep-breathe.				
5. After third deep breath, have patient inspire and hold air.				
6. Have patient expire forcefully against closed glottis, and then release air abruptly while flexing forward.				
7. Repeat for three deep coughs, or until mucus is expectorated.				
8. Auscultate lungs.				
9. Offer oral hygiene.				
10. Chart.				
11. Repeat hourly or as needed to clear lungs of secretions.				
Postural drainage (moderate positions)				
1. Instruct patient.				
2. Gather equipment.				
3. Position patient.				
4. Identify specific segments to be drained.				

	Unsatisfactory	Needs more practice	Satisfactory	Comments
5. Drain upper lobes. a. Have patient sit upright if possible.				
b. Have patient lean (45-degree angle) to right for five minutes.				
c. Have patient lean (45-degree angle) left for five minutes.				
d. Have patient lean forward (45-degree angle) for five minutes.				
e. Have patient lean backward (30- to 40-degree angle) for five minutes.				
f. Have patient lie on abdomen, back, and side, while horizontal.				
6. Drain lower lobes. a. Place patient in bed.				
b. Use pillows or bed gatch to elevate hips higher than head. (Head should be approximately 30 to 45 degrees below horizontal level.)				
c. Have patient lie in each position for five minutes, breathing deeply. (1) On left side with shoulders perpendicular to bed.				
(2) On left side with shoulders slanted backward at 45-degree angle from bed.				
(3) On back.				
(4) On right side with shoulders slanted backward at 45-degree angle from bed.				
(5) On right side with shoulders perpendicular to bed.				
(6) On abdomen with head turned to side.				
7. While still on abdomen, have patient cough to raise secretions.				
8. Return patient to comfortable position.				
9. Allow patient to rest.				
10. Chart.				

	Unsatisfactory	Needs more practice	Satisfactory	Comments
Percussion				
1. Place patient in appropriate position for postural drainage.				
2. Use cupped hands.				
3. Clap rapidly over area being drained.				
Vibration				
1. Place patient in appropriate position for postural drainage.				
2. Use flat hands placed firmly against chest wall.				
3. Vibrate hands against chest while patient exhales.				

QUIZ

Short-Answer Questions

1. Why is deep breathing necessary for the inactive or immobile patient?

    _____

2. What is the correct ratio of inspiration to expiration? _____

3. What is the purpose of postural drainage? _____

4. What five basic positions are used to drain the upper lobes?

    a. _____

    b. _____

    c. _____

    d. _____

    e. _____

5. What four positions are used to drain the left lower lobe?

    a. _____

    b. _____

    c. _____

    d. _____

6. What is the purpose of percussion and vibration? _____

7. What is the purpose of the incentive spirometer? _____

Module 34 Preoperative Care

MAIN OBJECTIVE

To prepare patients physically and psychologically for both anesthesia and surgery.

RATIONALE

An important factor that contributes to safe and successful surgery and an uneventful convalescence is the conscientious preparation of patients by the registered nurse. Remember that the patient is traumatized, not only by the surgical procedure, but by exposure to anesthetic agents as well. Preoperative care, therefore, must include adequate health teaching, physical preparation, and psychological support. Although portions of preoperative care may be undertaken by other members of the health care team, it remains the nurse's primary responsibility.

PREREQUISITES

1. Successful completion of the following modules:

    VOLUME 1
    Assessment
    Charting
    Medical Asepsis
    Basic Body Mechanics
    Hygiene
    Admission and Discharge
    Collecting Specimens
    Temperature, Pulse, and Respiration
    Blood Pressure

    VOLUME 2
    Respiratory Care Procedures

2. The following modules are not essential, but their successful completion will allow you to carry out more complete care for selected patients.

    VOLUME 1
    Administering Enemas

    VOLUME 2
    Gastric Intubation
    Irrigations
    Catheterization
    Administering Oral Medications
    Giving Injections

117

SPECIFIC LEARNING OBJECTIVES

	Know Facts and Principles	Apply Facts and Principles	Demonstrate Ability	Evaluate Performance
1. Initial preoperative planning and care				
a. Interview	List information to be obtained through preoperative interview	Given a patient situation, identify information indicating potential problem	Carry out preoperative interview correctly	Evaluate own performance using Performance Checklist
b. Teaching	State information to be included in preoperative teaching	Adapt teaching plan to meet individual patient's concerns	Carry out preoperative teaching correctly	Evaluate own performance using Performance Checklist
2. Preoperative skin preparation	State three objectives of preoperative skin preparation		Assist patient with preoperative bath or shower	
a. Timing shave		Given a time schedule for surgery, identify appropriate time for shave preparation		
b. Wet versus dry shaving	List advantages and disadvantages of wet and dry shaving			
c. Depilatories	List advantages and disadvantages of using chemical depilatories			

d. *Shaving procedure*	List equipment needed for preoperative shave	Given a patient situation, describe correct area to be shaved by naming perimeters	Correctly and safely complete preoperative shave	Evaluate shave by checking skin with strong light for hair removal and irritation. Evaluate own performance using Performance Checklist.
3. *Immediate preoperative care*	List aspects of physical care given during immediate preoperative period	In the practice setting, simulate immediate care of patient	Carry out immediate care of preoperative patient	Evaluate own performance using Performance Checklist.
4. *Checklist*	State information included on preoperative checklist	In the practice setting, complete preoperative checklist	In the clinical setting, complete patient's preoperative checklist	Evaluate with instructor

LEARNING ACTIVITIES

1. Review the Specific Learning Objectives.
2. Read the chapters on health teaching and hygiene, and the section on anxiety (in the chapter on mental health) in Ellis and Nowlis, *Nursing: A Human Needs Approach,* or comparable material in another textbook.
3. Review the material in your medical-surgical nursing textbook that relates to preoperative care.
4. Look up the module vocabulary terms in the glossary.
5. Read through the module.
6. In the practice setting:
    a. Set up a preoperative unit, using the Performance Checklist.
    b. Using a partner as a patient, practice performing the assessment interview. Include preoperative teaching and record your data.
    c. Have your partner evaluate your performance using the Performance Checklist.
    d. Reverse roles, and have your partner interview you and perform preoperative teaching.
    e. Evaluate your partner's performance.
    f. Observe the equipment used for the preoperative shave.
    g. Again, with your partner, role-play the immediate preoperative period, using the Performance Checklist as a guide.
    h. Have your partner evaluate your performance.
    i. Reverse roles, and repeat step g.
    j. Evaluate your partner's performance.
    k. Demonstrate making an operative bed.
7. In the clinical area:
    a. Perform initial preoperative planning and care.
        (1) Review your facility's procedure manual for initial preoperative planning and care.
        (2) Consult with your instructor when you think you are ready to perform initial preoperative planning and care.
    b. Perform preoperative skin preparation.
        (1) Review your facility's procedure for preoperative skin preparation, paying special attention to the areas to be shaved for designated surgeries.
        (2) Ask for an opportunity to observe a preoperative shave.
        (3) Consult with your instructor regarding an opportunity to do a preoperative shave. (Shaving for abdominal surgery is a wise choice for a beginning experience.)
    c. Perform immediate preoperative care.
        (1) Review your facility's procedure for giving immediate preoperative care.
        (2) Examine the checklist used.
        (3) Request an opportunity to give immediate preoperative care, including the completion of the checklist.

VOCABULARY

anesthesia
anesthesiologist
anesthetic
anesthetist
antiembolic stockings
antimicrobial
aspiration
complete blood count
depilatory
diuretic
endotracheal tube
epithelial
laparotomy
lather
NPO
perineal
TEDs
thoracotomy

PREOPERATIVE CARE

A patient can have either elective or emergency surgery. *Elective surgery* is performed at a time planned by the surgeon and patient; *emergency surgery* is performed when the patient's condition warrants immediate action. Your basic preoperative planning and care is essentially the same for both types of surgery, although you may have to omit certain portions or act more quickly when the surgery is done on an emergency basis.

Preoperative care varies from facility to facility. At points throughout the module, you may have to check the policies of the facility in which you practice and adapt your care to those policies.

The patient, on entering the unit, often has already been to the laboratory, where blood and urine samples for a complete blood count (CBC) and urinalysis (UA) have been collected. The consent-for-surgery form may have been signed and witnessed in the admitting office. See Module 10, Admission and Discharge, for general admitting procedure.

Initial Preoperative Planning and Care

1. Verify the type of surgery, the date and time surgery is scheduled, and the name of the surgeon. You can do this by checking the operative schedule form that comes to the unit from the operating room. A specific time will usually be listed, or the abbreviation TF may be used. This means your patient's surgery is "to follow" a previous procedure and the exact time is undetermined.
2. Check the preoperative orders. By reading over the orders on the doctor's order sheet, you get an idea of your responsibilities toward preparing the patient for surgery. Some surgeons use a stamp for their routine orders on a specific procedure and add any special orders for the individual patient.
3. Consult your facility's procedure book

regarding the type of surgery, the preparation needed, and the surgeon's preferences. Some facilities maintain a Kardex or file that lists surgeons' preferences.

4. Check the patient's chart for history and physical (H&P), CBC, and UA results, and the consent form. These must all be on the record before surgery, to protect the physician and hospital legally. In some facilities, it is permissible to go ahead with the surgery if the H&P is not on the record but has been performed and dictated. You may have to check on this. Surgery cannot proceed (except in a life-threatening emergency) without a properly completed consent form. Know your facility's policy regarding consent.
5. Arrange to complete the elements listed in step 4 if they are not on the record. Inform the laboratory or physician about any missing data.
6. Using the appropriate form, perform the assessment interview.
   a. *Verification of patient's identity* To practice safely, *always* validate the patient's identity.
   b. *General appearance and physical condition* It must be understood that a description of the patient's general appearance and physical condition is objective data. Enter the patient's height and weight.
   c. *Anxiety level* Communication with the patient during the interview will usually tell you something about the patient's level of anxiety.
   d. *Knowledge level regarding current surgery* Ask the patient what he or she knows about the surgery. The physician may have adequately explained the procedure, but, if not, you should give a general explanation. As with all health teaching, gear any necessary explanation to the level of the individual patient. Remember that explicit details can raise the

patient's anxiety level. Any specific points should be answered by the physician.

e. *Prior surgeries*   List all prior surgeries. Any previous surgery may have both physical and psychological consequences for the current surgery. Never assume that the patient who has had multiple surgeries needs less preparation or care.

f. *Smoking habits*   Note whether the patient is a smoker or nonsmoker. The lung tissue of a patient who smokes is more sensitive to anesthetic gases because of mild irritation. Discourage smoking just prior to surgery.

g. *Drug and alcohol intake*   List *all* medications that the patient is taking, including vitamin preparations and birth control pills. Some patients will not think to mention long-term medications, such as diuretics or daily birth control pills. Emphasize the importance of a complete list because anesthetic agents and other medications ordered react with the medications the patient is taking. Certain medications (for example, anticonvulsant drugs) will be continued throughout the operative period because interruption would cause adverse effects for the patient.

A reliable alcohol history is also essential. Heavy use of alcohol has multiple effects on the body that can change the patient's response to anesthesia and surgery.

h. *Family data*   Because the family is concerned about the patient, may be involved in the health teaching, and often cares for the patient after discharge, it is important to list the names and relationships of close family members on the form.

7. Encourage the patient to ask questions about the procedure, the policies of the hospital, or aspects of care. If you do not know the answers to specific ques-

tions, consult the proper resource person.

8. Provide emotional support. To add to the patient's confidence, demonstrate your own competence to care for the patient and help the patient learn what to expect. Refer to your basic text for techniques for handling anxiety.

9. Record the assessment data on the form used in your facility.

10. Perform preoperative teaching. Review once again the preoperative orders, so that you can give appropriate information. Know the principles of health teaching. Also, sometimes it is appropriate to include a member of the family when you do preoperative teaching. During the postoperative period, this person can then reinforce for the patient what has been taught.

a. *Preoperative routines*   Outline these routines for the patient in clear, understandable terms. You might choose to do this by systems, describing preoperative care of the GI tract, skin, and so on; or, you may choose to go through the preparation sequentially.

b. *Postoperative routines*   Explain what will be done with what frequency, and why.

(1) *Vital signs*   Blood pressure, pulse, and respiration are checked as often as every 15 minutes for early identification of any problems.

(2) *Dressing checks*   These are made to observe the kind and amount of drainage.

(3) *Progressive surgical diet*   List the usual progression—from ice chips, to clear liquids, to full liquids, to a soft diet, and finally to a regular diet.

(4) *Special procedures*   There may be specific procedures (irrigations, respiratory therapy, casting, brace fitting) for particu-

lar surgeries. Explain any special or unusual procedures that will be ordered.

c. *Pain management* All surgical patients want to be as free from pain as possible after surgery. By encouraging the patient before the surgery to be a participant in the plan for pain management, you relieve the patient's fear that pain will not be controlled. Tell the patient about available pain medications. Instruct the patient to alert a nurse *before* the pain becomes moderate or acute. Allay possible fears of overuse by explaining that, after the first few postsurgical days, the pain will subside and the medications will no longer be needed.

d. *Postoperative appliances, tubes, and equipment* Inform the patient of any equipment or appliances that will be in place after surgery. These might include a catheter, an IV infusion, or a suction apparatus.

When teaching steps e–g, first explain what you want the patient to do and why it is important; then, *demonstrate* for the patient, and, last, ask the patient to *return the demonstration.* Give positive feedback to the patient when the return demonstration is correct.

e. *Deep breathing and coughing* If the patient is going to have general anesthesia, the anesthetic agents and the immobility of surgery will cause the build-up of secretions in the lungs. Therefore, teach the patient how to deep-breathe and cough. (For instructions, consult Module 33; Respiratory Care Procedures.)

f. *Methods for moving* These methods include moving in bed and getting in and out of bed, as appropriate for the patient's postoperative condition and expected physician's orders. The purpose of teaching the patient to move with as little discomfort as possible

is to encourage the action. Turning in bed and getting in and out of bed prevent circulatory problems, stimulate the respiratory system, and decrease discomfort from gas. Review your medical-surgical text for the use of pillows for splinting, side rails for support, and body mechanics adaptations.

g. *Leg exercises* These exercises facilitate venous return in the lower extremities, and prevent stasis and clot formation. Three different exercises are most commonly taught:

(1) *Calf pumping* Instruct the patient to alternately dorsiflex and plantar flex the foot. This causes the calf muscles to contract and relax.

(2) *Quadriceps setting* Instruct the patient to alternately contract the anterior thigh muscles and allow them to relax.

(3) *Gluteal setting* Instruct the patient to alternately contract the posterior thigh and gluteal muscles and allow them to relax.

These exercises should be done ten times each hour as soon as possible after surgery. If appropriate to the patient's surgery, active range-of-motion exercises can be substituted for these isotonic exercises.

11. Note the visit by the anesthesiologist. The evening before surgery the patient is usually visited by the anesthesiologist or anesthetist, who (1) makes as assessment of the patient, (2) gives the patient information about the anesthetic that is to be given, and (3) writes the orders for the preoperative medication.

12. Carry out any preoperative procedures ordered.

a. Consult the appropriate modules if an enema, a douche, or irrigation is ordered.

b. Administer any sleeping medication ordered. It is important for the patient to understand that unfamiliar surroundings may prevent a good night's rest before surgery.

c. Explain that the patient will be given nothing by mouth after midnight. This is to be sure that the stomach is free of contents that could be vomited and aspirated. At midnight, remove the water pitcher from the patient's bedside and post an NPO sign.

Preoperative Skin Preparation

The effective preparation of the skin before an operation is an important aspect of the prevention of infection in the postoperative patient. Because the skin—the first line of defense against invasion by microorganisms—will be opened, additional measures to prevent the invasion of microbes are needed.

The main objective of preparing the skin is to remove dirt, oils, and microorganisms. A second objective is to prevent the growth of microorganisms that remain. A third objective is to leave the skin undamaged, with no irritation from the cleansing procedure.

BATH

In most facilities, the preoperative patient is asked to shower or bathe using an antimicrobial cleansing agent on the evening before or the morning of surgery. Whenever possible, the patient should shampoo at the time of the bath. The bath removes gross contamination, dirt, and body oils. The antimicrobial agent also leaves a residue on the skin that serves to decrease the overall bacterial count.

SCRUB OF THE SURGICAL SITE

On some occasions, a surgeon may order that a surgical site be scrubbed for a predetermined length of time (for example, five minutes) daily for several days before the surgery. This is most commonly done for elective orthopedic (bone) surgery because of the high risk of infection. The process results in a significantly lower bacterial count on the surgical site at the time of surgery. Because it is so time consuming and because infection is not as frequent and serious in other surgeries, it is not a routine procedure for most surgeries. A scrub procedure may also be ordered to be done after the preoperative shave.

SHAVE

Because microorganisms are found in large numbers on hairs, the removal of skin hair at and near the operative site cuts down the number of these organisms. The smooth skin can then be more completely cleaned. In order to have the skin as nearly sterile as possible, a shave preparation is routine before surgery.

Recent studies, however, have shown that, for some elected surgeries, preoperative shaving does not change the infection rate over no shaving. Based on this, certain facilities allow preoperative shaving on a selective basis.

Although in most settings the actual shave preparation is carried out by nursing assistants, the registered nurse is usually responsible for teaching the skill and for evaluating the thoroughness with which the procedure is done.

When to Shave   Although the timing can be ordered by the surgeon, it may be determined by hospital routine. If you have an opportunity to affect the planning, you should understand the differences in infection rate that result from changes in timing of the preoperative shave in relationship to the time of surgery. *Any time interval between the shaving and the actual surgery allows hair to begin to regrow and microorganisms to multiply.* Although the practice for many years was to perform the preoperative shave the evening before surgery, recent studies have demonstrated that the overall infection rate is reduced by moving the time of the shave closer to the time of surgery. In some hospitals, therefore, the shave is done early in the morning on the day scheduled for surgery. And, increasingly, hospitals are going a step further: in many, the preoperative shave is being done immediately before the surgery in a special preparation area or in the induction room in the operating room suite.

The question of infection rate is important, but also the procedure is less uncomfortable for the patient when the shave is performed as late as possible. It certainly relieves the patient of the discomfort associated with the regrowth of hair in those instances when surgery is canceled. And there are other advantages: it is more convenient for the staff to do all preoperative shaves in one area, saving time that would be spent moving from unit to unit; and lighting in a special area is usually better, which also makes the procedure easier.

Not all hospitals have the facilities to make this type of change in procedure, but where it is possible it is wise practice.

Wet versus Dry Shaving   Wet shaves are done using warm water and lather; dry shaves are done on dry skin. Most patients feel that the wet shave is more comfortable. The water and lather serve as lubricants to the razor, decrease the pull, and lessen the chance of nicks or cuts. In addition, the use of antibacterial soap is one more technique to decrease the skin count of microorganisms.

Recent evidence indicates that fewer epithelial cells are removed by using a dry shave. Also, the skin is clearly visible, making a very close shave possible. When you perform a dry shave, it is imperative that you use a sharp razor to avoid nicks and cuts. In fact, you may have to change the razor during the procedure if thick hair is being cut. You can use powder as a lubricant.

Usually, hospital policy determines whether a wet or dry shave is used, although the surgeon may also make the decision.

Depilatories   Depilatories are chemicals that destroy the hair below the skin level, causing the hair to break off and leaving the skin freer of hair than is possible with a razor. However, depilatories can irritate the skin, which would make surgery inadvisable. Therefore, depilatories are only in limited use.

To use a chemical depilatory, read the instructions *very* carefully and follow them exactly.

PROCEDURE FOR SHAVING

1. Verify the surgeon's order. Do not perform a shave preparation unless it has been ordered by a surgeon. The order may indicate the specific area to be "prepped," although, in many facilities, a standard routine is followed unless the surgeon specifically describes another preparation area. If the order simply reads, "Prep. for gastric surgery," you would have to refer to your facility's procedure book to identify the exact area to be prepped.

2. Plan the area to be shaved. Obviously, you will include the area of the incision itself, but you will also include a very large area beyond the incisional site. This is done to decrease the possibility of microorganisms' moving from unprepared areas to the surgical site. In addition, this provides a safeguard if the physician must enlarge the surgical area during the surgery beyond what was originally planned.

   Each facility where surgery is done will have identified the specific areas to be prepared for each type of surgery. The variation from facility to facility is slight. The areas presented here are for your information, but remember that you must consult the procedure book in your facility to verify them.

   a. *Head and neck surgeries*   If the scalp must be shaved, it is best to wait until the person has been anesthetized. Shaving the head can be psychologically traumatic. If it must be done earlier, you must provide a head covering to lessen the patient's embarrassment. Long hair may be saved for later use in a hairpiece, although the ready availability of wigs has made this a less frequent occurrence. Still, it is wise to ask the patient before you begin.

      Do not shave the eyebrows unless

expressly ordered by the surgeon. Eyebrows may not grow back in or may grow in an irregular manner. This can significantly alter a patient's appearance and should be avoided unless it is essential.

The prepared area extends from above the eyebrows over the top of the head, and includes the ears and both anterior and posterior areas of the neck (Figure 34.1). The face is not shaved.

b. *Lateral neck surgery* The prepared area extends from the midline of the back, from the scapula to a line level with the top of the ear, around the operative side, across the front of the neck, and to the top of the opposite shoulder. Anteriorly, the preparation area slants down from the top of the ear on the operative side across the chin line, and extends down below the clavicle across the thorax. (See Figure 34.2.)

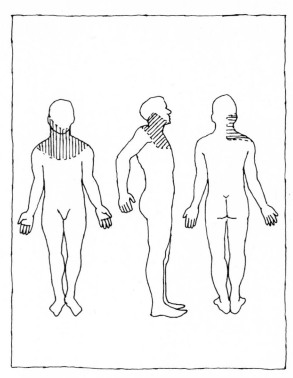

FIGURE 34.2   LATERAL NECK SURGERY

c. *Chest surgery* For a lateral thoracotomy, prep the chest from the center of the sternum, extending from the neck to the bottom of the rib cage. Continue the prep on the posterior side to the center of the back at the same level. The arm on the operative side is also prepped to the middle of the forearm. In some instances the prep is extended across the entire back and chest. (See Figure 34.3, part A.)

For a midline or sternal incision, the preparation extends from the neck to the pubic bone, and to the midaxillary line on each side (See Figure 34.3, part B.)

For access to the femoral artery, extend the preparation to include the area prepped for femoral artery surgery on the designated side. (See Figure 34.3, part C.)

d. *Abdominal surgery* The abdomen is prepared from a line level with the axillae to the pubic bone. The area

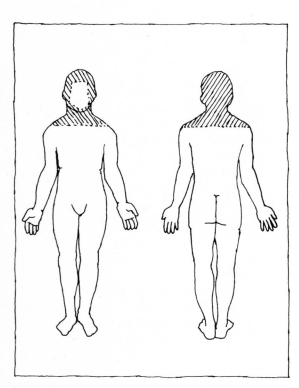

FIGURE 34.1   HEAD AND NECK SURGERY

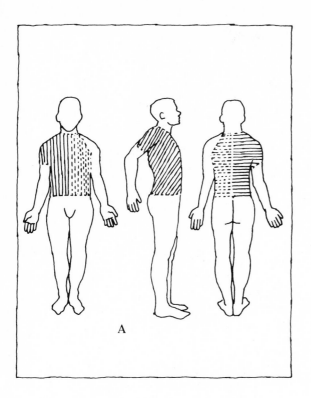

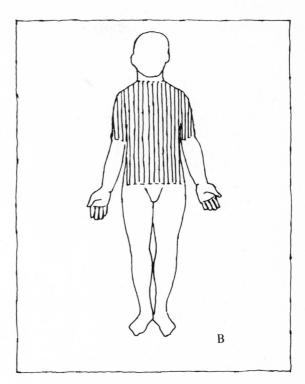

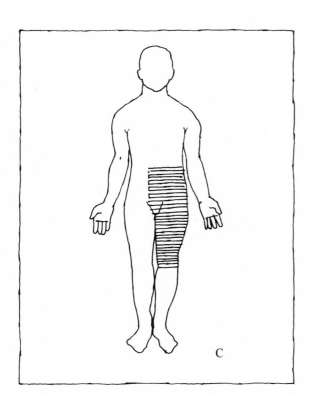

FIGURE 34.3   CHEST SURGERY   *A:* Lateral thoracotomy; *B:* sternal incision; *C:* femoral artery access needed.

extends on each side to the mid-axillary line (Figure 34.4).

e. *Perineal surgery*   The perineal preparation includes shaving all of the pubic area. The area begins above the pubic bone in the front and extends beyond the anus posteriorly. Shave the inner thighs approximately one third of the way to the knees. (See Figure 34.5.)

f. *Cervical-spine surgery*   Prep the back from the line level with the bottom of the ears down to the waist. Include the shoulders. The back area is prepped to the midaxillary line on each side. (See Figure 34.6.)

g. *Lumbar-spine surgery*   Prep the back from a line level with the axillae, down onto the buttocks, to the midgluteal level. The area extends to the midaxillary line on each side. (See Figure 34.7.)

h. *Rectal surgery*   Shave the buttocks

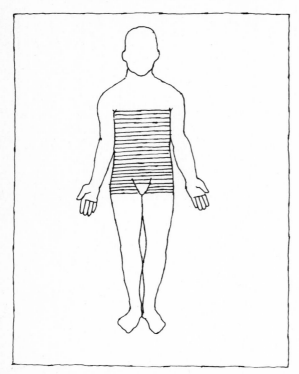

FIGURE 34.4   ABDOMINAL SURGERY

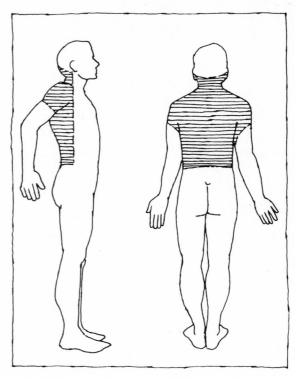

FIGURE 34.6   CERVICAL-SPINE SURGERY

from the iliac crest down the posterior thigh, to a line one third of the way to the knee. Include the anal area. The area extends to the midline on each side. (See Figure 34.8.)

i. *Flank incision* Prep from just beyond the midline anteriorly, around the designated side, to beyond the midline posteriorly. Include the axilla, from the upper level at the

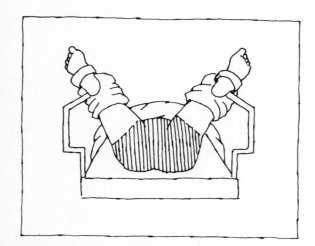

FIGURE 34.5   PERINEAL SURGERY

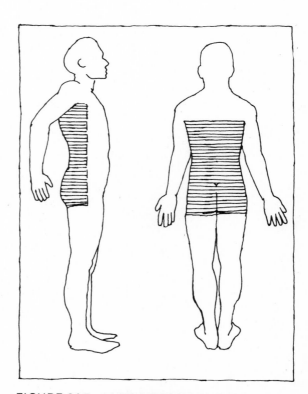

FIGURE 34.7   LUMBAR-SPINE SURGERY

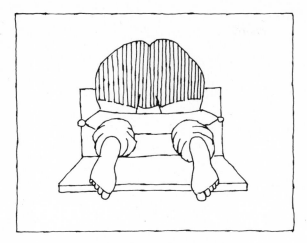

FIGURE 34.8   RECTAL SURGERY

nipple line in the front to the scapula in the back. Shave the back down to the middle of the buttocks. In the front, the pubic area and the upper thigh are shaved. (See Figure 34.9.)

j. *Hand and forearm surgery*   Prep the entire circumference of the arm, to the axilla. (See Figure 34.10.)

k. *Entire lower extremity surgery* Prep the entire leg, including the

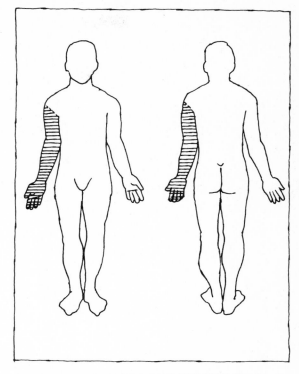

FIGURE 34.10   HAND AND FOREARM SURGERY

toes and the foot. Extend posteriorly up over the buttocks, and anteriorly over the pubis up to the umbilicus. (See Figure 34.11.)

l. *Lower leg surgery*   Prep the leg and foot, extending the area to midthigh. (See Figure 34.12.)

3. Obtain the necessary equipment. In most settings the preoperative shave is done using disposable equipment that is originally sterile. Although the procedure itself is a clean procedure, starting with sterile equipment ensures that new microorganisms from the hospital environment are not introduced to the patient's skin at this critical time. Where disposable equipment is not available, the reusable items are carefully cleaned and sent to central supply for resterilization.

a. You will need a good light source so that you can clearly see the area being shaved. Even the small hairs that are not generally noticeable must be removed, and these may not be visible if the light is dim.

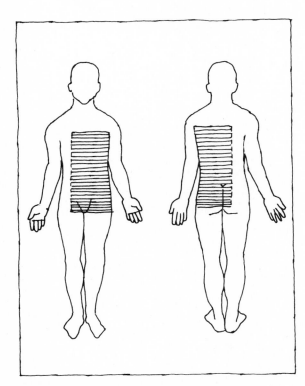

FIGURE 34.9   FLANK INCISION

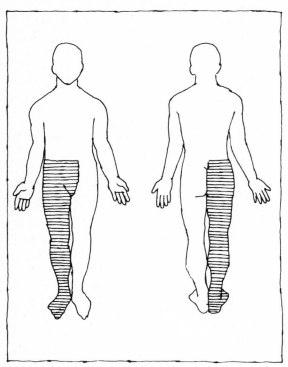

FIGURE 34.11   ENTIRE LOWER EXTREMITY SURGERY

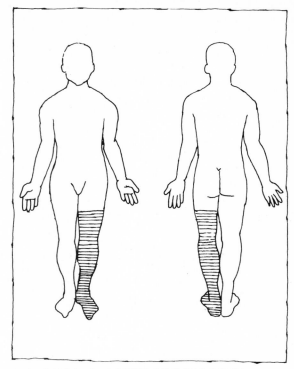

FIGURE 34.12   LOWER LEG SURGERY

b. You will need a bath blanket to drape the patient. Top linen is sometimes substituted for the bath blanket, but it can cause subsequent discomfort if small hairs drop in the bed or if the linen becomes wet or soiled.

c. You will need shaving equipment. A prepackaged shave preparation kit usually contains most of the necessary items, but be sure to check the label. If you are not using a prepackaged kit, obtain the following:
   (1) A small basin for warm water
   (2) An antibacterial soap for lather
   (3) A razor with a new blade
   (4) A small number of sterile gauze squares
   (5) An antibacterial cleansing agent
   (6) Cotton swabs

d. If the instructions for the shave preparation in your facility include covering the area with a sterile towel after shaving, then include this in the equipment.

4. Explain the procedure to the patient. Most patients are upset at the idea of the shave preparation. Therefore, carefully explain the exact nature and extent of the preparation.

5. Provide for the patient's privacy. In order to do a thorough job, you will have to expose the patient. But, make sure that the drapes and bed curtains are carefully closed.

6. Arrange for adequate lighting.

7. Wash your hands.

8. Use a bath blanket to drape the patient, to provide as much warmth and privacy as possible. Base the draping technique on the area to be exposed.

9. Shave the area to be prepared.
   a. Make sure the water is warm. This makes the patient more comfortable and produces better lather. The warm water also helps to soften the hair.
   b. Lather the area well. The suds soften the hair and also provide lubrication, so that the razor moves easily.

c. Shave carefully. Shaving against the grain provides for a closer shave. Use short strokes which are more easily controlled, and pull the skin taut to prevent nicks.

d. Rinse the razor frequently to remove hairs that have accumulated on the blade. These hairs could interfere with the cutting action of the razor.

e. Wipe off excess hair from the skin as it is removed. This allows you to see the skin clearly and allows the razor to operate more freely.

f. After all the hair has been removed, scrub the area with an antibacterial cleaner, keeping the cleansing agent in contact with the skin for five minutes. Check your facility's procedures, because some omit this step.

g. Clean any body orifice or crevice in the prep area (the umbilicus, the ear canals, under the fingernails) using cotton swabs.

h. Rinse the area with clean water.

i. Dry the skin, but do not rub vigorously. Vigorous rubbing can traumatize the skin.

j. Cover the area with a sterile towel if necessary.

10. Make the patient comfortable.
11. Dispose of the equipment as prescribed by your facility.
12. Wash your hands.
13. Record the prepared area on the patient's chart. Also record any breaks in the skin integrity.

Immediate Preoperative Care

1. Take the patient's vital signs and record. The blood pressure, pulse, and respirations may be increased because of anxiety, but if the patient's temperature is at all elevated, report this to the surgeon at once. An elevated temperature can mean a pending infection, and the surgeon will have to decide whether to proceed with the surgery. By recording the vital signs, you also establish a baseline for future measurement.

2. Administer or assist the patient with oral care. Oral care is necessary because the mouth tends to dry during the unconscious period with the administration of anesthetic gases. Caution the patient not to swallow water, but only to rinse the mouth. You may have to perform oral care for some patients.

3. Insert a nasogastric tube if ordered. (See Module 28, Gastric Intubation.)

4. Have the patient put on a clean gown, untied. If the gown is untied, it can be changed or removed easily when the patient is unconscious.

5. Have the patient void or insert a Foley catheter if ordered. The bladder is emptied to avoid incontinence or injury during surgery. If the surgery is of short duration, voiding is usually sufficient. If a Foley catheter is ordered, consult Module 39, Catheterization.

6. Remove colored nail polish, so that the anesthesiologist can observe the nail beds during surgery for circulatory assessment.

7. Remove and store the patient's contact lenses or glasses. Place these safely in a drawer where they will not fall to the floor.

8. Remove any makeup, so that skin color can be assessed during surgery.

9. Remove hairpins and hairpieces. These can cause pressure on the patient's scalp during the unconscious period or become dislodged.

10. Store the patient's dentures. Usually patients go to surgery without their dentures in place. However, some anesthesiologists prefer that dentures be kept in place to provide a better "seal" around the endotracheal tube that delivers the anesthetic agent.

11. If the patient has natural teeth or is a child, check for loose teeth that might be dislodged and aspirated during surgery.

12. Remove and store the patient's jewelry. Jewelry can be given to the family during surgery. Religious medals are often sent with the patient for comfort. If a

Nursing Unit Check List	Initial		Date _____		

	Yes	No		Yes	No
1. Pre-operative bath or shower			14. ALLERGIES		
2. Make-up removed					
3. Bobby pins, combs, hair pieces removed			15.　　　　　B/P		
4. Rings, jewelry, watch etc. (disposition)			16. Voided		
5. Prothesis 　　artificial eye　　in　　out 　　contact lens　　in　　out 　　pacemaker 　　other			17. Catheterized retention catheter		
6. Dentures (bridges, partial plates) 　　Removed　　　　Permanent			18. Urinalysis		
7. Loose teeth			19. Hematology		
8. Consent signed					
9. History & physical					
10. Note any skin lesions, burns, abrasions etc.					
11. Surgical prep			PATIENT IDENTIFICATION ON UNIT		

12. Apparent pre-operative mental condition
of patient

within normal limits		excited	
depressed		apprehensive	
irritable		other	

13. Where family will be during &
immediately after surgery.

A. Person from Surgery calling for patient
　　1. Ask for patient by name

　　2. Check patient's chart with someone
　　　on floor.

SIGNATURES: _____
　　　　　　　　　nursing unit

_____
　　　　　　　　　surgery personnel

BALLARD COMMUNITY HOSPITAL
Seattle, Washington

PRE-OPERATIVE CHECK LIST

FIGURE 34.13 PREOPERATIVE CHECKLIST
Courtesy Ballard Community Hospital, Seattle, Washington

patient does not want to have a wedding band removed, tape it in place to guard against loss.

13. Put antiembolic stockings (TEDs) on the patient if ordered. These compress the peripheral leg tissue, increasing venous return during the immobile period.

14. Ascertain the location of the patient's family or friends during surgical procedures, so that they can be reached in an emergency or can be informed when the patient moves to the recovery room.

15. Check the orders for preoperative medications.

16. Prepare medications as ordered and administer. More than one medication is usually given, and you must be certain that all drugs are compatible and measured acurately. (See Module 45, Giving Injections.)

17. Caution the patient to remain quietly in bed once medication has been given.

18. Put the side rails up for safety.

19. In some facilities, you might place the bed in the high position, so that the stretcher can be brought up to the side of the bed to transfer the patient. In most facilities, the bed is left down until the stretcher arrives.

20. Place the call bell within the patient's reach.

21. Wash your hands.

22. Complete the preoperative checklist (See Figure 34.13.) Check the form used in your facility. You should also chart the location of glasses, dentures, and jewelry.

23. Follow the proper procedure for patient identification as the patient leaves the unit. In most facilities, the operating room transport person reads the patient's identifying data off of the patient's armband while another hospital employee checks the chart. This is a legal precaution to verify identification.

24. Send the patient's chart and x rays with the patient. The surgeon may need to refer to them during surgery.

The objective evaluation of how well you have carried out preoperative care becomes apparent during surgery and the postoperative period. If the patient's surgery goes smoothly and the postoperative period is uneventful, much of the credit belongs to you—the nurse who has administered complete and well-planned preoperative care.

PERFORMANCE CHECKLIST

Long-term preoperative planning	Unsatisfactory	Needs more practice	Satisfactory	Comments
1. Verify the following: a. Type of surgery				
b. Date and time scheduled				
c. Surgeon				
2. Check preoperative orders.				
3. Consult your facility's references regarding type of surgery, preparation needed, and surgeon's preferences.				
4. Check patient's chart for the following: a. History and physical				
b. CBC results				
c. UA results				
d. Consent form				
5. Arrange for completion of above if not on record.				
6. Perform assessment interview, including the following: a. Verification of patient's identity				
b. General appearance and physical condition				
c. Anxiety level				
d. Knowledge level regarding current surgery				
e. Prior surgeries				
f. Smoking habits				
g. Drug and alcohol intake				
h. Family data				
7. Encourage patient to ask questions.				
8. Provide emotional support.				
9. Record assessment data.				
10. Perform preoperative teaching, including the following: a. Preoperative routines				
b. Postoperative routines (1) Vital signs				
(2) Dressing checks				
(3) Progressive surgical diet				
(4) Special procedures				

	Unsatisfactory	Needs more practice	Satisfactory	Comments
c. Pain management				
d. Postoperative appliances, tubes, and equipment				
e. Deep breathing and coughing (1) Explanation				
(2) Demonstration				
(3) Return demonstration				
f. Methods for moving (1) Explanation				
(2) Demonstration				
(3) Return demonstration				
g. Leg exercises (calf pumping, quadriceps setting, gluteal setting) (1) Explanation				
(2) Demonstration				
(3) Return demonstration				
11. Note anesthesiologist's visit.				
12. Carry out preoperative procedures.				
Preoperative skin preparation				
1. Assist patient with shower or bath using antimicrobial cleaner. (See Module 8, Hygiene.)				
2. Preoperative shave: a. Verify surgeon's order.				
b. Plan area to be prepped.				
c. Obtain equipment.				
d. Explain procedure to patient.				
e. Provide privacy.				
f. Arrange adequate lighting.				
g. Wash your hands.				
h. Drape patient.				
i. Shave patient. (1) Use warm water.				
(2) Lather well.				
(3) Shave against grain.				

	Unsatisfactory	Needs more practice	Satisfactory	Comments
(4) Rinse razor frequently.				
(5) Wipe off hair as removed.				
(6) Scrub with antibacterial cleaner if indicated.				
(7) Clean all body orifices and crevices.				
(8) Rinse with clean water.				
(9) Dry skin.				
(10) Cover with sterile towel if indicated.				
3. Make patient comfortable.				
4. Dispose of equipment.				
5. Wash your hands.				
6. Record on patient's chart.				
Immediate preoperative care				
1. Take vital signs and record.				
2. Administer or assist with oral care.				
3. Insert nasogastric tube if ordered.				
4. Have patient put on clean gown, untied.				
5. Have patient void or insert Foley catheter if ordered.				
6. Remove colored nail polish.				
7. Remove and store patient's contact lenses or glasses.				
8. Remove makeup.				
9. Remove hairpiece or hairpins.				
10. Store patient's dentures.				
11. If patient has natural teeth, check for loose teeth.				
12. Remove and store jewelry; tape wedding ring in place.				
13. Put antiembolic stockings on patient if ordered.				
14. Ascertain location of family during surgical procedure.				
15. Check order for preoperative medications.				
16. Prepare medications as ordered and administer.				

	Unsatisfactory	Needs more practice	Satisfactory	Comments
17. Caution patient to remain quietly in bed.				
18. Put side rails up.				
19. Place bed in high position if required.				
20. Place call bell in reach of patient.				
21. Wash your hands.				
22. Complete preoperative checklist, and chart location of glasses, dentures, and jewelry.				
23. Follow proper procedure for identification as patient leaves unit.				
24. Send chart and x rays with patient to operating room.				

QUIZ

Short-Answer Questions

1. What is the difference between elective and emergency surgery?

   _____

2. How does this difference affect your care? _____

3. List three activities you would teach a patient preoperatively.

   a. _____

   b. _____

   c. _____

4. Why is the patient usually placed on NPO at midnight the night before

   surgery? _____

5. List three objectives of preoperative skin preparation.

   a. _____

   b. _____

   c. _____

6. Why is the shave often done immediately before surgery?

   _____

7. What are two advantages of a wet shave?

   a. _____

   b. _____

8. List two reasons why vital signs are taken during the immediate preoperative period.

   a. _____

   b. _____

9. Name three aspects of immediate preoperative care that aid the anesthesiologist.

   a. _____

   b. _____

   c. _____

10. List two reasons why you should know the family's location during
    surgery.

    a. _____

    b. _____

Module 35 Postoperative Care

MAIN OBJECTIVE

To give postoperative care to surgical patients immediately upon their return from the recovery room and during the remainder of their hospital stay, with a view toward their comfort and safety, and the prevention of postoperative complications.

RATIONALE

Patients who have just returned from the recovery room are in most instances, dependent. They may depend on the nurse for all aspects of care after major surgery, or for only selected aspects of care after minor surgery. In either event, the nurse must make frequent and astute observations of these patients, to provide for their comfort and safety, to prevent the many potential complications, and to act appropriately when problems are identified.

PREREQUISITES

1. Successful completion of the following modules:

    VOLUME 1
    Assessment
    Charting
    Medical Asepsis
    Basic Body Mechanics
    Bedmaking
    Assisting with Elimination and
        Perineal Care
    Hygiene
    Intake and Output
    Moving the Patient in Bed and
        Positioning
    Range-of-Motion Exercises
    Ambulation
    Temperature, Pulse, and Respiration
    Blood Pressure

    VOLUME 2
    Inspection, Palpation, Auscultation,
        and Percussion

Respiratory Care Procedures

2. The following modules are not essential, but their successful completion will allow you to carry out more complete care for selected patients in the post-operative state:

VOLUME 1
Administering Enemas

VOLUME 2
Gastric Intubation
Administering Oxygen
Sterile Technique
Catheterization
Sterile Dressings
Oral and Nasopharyngeal Suctioning
Administering Oral Medications
Giving Injections
Preparing and Maintaining Intrave-
nous Infusions
Administering Intravenous Medica-
tions

SPECIFIC LEARNING OBJECTIVES

	Know Facts and Principles	Apply Facts and Principles	Demonstrate Ability	Evaluate Performance
1. *Postoperative nursing unit*	Discuss items to be included in postoperative nursing unit	Given a patient situation, state which items should be included in postoperative nursing unit	In the clinical setting, prepare unit to receive postoperative patient	Evaluate with instructor using Performance Checklist
2. *Initial observations*	List observations to be made immediately when postoperative patient arrives from recovery room	Given a patient situation, state appropriate initial observations	In the clinical setting, make complete initial observations on post-operative patient. Chart initial observations correctly.	Evaluate with instructor using Performance Checklist
3. *Information from chart*	State information to be obtained from chart after initial observations are made	Given a sample patient's chart, obtain appropriate information about patient, following recovery room period	In the clinical setting, check chart of post-operative patient for specific items of information after initial observations are made	Evaluate for completeness of information with instructor
4. *Potential complications*	Discuss observations, preventive actions, and treatment for potential postoperative complications	Given a patient situation, state appropriate observations and preventive actions	In the clinical setting, make appropriate observations and take appropriate actions to prevent postoperative complications	Evaluate own performance with instructor using Performance Checklist

LEARNING ACTIVITIES

1. Review the Specific Learning Objectives.
2. Read the section on hypothermia (in the section on neurological function) and the section on surgery and sexuality (in the chapter on sexuality) in Ellis and Nowlis, *Nursing: A Human Needs Approach,* or comparable material in another textbook.
3. Read the material in your medical-surgical nursing textbook that relates to postoperative care.
4. Look up the module vocabulary terms in the glossary.
5. Read through the module.
6. In the practice setting:
   a. Set up a post-op unit, using the Performance Checklist.
   b. Using another student as the patient, practice receiving your "patient" from the recovery room and making all of the appropriate initial observations. Use the Performance Checklist as a guide.
   c. Practice charting the information gathered in your initial observations, using the format used in your clinical facility.
7. In the clinical setting:
   a. Ask your instructor for an opportunity to assist a staff member in receiving a patient from the recovery room. Notice how the patient is moved. Compare your initial observations with those of the staff person.
   b. Ask your instructor to arrange for you to receive a patient from the recovery room under supervision. Compare your initial observations with those of your instructor.

VOCABULARY

atelectasis
dehiscence
evisceration
hemorrhage
Homan's sign
hypoventilation
intensive care unit (ICU)
paralytic ileus
pneumonitis
pulmonary embolus
purulent
recovery room (RR)
second intention healing
shock
singultus
thrombophlebitis

POSTOPERATIVE CARE

Immediately following surgery, the patient is usually taken to the recovery room (RR), where skilled care is provided by experienced nurses until the patient is recovered from the anesthetic and/or is able to respond to stimuli. The time spent in the recovery room is usually a minimum of one hour but can be considerably more. Patients who have had very complicated surgery may be taken to the intensive care unit (ICU) for a stay of several days after surgery.

In this module we deal with the care of patients upon their arrival back to the regular nursing unit. For a complete understanding of the complications mentioned, consult your medical-surgical nursing text.

Postoperative Nursing Unit

Before a patient is received from the recovery room, the room is prepared to facilitate efficient care. Make up the postoperative bed to receive the patient. (See Module 6, Bedmaking, page 67.) The postoperative bed should have extra protection at the head (a pad or bath towel) and in the middle (plastic drawsheet, pad, or Chux) to make changing easier in the event of vomiting or soiling.

Tissues, an emesis basin, equipment for taking vital signs, and an IV stand are usually standard equipment in the postoperative unit. A pencil and paper for making notes are also helpful. In addition, special equipment appropriate to the type of surgery the patient has undergone should be placed in the room to prevent disorganization at the time of the patient's arrival. This might include traction equipment for a patient who has undergone an orthopedic procedure, or a tracheostomy tray for a patient who has had thyroid surgery.

Initial Observations

When the patient arrives on the nursing unit, he or she is moved carefully from the stretcher to the postoperative bed. Rough or precipitous handling can contribute to sudden changes in vital signs, so be gentle. Leave in place the blanket that covered the patient en route to the unit, to help prevent chilling.

A recovery room nurse will usually have telephoned a report on the patient's stay in RR before the patient's arrival on the nursing unit. Using that information as a baseline, make the following initial observations:

1. Time of arrival on unit.
2. Responsiveness (to what does the patient respond and how does the patient respond, for example, to a name call).
3. Vital signs:
   a. Temperature
   b. Pulse
   c. Respirations
   d. Blood pressure
4. Skin:
   a. Color
   b. Condition (dryness or moisture)
5. Dressing:
   a. Clean
   b. Dry
   c. Intact
   Reach under patient to detect pooling of blood.
6. Presence of an intravenous infusion:
   a. Type of solution
   b. Amount left in bottle
   c. Drip rate
7. Presence of bladder catheter:
   a. Unclamped
   b. Connected to drainage bag or bottle
   c. Freely draining
   d. Characteristics and amount of urine
8. Presence of other drainage tubes:
   a. Unclamped
   b. Attached appropriately to bottle or suction
   c. Tubes not kinked or under patient
   d. Characteristics and amount of drainage
9. Safety and comfort:
   a. Side rails up
   b. Position appropriate for surgical procedure
   c. Presence of pain, nausea, or vomiting

All of the above items should be included in the note you enter on the patient's chart after the patient's arrival from the recovery room. Your facility may have a checklist for this purpose.

As soon as these observations have been made, you should check the chart for the following information (some of which may have been included in the verbal report from the recovery room nurse):

1. Operation performed
2. Postoperative diagnosis
3. Anesthetic agents used
4. Estimated blood loss (EBL)
5. Blood and/or fluid replacement given during surgery and recovery room stay
6. Type and location of drains
7. Vital signs when patient left recovery room (for use as a baseline)
8. Medications administered in the recovery room:
   a. Type
   b. Time
   c. Amount
9. Output:
   a. Urine
   b. Other drainage
   c. Vomitus
10. Physician's orders:[1]
    a. Frequency of vital signs
    b. Diet
    c. Activity
    d. Intravenous orders
    e. Medications (amount and frequency of pain and other medications)
    f. Laboratory and/or respiratory therapy orders
    g. Orders specific to type of surgery or other problems of patient

Some institutions employ an operating room nursing record that can be very useful to the nurse who is taking over the care of the patient on the nursing unit. (See Figure 35.1.)

[1] In most facilities, postoperative orders automatically cancel all previous written orders. These must be reordered by the physician following surgery if still wanted.

Ongoing Care

The ongoing care of the postoperative patient is largely preventive in nature. We present it here in chart form, using a systems approach.

Operating Room   Record

Pre-operative Diagnosis

_____
OPERATION

Date _____

Medications given in O.R. other than
those given with anesthesia

Drug & Dosage   Time   Method
_____
_____
_____

Catheter

Foley	Robinson	Other

Catheter in place when patient left O.R.   yes   no

Packing

Vaseline	Iodoform	Plain	Other

Location:

Drains

Penrose	Robinson	Hemovac	Other

Location:

Tubes

Levin	Chest	Gastrostomy	Other

Estimated blood loss

Blood ordered in surgery

Equipment (special)

Cautery used

Skin lesions etc.

SPECIAL COMMENTS

Culture	culture site

CONTAMINATED   YES   NO

SURGEON _____

ASSISTANT_____

_____
Circulation Nurse Signature

BALLARD COMMUNITY HOSPITAL
Seattle, Washington

OPERATING ROOM NURSING RECORD

FIGURE 35.1   OPERATING ROOM NURSING RECORD
Courtesy Ballard Community Hospital, Seattle, Washington

System	Complications	Observations	Preventive Actions	Treatment
1. Circulatory	a. Shock	External or internal hemorrhaging; drop in blood pressure; rapid weak pulse; cold, clammy skin	Avoid sudden movements; get patient up slowly; maintain IVs per physician's orders	Place flat with legs elevated; report changes in patient status to physician immediately; be prepared to administer medications, start oxygen, administer blood and/or intravenous fluids per physician's orders.
	b. Thrombophlebitis	Localized pain, heat, and swelling, usually in lower extremities; positive Homan's sign	Encourage early ambulation or bed exercises, active or passive; encourage fluids; provide elastic hose per physician's orders	Provide bed rest; apply hot moist packs; administer drug therapy per physician's orders.
2. Respiratory	a. Atelectasis	Rapid shallow breathing; diminished or enhanced breath sounds (auscultate)	Encourage to deep-breathe and cough (at least q.2h.); use suction if patient cannot cough out secretions; encourage fluids; encourage early ambulation	Administer respiratory therapy per physician's orders; turn, deep-breathe, and cough at least q.2h.
	b. Pneumonitis	Rapid noisy respirations; elevated temperature; increased pulse rate; restlessness; pain; cough	As for atelectasis	Administer respiratory therapy and antibiotics per physician's orders
	c. Pulmonary embolus	Rapid respirations; sudden chest pain; shortness of breath; anxiety; shock	Prevent thrombophlebitis (see above); *do not* massage lower extremities	Administer drug therapy per physician's order

3. Neural	a. Pain	Complaint of pain, grimacing; immobility (guarding wound); restlessness; blood pressure drop not accompanied by signs of blood loss	Administer pain medication *before* pain becomes severe; enhance pain medication with nursing measures (change of position, back rub, reassurance, information as to how long it will take pain medication to work); inspect for edema, tight dressings, or tight casts	Administer medication per physician's orders; splint when moving; move slowly
4. Integumentary	a. Wound infection	Local signs of infection (redness, heat, swelling, pain, purulent drainage); generalized signs of infection (fever, increased pulse, increased respiratory rate)	Keep dressing clean and dry; pay conscientious attention to care of patient's hygiene needs; change linen at least daily; follow strict aseptic technique when changing dressing; administer antibiotics per physician's orders	Administer antibiotics per physician's orders
	b. Dehiscence	Separation of skin edges	Apply abdominal binder (scultetus binder) per physician's orders	Keep sterile dressings over wound; notify physician (surgical reclosure may be needed or the wound may be left open to heal by second intention)

System	Complications	Observations	Preventive Actions	Treatment
	c. Evisceration	Complaint of "giving" sensation in area of incision; sudden leakage of fluid from wound; wound open with abdominal contents protruding	Apply abdominal binder per physician's orders	Cover open wound with sterile, warm saline packs; keep patient quiet; observe for signs of shock; notify physician; notify surgery (emergency surgical treatment usually required); stay with patient for psychological support
5. Gastrointestinal	a. Nausea and vomiting	Complaint of nausea; emesis	Urge patient to breathe in and out through mouth; keep area well ventilated and free from odors	Position patient on side to prevent aspiration; provide frequent oral care; give antiemetic medication prior to meals per physician's orders; NPO and nasogastric tube per physician's orders (for persistent vomiting)
	b. Abdominal distention	Complaint of discomfort; high-pitched bowel sounds present; drumlike distention of abdomen (palpate and percuss)	Encourage early ambulation	Continue to encourage active movement and ambulation; encourage hot fluids (ice can increase problem); administer rectal tube, return-flow enema (Harris flush), or medication per physician's orders; NPO and nasogastric tube per physician's orders (if paralytic ileus exists); administer medication to stimulate peristalsis per physician's orders

c. Constipation	Complaint of no bowel movement or small amounts of hard dry stool; abdominal discomfort; abdominal distention	Encourage early ambulation; encourage fluids; administer stool softeners per physician's orders. Administer enema per physician's orders (if no bowel movement in first four or five days); administer stool softeners per physician's orders
d. Hiccoughs (singultus)	Complaint of hiccoughs	Have patient rebreathe own carbon dioxide (inhaling and exhaling into paper bag held tightly over nose and mouth); administer medication per physician's orders
6. Genitourinary		
a. Urinary retention	Urine output (measure); bladder distention (palpate); complaint of discomfort	Attempt measures to encourage voiding; pass urinary catheter per physician's orders (if no voiding for 8 to 12 hours after surgery)
b. Urinary tract infection	Elevated temperature; cloudy and/or dark urine; burning on urination	Maintain adequate fluid intake; if catheter in place, give thorough catheter care. Encourage fluid intake; administer medications per physician's order

System	Complications	Observations	Preventive Actions	Treatment
7. Musculoskeletal	General muscle weakness	Weakness; dizziness; fatigue	Encourage early ambulation, or active or passive range of motion if ambulation not possible; encourage adequate nutrition	Same as preventive actions
8. Psychosocial	Depression and anxiety	Asocial behavior; malaise; listlessness; sleep disturbance	Encourage early ambulation; assist patient with personal needs; encourage patient's participation as appropriate; keep patient and patient's unit neat and free from odor; be available as listener; perform patient teaching	Same as preventive actions; also arrange psychiatric consultation per physician's orders (if depression persists)

PERFORMANCE CHECKLIST

	Unsatisfactory	Needs more practice	Satisfactory	Comments
Preparing the postoperative nursing unit				
1. Make postoperative bed. a. Extra protection at head				
b. Extra protection in middle				
2. Obtain necessary equipment. a. Tissues				
b. Emesis basin				
c. For vital signs: (1) Thermometer				
(2) Stethoscope				
(3) Blood pressure cuff				
(4) Sphygmomanometer				
d. IV stand				
e. Pencil and paper				
f. Special equipment				
Making initial observations				
1. Time of arrival on unit				
2. Responsiveness				
3. Vital signs: a. Temperature				
b. Pulse				
c. Respirations				
d. Blood pressure				
4. Skin: a. Color				
b. Condition				
5. Dressing: a. Clean				
b. Dry				
c. Intact				
6. Intravenous infusion: a. Type of solution				
b. Amount left in bottle				
c. Drip rate				

	Unsatisfactory	Needs more practice	Satisfactory	Comments
7. Bladder catheter: a. Unclamped				
b. Connected to drainage bag or bottle				
c. Freely draining				
d. Characteristics and amount of urine				
8. Other drainage tubes: a. Unclamped				
b. Attached appropriately to bottle or suction				
c. Not kinked or under patient				
d. Characteristics and amount of drainage				
9. Safety and comfort: a. Side rails up				
b. Appropriate position				
c. Pain, nausea, and vomiting				
Observations				

1. Circulatory
  a. Shock:
    (1) External or internal hemorrhaging				

(2) Drop in blood pressure				
(3) Rapid weak pulse				
(4) Cold, clammy skin				
b. Thrombophlebitis: (1) Localized pain, heat, and swelling, usually of lower extremities				
(2) Homan's sign				

2. Respiratory
  a. Atelectasis:
    (1) Rapid shallow breathing				

(2) Diminished or enhanced breath sounds (auscultate)				

	Unsatisfactory	Needs more practice	Satisfactory	Comments
b. Pneumonitis: (1) Rapid noisy respirations				
(2) Elevated temperature				
(3) Increased pulse rate				
(4) Restlessness				
(5) Pain				
(6) Cough				
c. Pulmonary embolus: (1) Rapid respirations				
(2) Sudden chest pain				
(3) Shortness of breath				
(4) Anxiety				
(5) Shock				
3. Neural a. Pain: (1) Complaint of pain				
(2) Grimacing				
(3) Immobility (guarding wound)				
(4) Restlessness				
(5) Blood pressure drop				
4. Integumentary a. Wound infection: (1) Local signs of infection (a) Redness				
(b) Heat				
(c) Swelling				
(d) Pain				
(e) Purulent drainage				
(2) Generalized signs of infection (a) Fever				
(b) Increased pulse				
(c) Increased respiratory rate				

	Unsatisfactory	Needs more practice	Satisfactory	Comments
b. Dehiscence: (1) Separation of skin edges				
c. Evisceration: (1) Complaint of "giving" sensation in area of incision				
(2) Sudden leakage of fluid from wound				
(3) Abdominal contents visible in wound				
5. Gastrointestinal a. Nausea and vomiting: (1) Complaint of nausea				
(2) Emesis				
b. Abdominal distention: (1) Complaint of discomfort				
(2) High-pitched bowel sounds				
(3) Drumlike distention (palpate and percuss)				
c. Constipation: (1) Complaint of no bowel movement or hard dry stool				
(2) Abdominal discomfort				
(3) Distention				
d. Hiccoughs (singultus): (1) Complaint of hiccoughs				
6. Genitourinary a. Urinary retention: (1) Urine output				
(2) Distended bladder (palpate)				
(3) Complaint of discomfort				
b. Urinary tract infection: (1) Elevated temperature				
(2) Cloudy and/or dark urine				
(3) Burning on urination				

	Unsatisfactory	Needs more practice	Satisfactory	Comments

7. Musculoskeletal
  a. General muscle weakness:
    (1) Weakness				

(2) Dizziness				
(3) Fatigue				

8. Psychosocial
  a. Depression and anxiety:
    (1) Asocial behavior				

(2) Malaise				
(3) Listlessness				
(4) Sleep disturbance				
Preventive actions				

1. Circulatory
  a. Shock:
    (1) Avoid sudden movements.				

(2) Get patient up slowly.				
(3) Maintain IVs as ordered.				
b. Thrombophlebitis: (1) Encourage ambulation or bed exercises.				
(2) Encourage fluids.				
(3) Provide elastic hose as ordered.				

2. Respiratory
  a. Atelectasis:
    (1) Encourage deep breathing and coughing.				

(2) Use suction if necessary.				
(3) Encourage fluids.				
(4) Encourage early ambulation.				
b. Pneumonitis: (1) As for atelectasis				
c. Pulmonary embolus: (1) Prevent thrombophlebitis.				
(2) Do not massage lower extremities.				

	Unsatisfactory	Needs more practice	Satisfactory	Comments

3. Neural
  a. Pain:
    (1) Administer pain medication *before* pain becomes severe.				

(2) Enhance pain medication with nursing measures. (a) Change of position				
(b) Back rub				
(c) Reassurance				
(d) Information (how long it will take medication to work)				
(3) Check for edema, tight dressings, or tight casts.				

4. Integumentary
  a. Wound infection:
    (1) Keep dressing clean and dry.				

(2) Attend to hygiene needs.				
(3) Change linen at least daily.				
(4) Follow strict aseptic technique when changing dressing.				
(5) Administer antibiotics as ordered.				
b. Dehiscence: (1) Apply binder as ordered.				
c. Evisceration: (1) Apply binder as ordered.				

5. Gastrointestinal
  a. Nausea and vomiting:
    (1) Urge patient to breathe in and out through mouth.				

(2) Keep room well ventilated and odor-free.				
b. Abdominal distention: (1) Encourage early ambulation.				
c. Constipation: (1) Encourage early ambulation.				
(2) Encourage fluids.				

	Unsatisfactory	Needs more practice	Satisfactory	Comments
6. Genitourinary				
a. Urinary tract infection:				
(1) Maintain adequate fluid intake.				
(2) Provide thorough catheter care.				
7. Musculoskeletal				
a. General muscle weakness:				
(1) Encourage early ambulation or ROM.				
(2) Encourage adequate nutrition.				
8. Psychosocial				
a. Depression and anxiety:				
(1) Encourage early ambulation.				
(2) Assist with personal needs.				
(3) Encourage patient's participation.				
(4) Keep patient and unit tidy and odor-free.				
(5) Listen.				
(6) Perform patient teaching.				

QUIZ

Short-Answer Questions

1. List four types of equipment that are usually included in the items gathered for a postoperative nursing unit.

    a. _____

    b. _____

    c. _____

    d. _____

2. List six general areas of concern that are included in the initial observation of the patient after his or her return from the recovery room.

    a. _____

    b. _____

    c. _____

    d. _____

    e. _____

    f. _____

3. If a bladder catheter is present when a patient returns from surgery, what four observations should you make?

    a. _____

    b. _____

    c. _____

    d. _____

4. Write a sample nursing note in the space below, using the format of your clinical facility. Include five items of information appropriate to any postoperative patient.

    _____

    _____

    _____

    _____

5. List seven of the items of information that are obtained from the patient's chart after the initial observations are made.

   a. _____

   b. _____

   c. _____

   d. _____

   e. _____

   f. _____

   g. _____

6. List two of the nursing actions that might help to prevent postoperative depression.

   a. _____

   b. _____

Module 36 Sterile Technique

MAIN OBJECTIVES

To identify situations where sterile technique is needed and to recognize breaks in technique when they occur.

To open a sterile pack, set up a sterile field, add sterile items or fluid to a sterile area, and put on sterile gloves.

RATIONALE

Strict sterile technique, or surgical asepsis, is needed frequently in nursing. It is used most extensively in operating and delivery rooms, but it is also essential in such nursing procedures as injections, catheterizations, dressings of open wounds, and intravenous therapy.

The purpose of sterile technique is to protect patients from possible infection. The nurse is responsible for identifying those situations in which sterile technique is needed and for carrying out sterile procedures in a precise manner.

PREREQUISITES

Successful completion of the following modules:

VOLUME 1
Assessment
Charting
Medical Asepsis

SPECIFIC LEARNING OBJECTIVES

	Know Facts and Principles	Apply Facts and Principles	Demonstrate Ability	Evaluate Performance
1. *Situations requiring sterile technique*	List common situations in which sterile technique is needed	Given a patient situation, identify what procedures require sterile technique	In the clinical setting, decide correctly when to use sterile technique	Evaluate decision with instructor
2. *Methods of sterilization*	Define *sterile*. List four common methods of sterilization and give an example of when each is used. State common ways to identify sterility.	Given a situation in which sterilization is needed identify appropriate process	Identify whether a package is sterile	Evaluate own performance using Performance Checklist
3. *Movement of microorganisms*	State six ways microorganisms move from one area to another. Identify methods used to maintain sterile field.	Given a situation in which a sterile field is used, identify any actions that would potentially contaminate it	Open sterile pack correctly. Add sterile objects to sterile field without contaminating them. Pour liquid into sterile container. Put on sterile gloves.	Evaluate own performance using Performance Checklist

LEARNING ACTIVITIES

1. Review the Specific Learning Objectives.
2. Read the chapter on nursing procedures and the chapter on infections, in Ellis and Nowlis, *Nursing: A Human Needs Approach,* or comparable chapters in another textbook.
3. Look up the module vocabulary terms in the glossary.
4. Read through the module.
5. Review the Performance Checklist.
6. In the practice setting:
   a. Open sterile packs.
   b. Add items to a sterile field.
   c. Pour liquids into sterile containers.
   d. Put on sterile gloves.
   Use the Performance Checklist as a guide.
7. When you believe you can perform correctly, select a partner.
   a. Have your partner observe your performance and evaluate you, using the Performance Checklist.
   b. Observe your partner and evaluate him or her, using the checklist.
   Repeat this exercise until you have mastered the skill.
8. Arrange with your instructor for a time to have your technique checked.

VOCABULARY

antiseptic
autoclave
contaminated
disinfect
disinfectant
microorganism
pathogen
spore
sterile
sterile technique
sterilize
surgical asepsis
transfer forceps

STERILE TECHNIQUE

Procedures Requiring Sterile Technique

Healthy intact skin and mucous membranes provide an effective barrier to microorganisms; but underlying tissue provides an excellent medium for their growth. Therefore, any time underlying tissues are exposed (through a wound or surgical incision), the tissue must be protected from the entry of microorganisms. This is done by using sterile technique.

Some internal body areas, such as the bladder and the trachea, are normally sterile. In order to maintain this status, sterile technique is used whenever such an area must be entered. And although the eyes are not normally sterile, sterile technique is used in any procedure relating to the eyes because they are susceptible to infection, and the consequences of even a minor infection in the eye can be serious.

Common situations in which sterile technique is used are catheterizations, changing surgical dressings, and preparing injections.

Methods of Sterilization

The ideal method of sterilization, not only would render an item free of all forms of life (including spores or vegetative forms), but would also not injure the item being sterilized, be relatively simple to use, and be inexpensive. Unfortunately, no single method of sterilization meets all these criteria for all items that must be sterilized.

In the modern hospital, many items arrive from manufacturers in presterilized packages. However, sterilization is still done for many items in central supply departments.

As a general staff nurse, you will most often be involved in sending items out for sterilization. It is often your responsibility to correctly wrap or label these items, for which you need some familiarity with the various types of sterilization processes available. If you were employed at a facility where you needed to carry out sterilization procedures, you would need more extensive education.

Any item to be sterilized must first be completely clean, no matter which method of sterilization is used. Among other reasons, protein often coagulates, providing a protective barrier for microorganisms that helps them to survive even the most careful sterilization procedure.

BOILING WATER

Boiling items in water is a very old sterilization method but is still valuable in certain situations. To use this method, the items must be completely covered and all surface areas must be exposed to the water. Timing is started only after a rolling boil has begun. Because it is difficult to maintain sterility while removing items from boiling water and drying them, this method is most often used for items, such as bedpans or emesis basins, that need sterilization between uses but need not be sterile during use. Some spore forms are not destroyed by boiling water.

STEAM

Steam, under pressure in an autoclave, is perhaps the most common sterilization procedure in use today. The high-pressure system enables the steam to reach a much higher temperature than is otherwise possible; and it is the temperature, not the pressure, that destroys microorganisms. The steam penetrates the cloth wrapper and soaks into nooks and crannies, providing complete contact and sterilization. Items should be left in an autoclave until they are cool and dry, so that the exterior of a wrapped package can be handled, maintaining the sterility of the contents.

SPORICIDAL CHEMICALS AND GAS

Certain items, such as instruments with gauges and dials, cannot be exposed to the high temperatures, moisture, or pressure of the autoclave without damage. These items can be immersed in sporicidal chemicals for sterilization. Plastics also cannot tolerate the autoclave, but they may react with chemicals or be so flexible that it is impossible to provide contact to all surfaces. For these items, exposure to ethylene oxide gas, commonly called *gas autoclaving,* is an effective sterilization method. However, this method requires expensive equipment.

IRRADIATION

A less common method of sterilization is exposure to cobalt 60 irradiation. This method can be used for all objects but is very costly.

INDICATORS

Indicators are used to ascertain that an item is sterile. They react to high temperature when exposed to it for a prolonged period of time. Indicators—in the form of special tape—are frequently used on packs. Dark lines appear on the tape after a package has been exposed to a temperature for time sufficient to sterilize the item. Small glass-tubing indicators, which contain a substance sensitive to heat are sometimes placed inside large packs to ensure sterility. The sterility of bottles of liquids is usually identified by the presence of a vacuum seal.

Every commercial product has some indicator of sterility. It is your responsibility to check the manufacturer's literature for this information, so that you can ascertain the sterility of an item before using it.

Avoiding Contamination

Microorganisms move through space on air currents. Thus, items that are exposed to the air for any prolonged period are considered contaminated. For this reason, it is important to minimize air movement or to control its direction through special ventilation to limit the movement of microorganisms. When a sterile field is open, do not shake drapes and clothing in the air and keep doors closed.

Microorganisms are transferred from one surface to another whenever a nonsterile object touches another object. Keep sterile objects at a distance from nonsterile ones to prevent the transfer of microorganisms. Any contact, no matter how brief, renders sterile items nonsterile. In order to preserve sterility, pick up sterile items with sterile gloves or with transfer forceps.

Microorganisms move from one object to another as a result of gravity when a nonsterile item is held above another item. For this reason, it is important to keep nonsterile objects, among them your own arm, from being over the sterile field.

Microorganisms travel rapidly along any moisture through a wicking action. Any time moisture connects a nonsterile surface to a sterile one, the sterile surface is considered contaminated.

Microorganisms move very slowly along a dry surface. If one side of a dry object is touched, that side is contaminated, but the opposite side is still considered to be sterile. When sterile forceps are picked up, the handle is immediately contaminated but the tips, which have not been touched, are sterile. Maintain a safety margin of approximately 1 inch around a contaminated portion.

Microorganisms are released into the air on droplet nuclei whenever a person breathes or speaks. In a situation where sterility is critical (the operating room), personnel wear masks to stop this source of contamination. In the general setting, a mask may not be worn, but avoid talking across a sterile field, turn your head away when speaking, and speak only when necessary in a sterile environment.

Because microorganisms are in constant motion in a variety of ways, sterile areas must be protected by providing wide margins for safety. Because you cannot guarantee what you cannot see, it is common practice to *consider anything that is out of sight to be unsterile.* A person's own back is considered unsterile, even when clothed in an originally sterile gown. Therefore, two persons in sterile gowns should always pass face to face or back to back, so that there is no danger of the sterile front touching the other person's unsterile back. Keep gloved hands in front of you, in your line of vision. Remember that all items below your waist or below table level are considered unsterile because they are out of full view.

The edge of any sterile field is potentially contaminated by microorganisms moving in from the outside. Therefore, keep sterile objects away from the edge of the field. Again, an inch is usually considered a minimum safety margin.

If a sterile field must be set up ahead of time or must be left after use has begun, cover it with a sterile drape of some type to prevent contamination. Use a single thickness of paper drape and a double thickness of cloth drapes.

Sterile Procedures

OPENING A STERILE PACK

Before sterilization, objects are wrapped so that they can be opened without contaminating the contents. The wrapper, when opened, provides a sterile field. Choose a flat, hard dry surface to prepare a sterile field. Clear a sufficient area, so that you have plenty of room to work. As a beginner, you will find you need at least a 12-inch-square field.

When you open a sterile package, remember not to reach over another sterile object. Grasp only the outside edge of the wrapper. In order to accomplish this, open the far flap first, then the side flaps, and finally the flap closest to you. The item can also be turned or you can walk around it. In some instances, you may reach around the object, but this is very difficult to do without contaminating the item.

Figure 36.1 shows the proper sequence for opening a sterile package.

ADDING ITEMS TO A STERILE FIELD

Objects   Whenever additional sterile items are added to a sterile field, care must be taken that contamination does not occur. Unwrap the items as for any sterile package and then pick them up from underneath the sterile covering. Gather the ends of the covering back around your wrist, forming a

sterile cover for your hand, and keep the ends from dragging. Commercially packaged sterile dressings usually come in packages that peel open. Remember that the ends you have grasped to peel back are contaminated and should not touch the dressing, nor should they be held over the sterile field. If one peeled-back side is folded *under*, it is possible to slide the dressing off over the sterile folded edge.

Place items well within the sterile field. Small items, such as gauze dressings, can be dropped from above the sterile field; large items can be put down carefully. You can use sterile forceps to remove an item from a package and to place it in the sterile field.

Liquids   To pour a liquid into a container in the sterile field, pour it from 6 to 8 inches above the receiving container, so that there is no possibility of the two containers touching. Always pour a small amount of the solution into a waste receptacle (to clean the lip of the container) before you pour the contents into the sterile receptacle.

If liquid is spilled onto the sterile field, that spot is considered contaminated if the moisture can soak through to the unsterile table beneath. Remember that microorganisms move rapidly through moisture. If the drape is impervious to fluid (many disposable drapes have a plastic layer) and the sterile liquid pools up on the surface, the area is still sterile.

PUTTING ON STERILE GLOVES

Sterile gloves should be put on without touching the outside of the gloves, so that contamination does not occur. Gloves are packaged in a uniform manner to facilitate this procedure.

Sterile gloves are sealed in a sterile package. Open the package in the same way you would open any other sterile package, unless it is a commercially prepared paper package. In that instance, instructions for opening are printed on the outside of the package.

Inside the sterile package, there is a folder containing the gloves. A small, folded-back

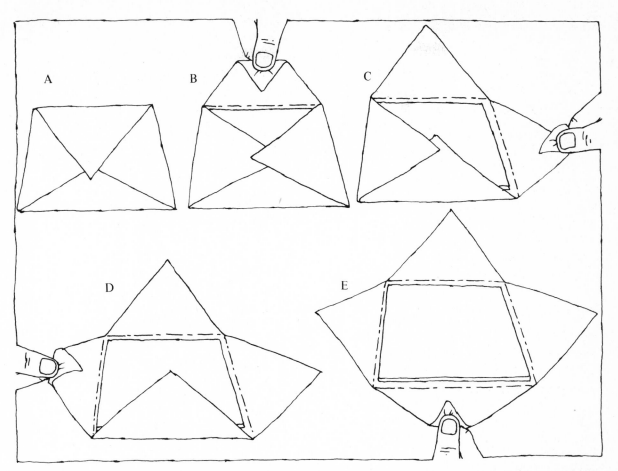

FIGURE 36.1   OPENING A STERILE PACKAGE   *A:* Unopened package; *B:* first flap opened; *C:* second flap opened; *D:* third flap opened; *E:* fourth flap opened, sterile object in center of sterile field.

margin is provided over each glove, so that you can open the folder without touching the gloves. The gloves in the package are arranged palm upward with the left glove on the left side and the right glove on the right side. A cuff of 2 to 4 inches is folded down over each glove. Figure 36.2 shows the correct sequence of opening and putting on sterile gloves.

Open one side of the folder, either left or right, touching only the center lower corner. Pick up the exposed glove with your opposite hand (the left glove with the right hand or the right glove with the left hand). Be sure to touch only the folded cuff, which is the *inside* of the glove. Then insert your free hand into the glove without touching skin to the outside of the glove. (The rhyme "sk*in* side to *in*side" can help you remember

this.) Be sure that you hold the glove well away from your body, and from the table or package, as you work. A common error is to brush the tips of the glove fingers against a nonsterile surface while manipulating, thus contaminating the gloves.

Open the second side of the folder with your bare hand, exposing the second glove. Pick up the glove with your gloved hand from under the cuff, which is the *outside* surface. Be sure to keep the thumb of the gloved hand rigidly extended outward or folded against the palm, so that you are not tempted to use it to grasp the other glove. Hold the glove under its cuff by your four gloved fingers. The cuff on the second glove protects the gloved hand from contamination by touching and also from microorganisms moving by gravity. Carefully maneuver

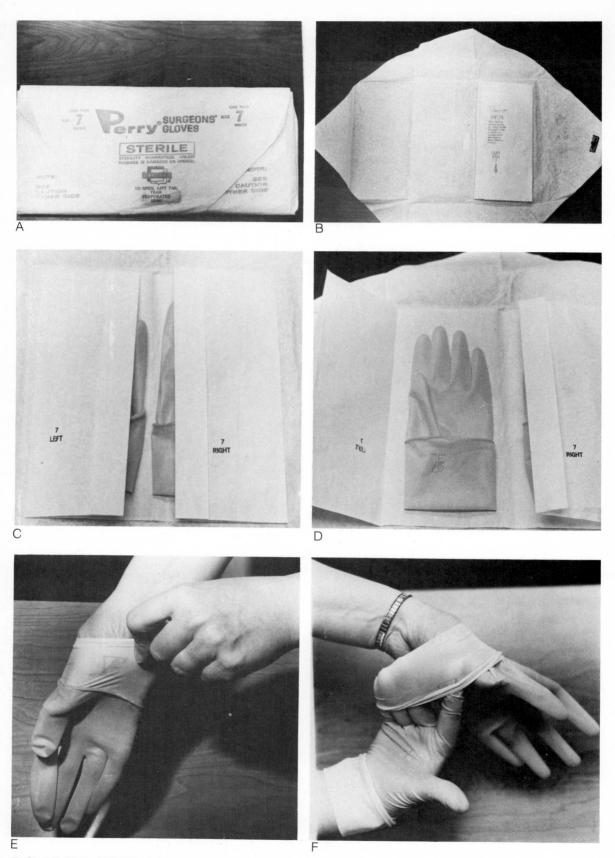

FIGURE 36.2 PUTTING ON STERILE GLOVES *A:* Obtain a sealed package of gloves; *B:* open the outer wrapper following the directions on the package; *C and D:* open the inner folder at the lower corner, without touching the gloves; *E:* pick up the right glove with your left hand, touching only the folded cuff, and put it on; *F:* grasp the left glove under the cuff and put it on.

Courtesy Ivan Ellis

the second hand into the glove. When both gloves are on, turn the cuffs up by flipping them, taking care not to roll the outside of the gloves onto skin.

Sterile gloves fit tightly and can be difficult to put on. Gloves are sometimes powdered to help them go on more easily. Also, you can powder or lubricate your hands before gloving, to make the process easier.

PERFORMANCE CHECKLIST

	Unsatisfactory	Needs more practice	Satisfactory	Comments
Arranging a sterile field				
1. Wash your hands.				
2. Separate items in sterile set.				
3. Keep sterile items over sterile field while moving.				
4. Place sterile items well within edge of sterile field.				
Opening a sterile set or pack				
1. Wash your hands.				
2. Do not cross your hand or arm over sterile area.				
3. Touch wrapper on outside only.				
4. Do not allow anything nonsterile to touch contents of pack.				
Adding material to sterile field				
1. Wash your hands.				
2. Open package away from sterile field.				
3. Drop sterile item onto sterile field, keeping hands as far from field as possible.				
4. Avoid reaching over field with arm as much as possible.				
Adding liquid to sterile field				
1. Wash your hands.				
2. Pour small amount over lip of bottle first, into waste receptacle.				
3. Pour from 6 to 8 inches above sterile container.				
4. Do not touch lip of bottle to container.				
5. Keep arm as far as possible from sterile field; avoid reaching over field if possible.				
Putting on sterile gloves				
1. Wash your hands.				
2. Open wrapper so that areas touched do not touch gloves.				
3. Pick up first glove, touching only inside surface (cuff).				

	Unsatisfactory	Needs more practice	Satisfactory	Comments
4. Put on first glove without allowing outside to touch anything else.				
5. Pick up second glove from under cuff with fingers (only) of gloved hand.				
6. Put on second glove touching only inside of second glove with bare hand.				
7. Turn up cuffs, touch gloved hand only to outside of other glove. Do not let outside of glove touch skin.				

QUIZ

Multiple-Choice Questions

_____ 1. The definition of *sterile* is

    a. the absence of all germs.
    b. the absence of disease-producing microorganisms.
    c. the absence of disease-producing microorganisms and their spores.
    d. The absence of all forms of life.

_____ 2. A precision instrument for measuring pressure must be sterilized. Which of the following methods would be suitable? (1) boiling water; (2) steam under pressure; (3) ethylene oxide gas; (4) sporicidal chemicals

    a. 1 and 3   c. 1 and 2
    b. 2 and 4   d. 3 and 4

_____ 3. A metal emesis basin must be sterilized. Which of the following techniques would work? (1) boiling water; (2) steam under pressure; (3) ethylene oxide gas; (4) sporicidal chemicals

    a. 1, 2, and 3   c. 1 and 2 only
    b. 2, 3, and 4   d. All of the above

_____ 4. Which of the following is the most common sterilization process in hospitals?

    a. Boiling water   c. Ethylene oxide gas
    b. Steam under pressure   d. Sporicidal chemicals

_____ 5. A plastic tubing to an instrument must be sterilized. The best method would be

    a. boiling water.   c. ethylene oxide gas.
    b. steam under pressure.   d. sporicidal chemicals.

_____ 6. In which of the following situations is sterile technique needed? (1) changing a dressing over a surgical wound; (2) changing a warm pack over an inflamed joint; (3) changing a dressing over an open decubitus ulcer; (4) changing a colostomy bag

    a. 1 and 2   c. 1 and 3
    b. 2 and 3   d. 3 and 4

_____ 7. We say the rhyme "skin side to inside" when we put on sterile gloves. From your knowledge of the basic rationale of sterile technique, this statement is

    a. correct   c. only partially correct.
    b. incorrect.   d. not relevant.

_____ 8. When adding objects to a sterile field, your arm should be

    a. anywhere convenient.
    b. as far from the sterile field as possible—at least 24 inches away.
    c. anywhere at least 12 inches above the table.
    d. kept to the side of the table, so as to not be above the sterile field.

True-False Questions

_____ 9. When a solution soaks through a sterile drape to an unsterile table beneath, the sterile drape is considered contaminated.

_____ 10. Persons in sterile gowns can pass one another in any manner because all surfaces of their gowns are sterile.

_____ 11. Articles dropped out of sight are considered contaminated.

_____ 12. It is permissible to reach over a sterile object with a bare arm so long as you do not touch it.

_____ 13. Sterile objects can be placed anywhere on the sterile field so long as they do not extend over the edge and contact an unsterile object.

Short-Answer Question

14. Give two examples of ways that sterility can be identified.

    a. _____

    b. _____

Module 37 Surgical Asepsis: Scrubbing, Gowning, and Gloving

MAIN OBJECTIVES

To scrub the hands and arms in a thorough manner in order to decrease the bacterial count, preparatory to participating in procedures that require surgical technique.

To don sterile gown and gloves correctly, so that outer surfaces remain sterile.

RATIONALE

Handwashing alone does not lower the count of normal flora on the hands, and this normal flora can produce infection when introduced into an open wound. During surgical procedures, deliveries, and invasive diagnostic procedures, sterile gloves are worn. However, gloves can break in the course of a procedure, so it is important that the hands be rendered as nearly free of microorganisms as possible. A gown too can become moist, allowing microorganisms to move from the arms to the gown's surface.

Surgical scrubbing lowers the total count of microorganisms on the hands and arms. It also removes dirt and oil from the skin, decreasing the ability of remaining microorganisms to multiply. Finally, it leaves a residue of antimicrobial cleansing agent on the skin, which further reduces the growth of microorganisms.

Gowns and gloves worn for sterile procedures must be put on in a way that ensures that nothing unsterile touches their outer surface. In order to maintain the highest standard of sterility, proper gowning and gloving technique is essential.

PREREQUISITES

Successful completion of the following modules:

VOLUME 1
Assessment
Medical Asepsis

VOLUME 2
Sterile Technique

177

SPECIFIC LEARNING OBJECTIVES

	Know Facts and Principles	Apply Facts and Principles	Demonstrate Ability	Evaluate Performance
1. *Purposes*	State three purposes of surgical scrub	Identify which persons in specific situation must perform surgical scrubs.		
2. *Scrubbing*				
a. *Equipment*	List equipment needed for surgical scrub and rationale for use		Obtain and set up needed equipment for surgical scrub	Check module to be sure all equipment is ready
b. *Types of scrub*	State two major bases for planning scrub procedure	Given a specific scrub procedure, identify major basis for planning procedure		
c. *Procedure*	List steps in scrubbing procedure	Explain rationale for each step in scrubbing procedure	Scrub using procedure outlined in module	Evaluate own performance using Performance Checklist. Verify procedure with observer.
3. *Gowning and gloving*	List steps for donning sterile gown. List steps of closed-glove technique. Identify that part of gown considered to be part of sterile field.	Identify situations in which gowning and gloving are necessary. Explain rationale for wearing gowns. Explain rationale for closed-glove technique.	Put on gown correctly. Put on sterile gloves correctly using closed-glove technique.	Evaluate own performance using Performance Checklist. Verify with observer that contamination did not occur.
4. *Guidelines for functioning in sterile attire*	List six guidelines for functioning in sterile garb	Identify reasons for guidelines	Preserve sterility of own garb. Identify contamination if it occurs and take immediate remedial action.	Evaluate own performance. Validate with observer.

LEARNING ACTIVITIES

1. Review the Specific Learning Objectives.
2. Look up the module vocabulary terms in the glossary.
3. Read through the module.
4. Read the scrub procedures of the facility where you practice, if available.
5. With a partner, in the practice setting:
   a. Look at the scrub equipment available.
   b. Compare it to what is suggested in the module.
   c. Adapt the equipment as needed. For example, if sink foot controls are not available, arrange for someone else to turn off the water or use a sterile towel to handle the faucets.
   d. Prepare the equipment, including a gown and gloves.
   e. Scrub your hands and arms using the Performance Checklist (or your facility's procedure) as a guide.
   f. Have your partner observe and evaluate your performance.
   g. Put on the sterile gown and gloves using the Performance Checklist as a guide.
   h. Have your partner observe and evaluate your performance.
   i. Reverse roles and repeat steps d–h.
   j. Repeat practice until you believe you have mastered these skills.
   k. Ask your instructor to check your performance.
6. Ask your instructor for an opportunity to observe in an area where scrubbing, gowning, and gloving are carried out.
7. In a discussion with the instructor, compare the procedure you learned with the one you observed. Identify strengths and weaknesses.
8. Ask your instructor for an opportunity to scrub in an area where appropriate and where you are prepared to undertake other activities.
9. Optional learning activities:
   a. Culture your hands before and after you scrub, to determine the effectiveness of the scrub.
   b. Apply lampblack to your hands before you scrub; then evaluate your own skill in removing it during the scrub.

VOCABULARY

antimicrobial
antiseptic
culture
disinfectant
lateral
medial
microorganism
normal flora
sterile
surgical asepsis

SURGICAL ASEPSIS

Scrubbing

Every facility has its own routine for performing a surgical scrub. The use of a specific routine ensures that each individual
maintains the same high standard. You
should always follow the procedure established by your facility or work to establish
an appropriate procedure if none exists.
What we present here are the general principles related to the surgical scrub, as well as
a sample procedure.

EQUIPMENT

A *nail-cleaning device,* either a metal nail
file or plastic nail cleaner, is always needed.
A separate one should be available for each
person. Wooden cleaning sticks (orange
sticks) are not recommended because it is
very difficult to sterilize wood.

The *scrubbing device* can be a special
sponge or a small soft-bristled brush. A
sponge is less irritating to the skin than is a
brush. The scrubbing device is sterile when
the procedure begins. In some facilities, two
sponges are used; one for the first half of the
scrub, and one for the second half.

Liquid antibacterial soap or detergent, in
a container that can be operated by a foot
control, is necessary. Many facilities provide
two types of cleansing agents, so that, if a
person is sensitive to one, the other can be
used. Some prepackaged, disposable scrub
sponges are impregnated with a cleansing
agent.

The *sink* must be large enough so that
both arms can be held over it and so that
water will not splash out. A *foot or knee
control for water* is also essential.

Before you begin to scrub, always open
the pack containing *sterile towels* for drying
after the scrub and set them out on a convenient table. Open the pack using appropriate sterile technique.

TYPES OF SCRUBS

Counted-Stroke Scrubs   In some facilities,
the prescribed routine for scrubbing includes

a specific pattern with a specified number of
strokes over each area. More strokes are used
over heavily folded or creviced areas (fingernails, knuckles), fewer strokes are used over
smoother areas (arms). The counted-stroke
method ensures complete and thorough
coverage of the area, no matter how rapidly
the scrubbing is done.

Timed Scrubs   In other facilities, the procedure requires that each area be scrubbed for
a specified time. Even so, a planned pattern
of scrubbing should be used to ensure that
no area is missed. The advantage of timed
scrubs is that they ensure optimum contact
with the antibacterial cleansing agent. Some
facilities use a combination of counted-
stroke and timed scrubs.

The timed scrub is commonly done for 10
minutes, 5 minutes on each arm. When
scrubbing between cases, use a total of 3
minutes, 1½ minutes on each arm. The 5-
minute scrub, 2½ minutes for each arm, is
commonly done if you are scrubbing for the
second time in 24 hours.

PROCEDURE

1. Prepare yourself for the scrub.
   a. Put on the scrub garments used in
      your facility.
   b. Put on shoe covers, a hair covering,
      and a mask (See Figure 37.1.)
   c. Clip your fingernails and remove
      polish. (Do not scrub if your skin is
      cut or blemished.)
2. Prepare the equipment.
   a. Set out the sterile towel pack and
      open it.
   b. Set out two sponges or brushes using
      sterile technique.
   c. Set out the nail cleaner using sterile
      technique.
   d. Check cleansing agent.
   e. Turn on the water and adjust the
      temperature so that it is comfortably
      warm. (Warm water emulsifies fats
      more effectively than does cold; and
      hot water is very hard on the skin.)
3. Position yourself over the sink, holding
   your hands higher than your elbows, so

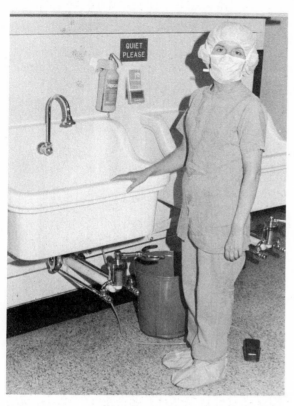

FIGURE 37.1   SCRUB ATTIRE
Courtesy Ivan Ellis

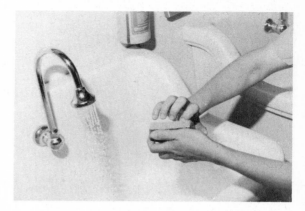

FIGURE 37.2   BRUSHING THE CORNERS OF
THE NAILS
Courtesy Ivan Ellis

that water will drain off the elbows. (This leaves your fingers the cleanest part of the hands when you are finished.)

4. Wash your hands. Use the cleansing agent and wash well above the elbows. Rinse thoroughly from the hands toward the elbows.

5. Relather your hands.

6. Using the nail cleaner, clean carefully under each nail (the subungual area). Rinse the cleaner after each finger, so that soil is not carried from one finger to the next.

7. Carefully pick up one brush or sponge. Wet it and add cleansing agent as necessary. (Add water and cleansing agent throughout the scrub to maintain a lather.) Use the following pattern for the right hand and arm:

   a. Brush the fingernails first using six strokes across each area. First brush directly across the ends of the fingernails; then slant the fingers to brush across the lateral corners (Figure 37.2) for six strokes; then slant the fingers to brush across the medial corners for six strokes.

   b. Brush six strokes across over the back of the fingers and the knuckles.

   c. Brush the thumbnail using six strokes across each corner and six strokes across the end.

   d. Brush across the back of the thumb for six strokes.

   e. Spread the fingers apart. Brush the lateral aspect of each finger with three strokes. Then, go back the other way brushing the medial aspect of each finger with three strokes.

   f. Close the fingers and brush the palmar surfaces of the fingers and the palm of the hand, using three circular strokes over each area.

   g. Brush around the wrist and up the arm (Figure 37.3), using three circular strokes over each area. Brush to a brush-width above the elbow.

8. Leave the lather on the arm to allow maximum antibacterial activity.

9. Carefully transfer the brush to the other hand.

10. Scrub the second (left) arm using the pattern in step 7. This finishes one cycle, or round.

11. Rinse the first hand and arm just before you start to scrub for the next round. You will rinse the second hand and

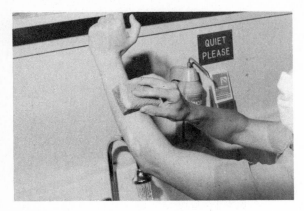

FIGURE 37.3   SCRUBBING THE ARMS
Courtesy Ivan Ellis

arm just before you start to scrub them. Rinse from the fingertips to the elbows, allowing the water to flow off the elbows. Keep your hand higher than your elbow and be careful not to touch the sink. (See Figure 37.4.)

12. Do the prescribed number of cycles. A cycle of this type done quickly and efficiently takes approximately one minute. Ten cycles (ten minutes) are commonly done as an initial scrub. Five cycles (five minutes) are done for the second scrub within 24 hours. Three cycles (three minutes) are adequate between cases if you do not leave the surgical unit.

13. When two sponges are used, do half the cycles with one sponge and then discard it; finish with the second one. Usually, two sponges are used only if ten cycles are necessary, although in some facilities, all cycles are done on one hand and arm using one sponge. Then, the second sponge is used to do all the cycles on the second arm.

14. When all the cycles have been finished, dispose of the brush by dropping it in the sink or receptacle.

15. Rinse both arms thoroughly, keeping your fingers up.

16. Keep your hands up and in front of you, and walk to the table where the towels are kept. If you must go through closed doors, back through. Allow your arms to drip. (See Figure 37.5.)

17. Dry your hands and arms.
    a. Pick up the sterile towel by one end.
    b. Allow the towel to unfold.
    c. Place one hand under half of the towel. Use that half to blot the opposite hand dry (Figure 37.6). Start at the fingers and move gradually up the arm.

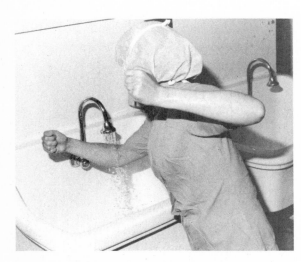

FIGURE 37.4   RINSING THE ARMS   Keep the hand higher than the elbow.
Courtesy Ivan Ellis

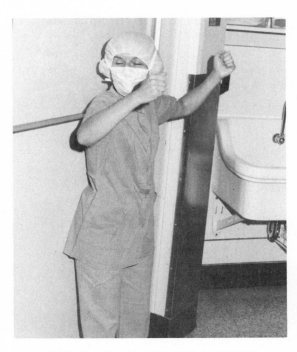

FIGURE 37.5   WALKING WITH ARMS UP
Courtesy Ivan Ellis

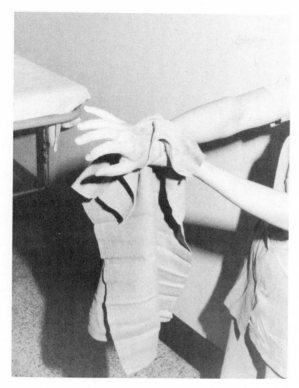

FIGURE 37.6 DRYING THE HANDS AND ARMS
Courtesy Ivan Ellis

You will need an assistant to safely put on a sterile gown, and your assistant will need sterile forceps.

The closed-glove technique, which is described in step 7, below, is in widespread use because it provides a way to don gloves without the possibility of their being touched on the outside by the bare hand. You will don the right glove first, and then the left glove. (Open-glove technique was described in Module 36, Sterile Technique.)

1. Pick up the sterile gown carefully by its neck edge.
2. Hold the gown in front of you and allow it to unfold (Figure 37.7).
3. Identify the back opening and the front of the gown.
4. Work your hands and arms carefully into the gown and into the sleeves, as far as the seam between the sleeve and the cuff. Take your time and proceed

d. Use the other half of the towel to blot the second arm dry. Again start at the fingers and move up the arm.
e. Push the cuticle of your fingernails back with the towel as you dry your hands. This helps to prevent ragged cuticle edges, decreasing the chance of harboring bacteria.

You are now ready to put on a sterile gown and gloves.

Gowning and Gloving

Open the packs in which the sterile gown and sterile gloves are wrapped at the same time you open the sterile towel pack. In fact, these items may all be wrapped in one package.

After you have scrubbed and dried your hands, you are ready to put on a sterile gown. Remember to keep your hands above your waist and higher than your elbows at all times. Gowning is a two-person procedure.

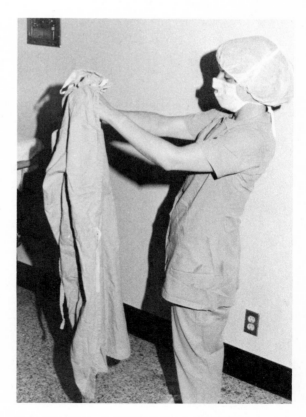

FIGURE 37.7 PUTTING ON A STERILE GOWN
Courtesy Ivan Ellis

slowly. Do *not* push your hands out through the ends of the sleeves.

5. Turn your back to your assistant, who will now grasp the *inside* of the back, pull it securely onto your shoulders, and tie the neck and back waistline ties.

6. Leave the front waistline tie tied in front of you.

7. Using the closed-glove technique, put on the sterile gloves.

 a. With your left hand still inside the gown, pick up the folded edge of the right glove.

 b. Hold your right hand out, with the palm up, still *inside* the sleeve.

 c. Lay the right glove on the right palm (which is still inside the sleeve). Position it with the glove fingers pointing toward the elbow and the cuff end pointing toward the finger-tips. The thumb of the glove should be over the thumb of your right hand. (See Figure 37.8.)

 d. Use your right hand (which is still inside the gown sleeve) to grasp the bottom fold of the cuff end of the right glove. You are touching sterile gown to sterile gown.

 e. With your left hand (which is still inside the gown sleeve), grasp the right glove cuff by the top fold of

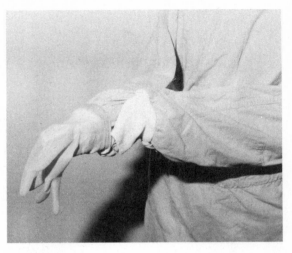

FIGURE 37.9   PULLING ON THE FIRST GLOVE
Courtesy Ivan Ellis

the cuff end and pull the right glove cuff up and over the right gown cuff. (See Figure 37.9.)

 f. Adjust the right glove cuff over the right gown cuff as necessary, keeping the left hand inside the gown.

 g. Work your right hand down into the glove. If the fingers are not in place, don't worry. You can correct them when both gloves are on.

 h. Pick up the left glove with the gloved right hand.

 i. Hold your left hand, palm up, inside the gown sleeve.

 j. Place the left glove on the left palm (which is still inside the gown), with the glove fingers pointing toward the elbow and the cuff end pointing to-ward your fingertips. Position the glove thumb over the left thumb of your hand.

 k. Use your left hand (which is still inside the sleeve) to grasp the bot-tom fold of the cuff end of the left glove.

 l. Grasp the top fold of the cuff edge with the gloved right hand and pull the glove cuff up and over the gown cuff (Figure 37.10).

 m. Work your left hand down into the left glove.

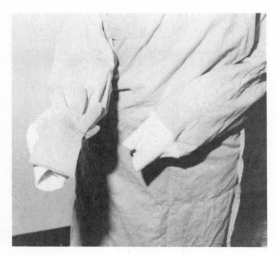

FIGURE 37.8   POSITIONING THE GLOVE
Courtesy Ivan Ellis

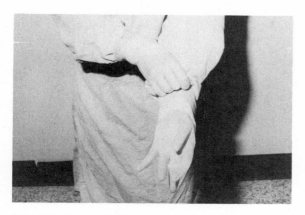

FIGURE 37.10   PULLING ON THE SECOND GLOVE
Courtesy Ivan Ellis

n. Turn up and adjust the cuffs of both gloves (Figure 37.11).
o. Pull the glove fingers out at the ends to reposition your fingers if necessary.
8. With your gloved hands, untie the front waist tie of your gown.
9. Hold the ends carefully, keeping them above your waist.
10. Hold the shorter tie in one hand.
11. With the other hand, hold the longer tie out for your assistant to grasp with sterile forceps.
12. While your assistant is holding the tie, turn around carefully, wrapping the gown around you as you turn (Figure 37.12). This completely covers your back with

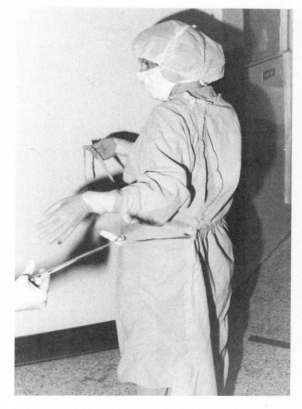

FIGURE 37.12   TYING THE GOWN
Courtesy Ivan Ellis

the sterile gown. Be sure you are well away from all equipment when you turn.
13. Retrieve the tie from your assistant and tie the two ties together in the front.

You are now prepared to handle sterile equipment. (See Figure 37.13.)

Guidelines for Working in Sterile Attire

1. *Everything below the waist or table height is considered nonsterile.* Therefore, keep your hands above your waist and keep sterile equipment on top of the tables. When you are waiting, it is often convenient to clasp your gloved hands together in front of you to protect them.
2. *Your back is considered potentially contaminated because you cannot see what happens to it.* Do not turn your

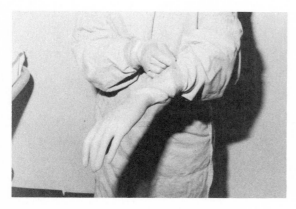

FIGURE 37.11   ADJUSTING THE CUFF
Courtesy Ivan Ellis

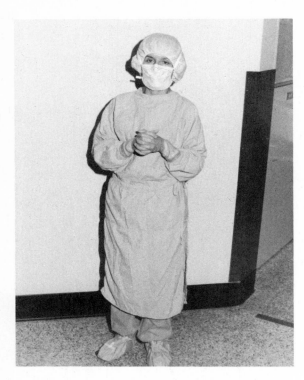

FIGURE 37.13 COMPLETELY GOWNED AND
GLOVED
Courtesy Ivan Ellis

back on any sterile area. Always pass it
with your face toward the sterile area.

3. Also, for the same reason, when passing
    another person in sterile attire, pass
    either face to face or back to back. If
    you must stand behind someone, fasten
    a sterile towel over that person's back.

4. *Sterility is a matter of certainty, not
    conjecture.* If you even suspect that a
    part of your attire has been contam-
    inated, notify the appropriate person
    (circulating nurse, perhaps) for assist-
    ance in changing.

5. *Moisture allows microorganisms to wick
    quickly and easily from one area to
    another.* If your attire becomes wet,
    consider it contaminated, and change it
    or cover it.

6. *Contamination often occurs accident-
    ally.* To prevent this, whenever you
    move close to anyone, warn them verb-
    ally. Do not take it for granted that
    they will see you.

PERFORMANCE CHECKLIST

Scrubbing	Unsatisfactory	Needs more practice	Satisfactory	Comments
1. Prepare yourself. a. Put on scrub garments.				
b. Cover hair and shoes, and put on mask.				
c. Care for your fingernails.				
2. Prepare equipment. a. Open towel pack.				
b. Set out brushes or sponges.				
c. Set out nail cleaner.				
d. Check cleansing agent.				
e. Turn on water in sink.				
3. Position self with hands higher than elbows.				
4. Wash your hands to above elbows and rinse thoroughly.				
5. Relather your hands.				
6. Clean the nails, rinsing after each finger.				
7. Scrub using the appropriate pattern. a. Fingernails (six strokes over each area)				
b. Backs of fingers and knuckles (six strokes)				
c. Thumbnail (six strokes over each area)				
d. Back of thumb (six strokes)				
e. Lateral and medial aspect of fingers (three strokes over each area)				
f. Palm (three circular strokes over each area)				
g. Wrist and arm (three circular strokes over each area)				
8. Leave lather on first hand and arm.				
9. Transfer brush to other hand.				
10. Scrub second arm and hand using same pattern.				
11. Rinse first hand and arm, from fingertips to elbow, before starting second cycle.				
12. Do prescribed number of cycles.				
13. Change brush or sponge after five cycles if ten are being done.				
14. After all cycles are complete, drop brush in sink.				
15. Rinse both hands and arms, keeping fingers up.				

	Unsatisfactory	Needs more practice	Satisfactory	Comments
16. Move toward towels, keeping hands up and in front of you.				
17. Dry your hands and arms. a. Pick up sterile towel.				
b. Allow towel to unfold.				
c. Use half to dry first hand and arm.				
d. Use second half to dry second hand and arm.				
e. Push cuticles back as you dry.				
Gowning and closed gloving				
1. Pick up gown by neck edge.				
2. Allow gown to unfold.				
3. Identify back opening and front of gown.				
4. Work hands and arms into gown to seam between gown and cuff.				
5. Turn your back to assistant for securing gown at neck and back.				
6. Leave front tie tied.				
7. Using closed-glove technique, put on sterile gloves. a. Use left hand inside gown to pick up folded edge of right glove.				
b. Hold right hand, palm up, inside gown.				
c. Position right glove on right palm.				
d. Use right hand inside gown to grasp bottom fold of cuff.				
e. Use left hand inside gown to pull right glove cuff over right gown cuff.				
f. Adjust right glove over right gown cuff.				
g. Work right hand into glove.				
h. Using gloved right hand, pick up left glove.				
i. Hold left hand, palm up, inside gown.				
j. Position left glove over left palm.				
k. Use left hand inside gown to grasp fold of glove cuff.				
l. Use gloved right hand to grasp top of fold and pull glove cuff over gown cuff.				

	Unsatisfactory	Needs more practice	Satisfactory	Comments
m. Work left hand into glove.				
n. Turn up and adjust cuffs.				
o. Reposition fingers as needed.				
8. Untie front waist tie.				
9. Hold ends above waist.				
10. Hold shorter tie in one hand.				
11. Hold longer tie out for assistant to grasp with sterile forceps.				
12. Turn around carefully, wrapping gown around you.				
13. Retrieve tie from assistant, and tie two ties in front.				
Working in sterile attire				
1. Keep your hands in front of you and above waist level.				
2. Do not turn your back on sterile field.				
3. Pass front to front or back to back with others in sterile attire.				
4. Change attire when contaminated.				
5. Change or cover attire if wet.				
6. Warn others of your movements.				

QUIZ

Short-Answer Questions

1. List three purposes of a surgical scrub.

    a. _____

    b. _____

    c. _____

2. Why is a wooden nail cleaner not recommended? _____

3. In what areas should a larger number of scrub strokes be used?

    _____

4. Why would you want a residue of antibacterial cleansing agent to

    remain on the skin? _____

5. Why are hands held higher than the elbows for a surgical scrub?

    _____

6. What is the advantage of the closed-glove technique? _____

7. List three situations in which a nurse would be required to don a sterile
    gown and gloves.

    a. _____

    b. _____

    c. _____

Module 38 Irrigations

MAIN OBJECTIVE

To know the purpose of an irrigation, to plan the correct technique needed to accomplish that purpose, and to carry out the irrigation safely.

RATIONALE

Irrigations are used to clean a body part (by removing secretions and microorganisms) and to deliver medications to various parts of the body. There are many similarities in the way these irrigations are done, but the differences are critical. The nurse must be able to plan an appropriate procedure and to carry it out correctly.

PREREQUISITES

1. Successful completion of the following modules:

    VOLUME 1
    Assessment
    Charting
    Medical Asepsis
    Intake and Output

2. The following may be needed for some irrigations:

    VOLUME 2
    Sterile Technique
    Sterile Dressings
    Administering Oral Medications

193

SPECIFIC LEARNING OBJECTIVES

	Know Facts and Principles	Apply Facts and Principles	Demonstrate Ability	Evaluate Performance
1. *Purposes*	List two general purposes for irrigation	In a specific situation, identify purpose of irrigation	Identify purpose of irrigation before proceeding	
2. *General concerns* *a. Clean versus sterile technique* *b. Safety*	Identify irrigations that require sterile technique. List factors in irrigation that may irritate or damage tissue.	Given an example of an irrigation, determine whether clean or sterile technique is needed	In the clinical area, use correct technique for situation. Use correct pressure, solution and temperature for irrigation.	Evaluate own performance using Performance Checklist
3. *Performing irrigation*	State procedure for each irrigation discussed in module	Modify procedure for individual situation. Explain procedure to patient.	Carry out specific irrigation correctly	Evaluate own performance using Performance Checklist
4. *Observations*	State important observations to be made during irrigation	Identify observations that are most critical for particular situation	Make appropriate observations while performing irrigations	Evaluate appropriateness of observations with instructor
5. *Recording*	State what needs to be recorded	Given an example of an irrigation, identify what should be recorded	Chart appropriate information on patient's record	Evaluate using Performance Checklist

LEARNING ACTIVITIES

1. Review the Specific Learning Objectives.
2. Read the chapter on dependent nursing functions in Ellis and Nowlis, *Nursing: A Human Needs Approach,* or a comparable chapter in another textbook.
3. Look up the module vocabulary terms in the glossary.
4. Read through the module.
5. Arrange for time to practice irrigations.
6. In the practice setting:
   a. Review the equipment available for irrigations.
   b. Identify the various types of syringes and any prepackaged sets for specific types of irrigations.
   c. Try using each piece of equipment to make sure you understand its function and can handle it.
   d. Review the charting of irrigations in sample situations.
7. In the clinical area:
   a. Seek opportunities to observe irrigations done by others.
   b. Perform irrigations with supervision.

VOCABULARY

asepto syringe
canthus
cerumen
concentration of solution
douche
exudate
instill
irrigate
mucus
Toomey syringe

IRRIGATIONS

Irrigations are done for two general purposes. The first is to clean. Large amounts of fluid can be used to remove secretions, clots, foreign matter, and microorganisms. The fluid used may be one that simply flushes particles away or it may contain special cleansing agents.

A second purpose is to instill medication. This may be an antibacterial agent, a soothing agent, or an agent that exerts another specific therapeutic effect, such as changing acidity. Sometimes an irrigation serves both these purposes at the same time. (Consult Module 44 regarding instilling medications.)

Techniques

Sterile technique must be used on all areas of the body that are normally sterile. These include the bladder, the kidney pelvis, and open wounds. Sterile technique is also used for irrigations involving the eye because of the potential for serious injury from even a minor eye infection.

Clean technique is used for all other irrigations. These include irrigations of the throat, ear, vagina, bowel, and stomach. However, in an instance of surgery on any of these organs, sterile technique is needed.

Safety

Most body tissue is very sensitive to excessive pressure. Fluid under pressure can cause spasms of an organ such as the bladder and actual tissue damage to a structure as sensitive as the eye. Therefore use gentle pressure only. If the patient feels discomfort, reduce the pressure. Remember that by decreasing the height of the container you decrease the pressure.

Medications or chemicals used may also irritate or cause tissue reaction. This is especially true if the wrong concentration is used for a particular tissue. For example, a benzalkonium chloride solution, suitable for use on instruments, is far too strong for mucous membranes. Therefore, carefully check both the type and concentration of solution used.

Most irrigations are done with solutions at room temperature. To increase the patient's comfort, solutions can be warmed to body temperature. Do not use extreme temperatures, however: very high temperatures can burn tissues; low temperatures can produce a shocklike reaction as the body attempts to maintain homeostasis.

Patient Teaching

As in all procedures, teaching the patient about it and what to expect is essential. This allows the patient to participate in the care as much as possible.

To begin, find out what the patient knows; then explain what the patient does not yet understand. If an irrigation has been done previously, it is important that you find out what the previous procedure was. It may upset the patient to have each nurse proceed in a different manner. The irrigation technique should be noted in the nursing care plan to facilitate continuing care.

Allow time for the patient to ask questions and to express personal feelings about the procedure. Many irrigation procedures produce anxiety and you will have to take action to decrease the patient's anxiety by listening and expressing concern.

Observation

During an irrigation, it is important that you observe the area being irrigated as much as possible. Of course, certain internal areas cannot be observed directly, but the opening into the area can be observed. Notice any drainage or exudate, and describe the amount, color, consistency, and odor of it. Also, observe the irrigation returns for secretions that may be washed out with the fluid.

Charting

When you chart, note the area that was irrigated, the type and amount of solution used, the time of irrigation, as well as the patient's response to the procedure.

All fluid that is used for irrigating should be returned. If the fluid fails to return, note that fact in the chart and record the amount retained on the intake worksheet.

General Procedure

1. Check the orders to verify the following:
   a. Patient's name
   b. Type of irrigation
   c. Amount, temperature, type, and concentration of solution
2. Identify the patient. As in any nursing procedure, positive identification is essential.
3. Explain the procedure to the patient.
4. Wash your hands.
5. Gather all the necessary equipment. (See Figure 38.1.) Depending on whether the irrigation is clean or sterile, the following items are usually needed:
   a. The solution
   b. An irrigating device (asepto, Toomey, or ear syringe, as shown in Figure 38.2; a container with attached tubing)
   c. A receptacle for used irrigating fluid
   d. Protective padding (towels or disposable waterproof pads to keep the patient and the environment dry)
6. Position the patient as needed for the irrigation.
7. Drape the patient to provide privacy and warmth.
8. Place the protective padding where needed.
9. Carry out the specific irrigation according to the procedures below.
10. Leave the patient dry and comfortable.
11. Dispose of the used equipment following the policy of your facility. If it is reusable, you may have to thoroughly wash it; if it is disposable, you may have to discard it in a specific place.
12. Wash your hands.
13. Record.
    a. Type of irrigation
    b. Type, concentration, and amount of fluid used
    c. The appearance and odor of any secretions washed away
    d. Results of the procedure
    e. The patient's response to the procedure

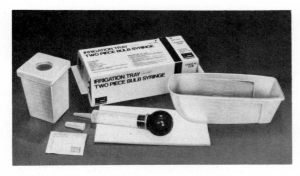

FIGURE 38.1   IRRIGATION SET
Courtesy American Hospital Supply Corp., Evanston, Illinois

Bladder and Catheter Irrigation

The terms *bladder irrigation* and *catheter irrigation* are often used interchangeably. Actually, they are not the same, so when either is ordered you should check carefully as to the purpose of the irrigation. A catheter irrigation is to keep the catheter patent; a bladder irrigation is to clean or medicate the bladder itself. Much of the technique is

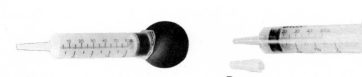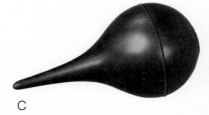

| A | B | C |

FIGURE 38.2   TYPES OF SYRINGES USED FOR IRRIGATIONS   *A:* Asepto syringe, *B:* Toomey syringe; *C:* ear syringe.
Courtesy American Hospital Supply Corp., Evanston, Illinois

identical for both procedures, and both procedures require sterile technique.

An open or closed technique can be used for intermittent irrigations. Today, the closed technique is being used increasingly in order to maintain the urinary drainage as a closed system, preventing the introduction of microorganisms that might cause infection. (For a further discussion of catheter care, see Module 39, Catheterization.)

CLOSED TECHNIQUE

This method can be carried out in three different ways. Two of them are described below. A third closed technique, three-way irrigation, will be described later.

Y-Connector and Fluid Reservoir   The first is through the use of a Y-connector on the catheter and a fluid reservoir. A sterile Y-connector is placed between the catheter and the drainage tubing. A large bottle or

bag of sterile irrigating solution is hung on an IV standard with a sterile tubing attached. This is the same setup used for the solution for a three-way irrigation. (See Figure 38.3.) The fluid tubing is attached to the Y-connector.

1. Gather the necessary equipment.
2. Clamp the drainage tubing from the catheter.
3. Open the fluid tubing from the container.
4. Allow the prescribed amount of fluid to flow into the bladder. Remember that you will be filling the bladder, so you have to watch carefully. Do not allow too much fluid to enter. If the amount is not specified, use between 50 and 100 ml.
5. Close the fluid tubing.
6. Open the drainage tubing and allow the fluid to flow into the catheter drainage bag.

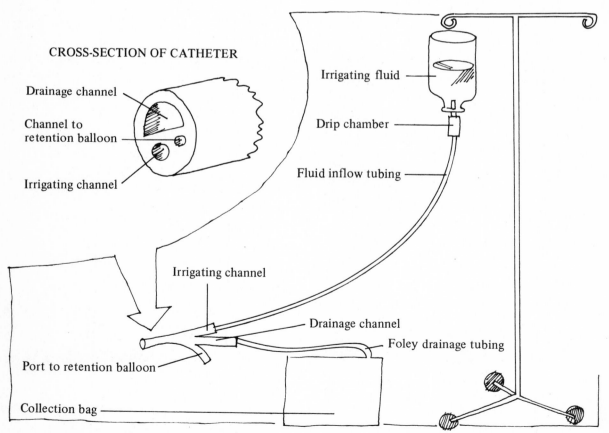

CROSS-SECTION OF CATHETER

Drainage channel

Channel to retention balloon

Irrigating channel

Irrigating fluid

Drip chamber

Fluid inflow tubing

Irrigating channel

Drainage channel

Foley drainage tubing

Port to retention balloon

Collection bag

FIGURE 38.3   THREE-WAY IRRIGATION SETUP

7. Observe the fluid returning.

8. Record the fluid used for irrigation as intake, or subtract it from the output later, whichever is the policy of your facility.

Syringe-and-Needle Method The second way to irrigate the catheter through a closed system is to use the syringe-and-needle method.

1. Gather the necessary equipment.
   a. 20- to 30-ml syringe with needle
   b. Alcohol wipe
   c. Solution ordered

2. Draw up the solution into the syringe using sterile technique. (See Module 45, Giving Injections, pages 312–313, for techniques for filling the syringe.)

3. Use the alcohol wipe to clean the entry port on the drainage tubing. This is a soft, resealable-rubber area. If the drainage tubing does not have an entry port, use the portion of the Foley catheter distal to the entry to the balloon as an entry area.

4. Insert the needle into the entry port.

5. Clamp the tubing distal to the needle entry area.

6. Inject the fluid into the catheter.

7. Remove the needle.

8. Release the catheter and allow the fluid to drain into the drainage bag.

9. Observe the fluid returning.

10. Repeat as necessary to use the amount of fluid ordered.

11. Note the amount of fluid used for the irrigation on the intake and output worksheet according to the policy of your facility.

OPEN TECHNIQUE

1. Gather the necessary equipment.
   a. Sterile irrigation set (asepto syringe, container for irrigating fluid, drainage receptacle, alcohol wipe.)
   b. Solution. (Normal saline is commonly used, however, acidifying or antibacterial solutions can also be ordered.)

2. Open the set, maintaining sterile technique. You can touch the exterior of the fluid container, the exterior of the receptacle, and the bulb of the syringe, to set them up conveniently.

3. Pour the solution from the original bulk container into the irrigating bottle.

4. To reduce the possibility of contamination, clean the junction of the catheter and drainage tubing before disconnecting them. Some sets contain a sterile cleansing wipe in a foil package for this purpose. If the set does not contain one, obtain separately.

5. Disconnect the catheter from the drainage tubing, and hold the catheter end over the drainage fluid receptacle. Many of these receptacles are made with a notched end to hold the catheter firmly, so that it doesn't touch anything.

6. Protect the end of the drainage tubing from contamination. There are many ways to do this. For example, you can fold a sterile gauze square over the end of the drainage tubing and secure it with a rubber band. (Some nurses are able to hold this end carefully while performing the irrigation, but we do not recommend this for beginners.) Or, you can slip the end of the drainage tubing inside the foil package that contained the cleansing wipe (it is sterile inside) and secure it with a rubber band.

   Also, a sterile drainage tubing cap may be included in the set or may be available packaged separately.

7. Instill the fluid.
   a. For a catheter irrigation:
      (1) Fill the asepto syringe with 30 to 60 ml solution.
      (2) Insert the tip of the asepto into the catheter and instill the fluid with gentle pressure.
      (3) Pinch the catheter closed and hold it closed while you withdraw the syringe.
      (4) Allow the fluid to drain into the drainage receptacle.
      (5) Observe the drainage for color and sediment.

   (6) Repeat this procedure until the
        catheter is clear of sediment.
    Do not aspirate the fluid into the
    asepto syringe because it can trau-
    matize the bladder lining or even
    collapse the bladder.
  b. For bladder irrigation:
    (1) Instill the ordered fluid into the
        bladder.
    (2) Clamp the tubing, so that the
        solution remains in the bladder
        for several minutes.
    (3) Allow the fluid to drain out.
8. Reconnect the catheter to the drainage
   tubing.

THREE-WAY IRRIGATION

Insert a special three-way catheter when this type of irrigation is needed. (See Figure 38.3.) There is a channel in the catheter for fluid to be instilled, as well as the usual channels for drainage and for inflating the balloon in the bladder. This type of irrigation is most frequently done after surgical procedures on the bladder.

1. Gather the necessary equipment.
   a. IV standard
   b. Solution
   c. Tubing
2. Hang a reservoir of the ordered sterile fluid, which looks much like an intravenous solution, from an IV pole.
3. Expel all air from the tubing before you attach it.
4. Attach the tubing to the inflow channel of the catheter.
5. Attach the other channel of the catheter to the drainage tubing.
6. Regulate the irrigation as a continuous drip with a clamp on the tubing.

   The physician may order a specific rate of flow in milliters per hour or may simply order that a slow continuous drip be used. The nurse is responsible for monitoring and maintaining this flow. (See Module 46.) Larger quantities of fluid can be run through as needed to keep the catheter open and the bladder free of debris.

   The most critical concern is that large quantities of fluid not be put into the bladder if the drainage tubing is clogged or inadvertently clamped. This causes severe pain and could rupture the patient's bladder. Therefore, closely watch the output of the catheter to see that it corresponds to the amount of fluid being instilled plus any other intake.

   All fluid instilled must be accounted for on the patient's intake and output record. It can be included as part of the intake, or a separate record of the fluid instilled can be kept and subtracted from the urinary output when that is measured. Follow the policy of your facility.

Irrigating the Ear

Before irrigating an ear, it must be examined with an otoscope. This may have been done by the physician, but, if not, you should do it. If the tympanic membrane (eardrum) is not intact, *do not* irrigate the ear. The fluid could enter the middle ear and cause an infection.

   An ear syringe is usually used to instill the fluid, although some facilities use a Water Pik on low pressure. This is a clean procedure.

1. Gather the necessary equipment.
   a. Ear syringe or Water Pik
   b. Emesis basin
   c. Clean towels
   d. Solution
2. Position the patient so that he or she is sitting or lying with the head tilted toward the side to be irrigated.
3. Place the basin under the patient's ear.
4. Place a towel across the patient's shoulder.
5. Fill the syringe with fluid.
6. Direct the tip of the syringe toward the top of the patient's ear canal (Figure 38.4), so that a circular current is set up with fluid flowing in along the top and out along the bottom. This will float out cerumen or foreign material. Be careful: severe discomfort and dizziness can result from fluid directed onto the eardrum.

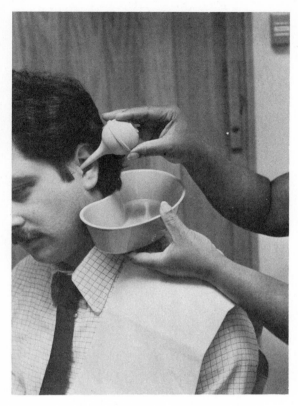

FIGURE 38.4   IRRIGATING THE EAR
Courtesy Lawrence Cherkas

7. Irrigate until either the ear canal is clean or the ordered volume is used.
8. Dry the ear with a clean sponge or towel.
9. Assist the patient to a comfortable position on the affected side, to drain out excess fluid.
10. Record procedure.

Irrigating the Eye

This is a sterile procedure. Use a sterile syringe and sterile fluid. If both eyes are to be irrigated, use separate sets for each eye to prevent cross-contamination.

1. Gather the necessary equipment.
   a. Sterile syringe
   b. Sterile solution
   c. Emesis basin
   d. Sterile cotton balls
2. Position the patient in the supine position. Turn the patient's head to the side of the eye that is to be irrigated. (The patient can be seated with the head tilted back and supported.)
3. Place an emesis basin beside and below the eye.
4. Hold the eye open with the thumb and forefinger of your nondominant hand. (Resting your hand on the patient's forehead may make this easier.)
5. Fill the syringe with fluid.
6. Gently release the fluid onto the eye at the inner canthus, allowing it to flow across the eye and then into the basin. *Do not touch the irrigator to the eye.* Keep the tip close to the eye so that fluid pressure is not increased by the height of the fluid container.
7. Continue this procedure until the eye is clean or until the fluid ordered has been used.
8. Dry the eyelid, wiping it from the inner canthus to the outer canthus, using a sterile cotton ball. Use each cotton ball only once, and discard.
9. Record the procedure.

LARGE-VOLUME EYE IRRIGATION

For large-volume irrigation, (1,000 ml) use a sterile IV container with IV tubing.

1. Adjust the IV standard to its lowest height.
2. Hang the solution on the IV standard.
3. Fill the tubing with fluid.
4. Eliminate the air from the tubing.
5. Position the patient with a drainage basin by the eye. If the fluid is to be given continuously, it is wise to have a large bath basin available, to empty the drainage basin part way through the irrigation. This prevents it from overflowing onto the patient.
6. Open the control valve or clamp on the IV tubing and allow the fluid to flow slowly across the eye. A continuous flow is important, but the pressure should never cause discomfort. It may be necessary to hold the eye open to allow the fluid to flow directly onto the eye itself rather than onto the eyelid.

Nasogastric Tube Irrigation

Clean technique is used except when there has been surgery on the stomach, in which case sterile technique may be required.

1. Obtain the necessary equipment.
   a. A conventional syringe with an adapter, an asepto syringe, or a Toomey syringe
   b. Solution. (Normal saline is preferred because it reduces electrolyte depletion.)
   c. An emesis basin
2. Disconnect the nasogastric tube from the connecting tube.
3. Fill the syringe with the fluid.
4. Gently instill approximately 30 ml fluid into the tubing. If the fluid will not enter the tubing, the outlet eyes may be against the mucosa. Untape the tube from the nose and moving it in and out gently (not over 1 inch either way). This can release the end of the tube and allow you to proceed with the irrigation. Be sure to retape the tube before you continue with the procedure.
5. Aspirate the fluid back and discard it in the basin. If the fluid does not return after several attempts at aspiration, instill another syringe of fluid; however, do not continue to instill fluid if none is returning. Report the situation to the nurse in charge.

   In some facilities the fluid is not aspirated. After instillation, the tubing is reconnected and the suction machine aspirates the fluid. The fluid must then be added to the intake record or a separate record is maintained of the irrigating fluid and that amount is subtracted from the suction amount when output is figured. Follow the policy of your facility.
6. Repeat the procedure, instilling and aspirating fluid, until the tubing is cleared of clotted material or thick mucus.
7. Reconnect the tubing to the suction machine. If the suction does not appear to be functioning and you have cleared the nasogastric tube, the tubing to the machine itself may be clogged. Squeeze this tubing between your fingers to loosen the material and allow the machine to clear the tubing. (See Module 28, Gastric Intubation, for the care of a patient with a nasogastric tube in place.)
8. Record the procedure.

Vaginal Irrigation

This procedure is also called a *vaginal douche.* Clean technique is used.

1. Gather the necessary equipment.
   a. A douche set with a special douche tip (Figure 38.5)
   b. Solution (approximately 1,000 ml), at body temperature
   c. An IV standard. (Although it is possible to hold the fluid container during the procedure, you will find that it is very inconvenient to try to do so.)
   d. A waterproof pad
   e. A bedpan
   f. Tissues
2. Have the patient void before beginning.
3. Position the patient flat on her back in bed. If the patient sits up, fluid will

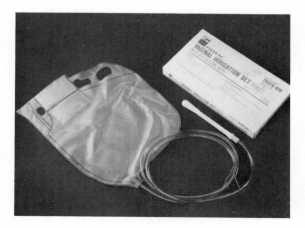

FIGURE 38.5   VAGINAL IRRIGATION SET
*Courtesy American Hospital Supply Corp.,
Evanston, Illinois*

drain out too quickly and not contact all the tissue.

4. Place a waterproof pad under the patient's hips to protect the bed.
5. Place a bedpan under the patient.
6. Drape the patient in the dorsal recumbent position with the perineal area exposed.
7. Wash the patient's perineal area if necessary.
8. Fill the fluid container.
9. Hang the container on the IV standard 18 to 24 inches above the vagina.
10. Run the fluid through the tubing to clear the air.
11. Moisten the douche tip to lubricate it.
12. Run a small amount of fluid over the patient's labia to check that the temperature of the solution is comfortable.
13. With the tubing clamped, insert the tip 3 to 4 inches into the vagina, at an angle toward the base of the spine.
14. Unclamp the tubing and allow the fluid to flow.
15. Rotate the tip.
16. Remove the tip.
17. Help the patient to sit on the bedpan.
18. Provide tissue for drying the perineun.
19. Record the procedure.

Irrigating Wounds

Always use sterile technique for wound irrigations.

1. Gather the necessary equipment. This will vary according to the wound, but, commonly, you will need the following:
   a. An irrigating set (asepto syringe, solution container, receptacle for used solution). A special Water Pik is used to irrigate seriously contaminated traumatic wounds. However, these are most often used in the emergency room or in the operating room.
   b. Sterile gloves (if the wound is to be touched)
   c. Materials for applying a new sterile dressing (including gauze squares)
   d. Solution (as ordered by the physician)
   e. Padding
2. Open the sterile pack and pour the sterile fluid into the container.
3. Remove the sterile dressing, using gloves if the wound is draining.
4. Position the patient so that the solution will flow from the upper end of the wound to the lower, and then into the receptacle.
5. Position the receptacle.
6. Position the padding.
7. Fill the syringe with fluid.
8. Put on a sterile glove if it is necessary to touch the wound. The gloved hand is then used to touch the wound; the ungloved hand is used to manipulate the equipment.
9. Direct the fluid onto all parts of the wound, paying particular attention to areas with exudate or drainage.
10. Irrigate until no exudate is present, until solution returns clear, or until ordered volume has been used.
11. Use a sterile gauze square to dry the area.
12. Redress the wound using sterile technique. (See Module 40, Sterile Dressings.)
13. Record the procedure and observations of the wound.

PERFORMANCE CHECKLIST

General procedure	Unsatisfactory	Needs more practice	Satisfactory	Comments
1. Check orders to verify: a. Patient's name				
b. Type of irrigation				
c. Amount, temperature, type, and concentration of solution				
2. Identify patient.				
3. Explain procedure to patient.				
4. Wash your hands.				
5. Gather appropriate equipment a. Solution (Check temperature.)				
b. Irrigating device				
c. Receptacle for used fluid				
d. Protective padding.				
6. Position patient.				
7. Drape patient.				
8. Place protective padding.				
9. Carry out specific irrigation.				
10. Leave patient dry and comfortable.				
11. Dispose of equipment correctly.				
12. Wash your hands.				
13. Record procedure. a. Type of irrigation				
b. Type, concentration, and amount of solution				
c. Description of excretions or exudate, including odor				
d. Result of procedure				
e. Patient's response				
Bladder and catheter irrigation: Closed technique				
1. Y-connector and fluid reservoir a. Use sterile technique.				
b. Gather necessary equipment.				
c. Clamp drainage tubing.				
d. Open fluid tubing.				
e. Allow fluid to flow into catheter.				

	Unsatisfactory	Needs more practice	Satisfactory	Comments
f. Close fluid tubing.				
g. Open drainage tubing.				
h. Observe fluid return.				
i. Record fluid as necessary.				
2. Syringe-and-needle method a. Use sterile technique.				
b. Gather necessary equipment. (1) 20- to 30-ml syringe				
(2) Alcohol wipe				
(3) Solution ordered				
c. Draw up solution into syringe.				
d. Clean entry port or distal portion of catheter with alcohol wipe.				
e. Insert needle into entry port or catheter wall.				
f. Clamp drainage tubing distal to needle.				
g. Inject fluid.				
h. Remove needle.				
i. Release catheter.				
j. Observe fluid return.				
k. Repeat as necessary.				
l. Record fluid as necessary.				
Bladder and catheter irrigation: Open technique				
1. Use sterile technique.				
2. Gather necessary equipment. a. Sterile irrigation set				
b. Solution				
3. Open set.				
4. Pour solution into irrigating bottle.				
5. Clean juncture of catheter and drainage tube.				
6. Separate tubing, not allowing catheter to touch anything.				
7. Cover end of drainage tubing to preserve sterility.				

	Unsatisfactory	Needs more practice	Satisfactory	Comments

8. Instill fluid slowly.
  a. Catheter irrigation:
    (1) Insert syringe tip into catheter and exert gentle pressure to instill fluid.				

(2) Pinch catheter closed.				
(3) Allow fluid to drain.				
(4) Observe drainage for sediment.				
(5) Repeat until fluid is clear.				
b. Bladder irrigation: (1) Instill ordered fluid.				
(2) Clamp tubing, holding solution in bladder for several minutes.				
(3) Allow fluid to drain.				
9. Reconnect catheter to drainage tubing.				
10. Record fluid as necessary.				
Bladder and catheter irrigation: Three-way irrigation (Continuous drip and cleaning)				
1. Use sterile technique.				
2. Gather necessary equipment. a. IV standard				
b. Solution				
c. Tubing				
3. Set up pole, fluid container, and tubing.				
4. Clear air from tubing by filling with fluid.				
5. Attach to inflow tube on three-way catheter.				
6. Make sure outflow tube is open.				
7. Regulate flow: a. For continuous drip, regulate drip rate.				
b. For cleaning: (1) Open inflow tubing to continuous stream.				
(2) Continue flow until outflow is free of clots and sediment.				
(3) Reclamp tubing.				
8. Record fluid as necessary.				

Irrigating the ear

	Unsatisfactory	Needs more practice	Satisfactory	Comments
1. Check to see that ear has been examined.				
2. Use clean technique.				
3. Gather necessary equipment. a. Ear syringe or Water Pik				
b. Emesis basin				
c. Clean towels				
d. Solution				
4. Tilt patient's head to side.				
5. Place receptacle under ear.				
6. Place towel across shoulder.				
7. Fill syringe.				
8. Direct tip of syringe against top of ear canal.				
9. Continue irrigation until ear is clean.				
10. Dry ear.				
11. Position comfortably for drainage.				
12. Record procedure.				

Irrigating the eye

	Unsatisfactory	Needs more practice	Satisfactory	Comments
1. Use sterile technique. Do not touch irrigator to eye.				
2. Gather necessary equipment. a. Sterile syringe				
b. Sterile solution				
c. Emesis basin				
d. Sterile cotton balls				
3. Position patient in dorsal recumbent position with head turned toward eye to be irrigated.				
4. Place emesis basin.				
5. Hold eye open.				
6. Fill syringe with fluid.				
7. Release fluid with gentle pressure, from inner to outer canthus.				
8. Continue irrigation until eye is clear or all solution is used.				

	Unsatisfactory	Needs more practice	Satisfactory	Comments
9. Dry eye from inner to outer aspect.				
10. Record procedure.				
Note: If both eyes are done, treat each as separate irrigation.				
Nasogastric tube irrigation				
1. Use clean technique. Use sterile technique if patient has had stomach surgery.				
2. Obtain necessary equipment. a. Syringe				
b. Solution				
c. Emesis basin				
3. Disconnect nasogastric tube from suction machine.				
4. Fill syringe.				
5. Gently instill approximately 30 ml.				
6. Aspirate fluid back, and discard or reconnect to suction machine.				
7. Repeat as necessary.				
8. Reconnect to suction.				
9. Record procedure.				

Vaginal irrigation (douche)	Unsatisfactory	Needs more practice	Satisfactory	Comments
1. Use clean technique.				
2. Gather equipment. a. Douche set with douche tip				
b. Solution (1,000 ml at body temperature)				
c. IV standard				
d. Waterproof pad				
e. Bedpan				
f. Tissues				
3. Have patient void.				
4. Position patient flat on back.				
5. Place waterproof pad.				
6. Place bedpan under patient.				
7. Drape in dorsal recumbent position.				
8. Wash perineal area if needed.				
9. Fill fluid container.				
10. Hang on IV pole 18 to 24 inches above vagina.				
11. Fill tubing with fluid, clearing air.				
12. Moisten tip to lubricate.				
13. Run fluid over patient's labia to check temperature.				
14. Insert tip 3 to 4 inches, angled toward base of spine.				
15. Unclamp tubing and allow fluid to flow.				
16. Rotate tip.				
17. Remove tip.				
18. Help patient to sit on bedpan.				
19. Provide tissue for drying perineum.				
20. Record procedure.				

Irrigating Wounds	Unsatisfactory	Needs more practice	Satisfactory	Comments
1. Use sterile technique.				
2. Gather necessary equipment. a. Irrigating set				
b. Sterile gloves				
c. Dressing materials				
d. Solution				
e. Padding				
3. Open sterile pack and pour sterile fluid.				
4. Remove sterile dressing, using gloves if necessary.				
5. Position patient.				
6. Position receptacle.				
7. Place padding.				
8. Fill syringe.				
9. Put on one sterile glove if wound must be touched.				
10. Direct fluid onto all parts of wound.				
11. Continue irrigation until clean or ordered volume is used.				
12. Dry area.				
13. Redress wound using sterile technique.				
14. Record procedure.				

QUIZ

Short-Answer Questions

1. List two major purposes of irrigation.

   a. _____

   b. _____

2. Mrs. Jones has had bladder surgery. An irrigation with an antibacterial medication, nitrofurantoin, has been ordered. This irrigation is probably for which of the above purposes? _____

3. Name a type of irrigation in which sterile technique is essential.

   _____

4. Name a type of irrigation in which clean technique is safe.

   _____

5. List three factors in an irrigation that can cause irritation or damage tissue.

   a. _____

   b. _____

   c. _____

6. After prostate surgery, Mr. Jefferson has a continuous three-way irrigation setup. What is the most critical safety concern with this irrigation?

   _____

7. Under what circumstances should an ear *not* be irrigated? _____

   _____

8. Why is it not appropriate to administer a vaginal douche while the patient sits on a toilet? _____

   _____

Module 39 Catheterization

MAIN OBJECTIVES

To insert a urinary catheter using correct sterile technique.

To establish, maintain, and discontinue continuous urinary drainage when appropriate.

RATIONALE

Patients' bladders are catheterized for a variety of diagnostic and therapeutic reasons. It is the nurse's responsibility to carry out this task. Because the inside of the bladder is sterile and provides direct access to the kidneys, the primary concern must be the prevention of contamination of the bladder.

It is also the nurse's responsibility to know the anatomy of the urinary system, so that the urethra is not damaged in the catheterization process. Once the catheter is in place, the nurse must establish correct drainage, if appropriate, and teach patients what they need to know to relieve their anxiety and to participate in their own care.

PREREQUISITES

1. Successful completion of the following modules:

   VOLUME 1
   Assessment
   Charting
   Medical Asepsis

   VOLUME 2
   Sterile Technique
2. A review of the anatomy of the urinary system

SPECIFIC LEARNING OBJECTIVES

	Know Facts and Principles	Apply Facts and Principles	Demonstrate Ability	Evaluate Performance
1. *Patient concerns*	State usual concerns of patient regarding catheterization	Given a patient situation, identify what concerns have and have not been met	Prepare patient by teaching. Provide privacy and drape. Provide time for patient's questions. Leave patient comfortable.	Evaluate own performance using Performance Checklist
2. *Procedure*	List common ways contamination occurs in catheterization. Identify all items needed for catheterization and their purpose. State usual length of urethra in male and female. State rationale for sterile technique. Identify and explain principles of sterile technique used in catheterization.	Describe proper way to clean external meatus. Given a patient situation, state how to expose urinary meatus. Given a patient situation, state how far to insert catheter.	In the practice lab, correctly set up equipment and arrange sterile field for catheterization. Carry out catheterization without contamination. Correctly identify meatus. Insert catheter correct distance.	Evaluate own performance using Performance Checklist

3. *Maintaining continuous drainage*	List major concerns related to continuous drainage	Given a patient situation, identify errors in continuous drainage setup	Assess patient with continuous drainage to identify problem. Correct errors in continuous drainage setup.	Evaluate own performance using Performance Checklist
4. *Removing a Foley catheter*	Describe procedure for removing Foley catheter	Plan teaching regarding Foley catheter removal	Teach patient regarding removal of Foley catheter. Remove Foley catheter correctly.	Evaluate own performance using Performance Checklist
5. *Recording*	List observations to be recorded	Given a patient situation, identify information that should be recorded. Write nurses' note that would be appropriate for situation.	Record catheterization in appropriate places on patient chart	

LEARNING ACTIVITIES

1. Review the Specific Learning Objectives.
2. Read the section on the urinary system (in the chapter on elimination) in Ellis and Nowlis, *Nursing: A Human Needs Approach,* or comparable material in another textbook.
3. Look up the module vocabulary terms in the glossary.
4. Review the anatomy of the urinary system.
5. Read through the module.
6. In the practice setting:
   a. Obtain a catheterization set.
   b. Open the set properly, noting the arrangement of all equipment. If more than one type or brand of equipment is available, compare the different sets.
   c. Repack the set as it was originally.
   d. Using the Performance Checklist as a guide, go through the entire procedure, improvising an area to represent a patient (pillows will work for this). Repeat the procedure until you feel comfortable with the equipment and you remember the steps.
   e. With a partner, arrange for a time to use a practice model.
   f. Take turns going through the procedure and evaluate one another's performance using the checklist.
   g. Have your supervisor evaluate your performance.
7. In the clinical setting:
   a. Consult with your clinical instructor regarding an opportunity to perform a catheterization under supervision.
   b. Evaluate your own performance using the Performance Checklist.
   c. Consult your instructor regarding your performance.

VOCABULARY

catheter
catheterization
Foley catheter
foreskin
meatus
penis
perineum
straight catheter
urethra
void

CATHETERIZATION

A catheter drains urine from the bladder or instills solution into the bladder. Because the bladder is normally sterile, it is important to use careful sterile technique in the procedure. Urinary-tract infections are very common in those who have indwelling catheters; and even a single catheterization carries with it the danger of contaminating the bladder. Although bladder infections can be serious in themselves, they can also lead to infections of the kidneys.

Preparing the Patient

Many patients are upset by catheterization, fearing pain and discomfort. However, there is also an emotional reaction to any procedure related to the genito-urinary system—one that involves penetration of the body. Feelings of embarrassment and the loss of privacy are especially prominent in this procedure. In preparing the patient, use a calm, businesslike manner to relieve some of the patient's anxiety. Explain the procedure completely and what the patient will experience. Give the patient an opportunity to ask questions and express concerns. Pay careful attention to privacy by closing doors, draping, and keeping all parts of the patient's body covered except the area that must be exposed. These actions show your concern for the patient's privacy and should alleviate some of his or her distress.

Equipment

A catheterization set contains the basic equipment needed for the task. (See Figure 39.1.) There may be some variation from one brand to another, but usually the following items are included:

1. Sterile wrapper. When opened, the inside of the wrapper provides a sterile field, and the outside is usually impervious to moisture.
2. Sterile gloves. These are usually on top so that all other items can be set up using sterile technique. As a beginner,

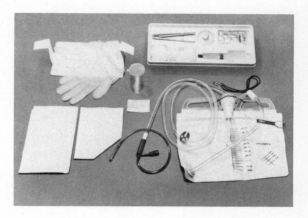

FIGURE 39.1   FOLEY CATHETERIZATION SET
Courtesy American Hospital Supply Corp., Evanston, Illinois

you may want to have an extra pair of gloves on hand.
3. Sterile drapes. Two drapes are usually provided. One is a plain drape to slide under the female patient or to spread out under the penis. The other drape is often fenestrated (has a hole in it). This drape is placed over the perineum with the opening over the meatus for a female patient or around the penis of a male patient. Occasionally, the first of these drapes is on top of the gloves.
4. Sterile cleansing swabs. These may be cotton balls or swabs with a short handle attached.
5. Thumb forceps (also called *pickups*). You will need these to handle the cotton balls without contamination.
6. Cleansing solution. A water-soluble iodine preparation is an excellent antibacterial agent for this purpose. Benzalkonium chloride (Zephiran) is also used.
7. Prefilled syringe. This is used to fill the retention balloon of a Foley catheter. It contains sterile water.
8. Water-soluble lubricant. This is used to lubricate the catheter.
9. Specimen container and label if necessary.
10. Safety pin and rubber band. These are used to secure the tubing to the bed if the catheter is to remain in place. If

they are not in the set, you will have to obtain them separately.

11. Catheter. Either a plain catheter or a Foley catheter can be used. They come in a variety of sizes. Number 16 French is the most common size for an adult patient. A Foley catheter is used when continuous drainage is needed.

12. Drainage tubing and collecting bag. These are sometimes packaged with a Foley catheter set.

Procedure

1. CHECK THE ORDERS

Be sure the correct procedure is being done for the correct patient. Also, determine the need for a specimen. If there is any doubt, you can always collect one and then discard it if it is not needed. You also must know whether the catheter is to be removed or whether a Foley catheter is needed for continuous drainage.

2. GATHER THE EQUIPMENT

If the catheter is ordered for one time only (to remove urine or to instill solution) use a straight catheter for the procedure and then remove it. If the urine is to drain continuously, connect a Foley catheter (as ordered) for continuous or constant drainage (CD). In addition to the catheterization set, you need a good light (a flashlight or gooseneck lamp will work well) and a bath blanket or sheet to drape the patient.

3. WASH YOUR HANDS

4. PREPARE THE PATIENT

First, explain the procedure to the patient and answer all questions. Pull the bed curtains and position the patient.

For a female, the dorsal recumbent position with knees elevated and spread (Figure 39.2) is usually most convenient. Sometimes it is more comfortable for the patient to have her knees supported with pillows. Drape the bath blanket so that both legs are covered and only the perineum is exposed. If the patient cannot assume the dorsal recumbent position, a Sim's position can be used (Figure 39.3).

Arrange the light so that the perineum can be seen easily. If the perineal area is soiled, perform perineal care with soap and water before you begin. For the male, the supine position is appropriate (Figure 39.4).

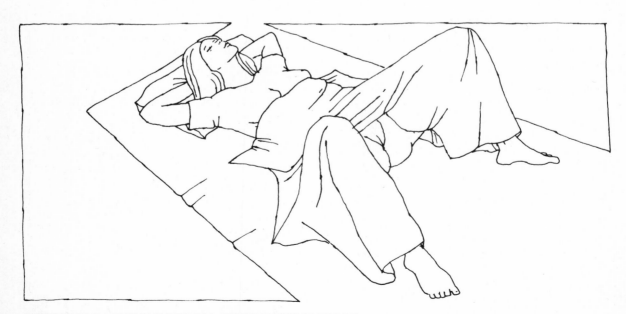

FIGURE 39.2   FEMALE DORSAL RECUMBENT POSITION

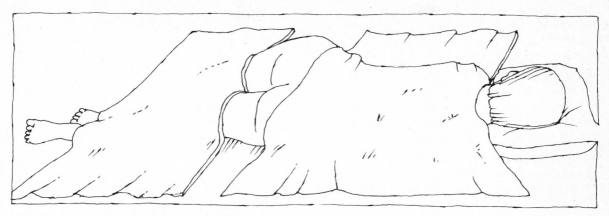

FIGURE 39.3   FEMALE SIM'S POSITION

Expose only the penis and a small surrounding area. (See Module 7, Assisting with Elimination and Perineal Care, page 84.)

5. SET UP THE EQUIPMENT

Open the package and arrange the sterile field in a convenient location (on an overbed table, at the foot of the bed for the female patient and beside the bed for the male patient). Set up a receptacle for soiled cleansing swabs. The plastic bag that contained the set, a bedside bag, or several paper towels stacked together can be used for this purpose. If the drainage bag is in a separate package, open it and attach it to the bed at this time.

If a sterile drape is on top of the set, grasp it by one corner and open it with care, touching only the underneath side and the edges. Keeping your hands under the drape, ask the female patient to lift her hips and carefully slide the drape under the hips slightly, so that the upper side between the patient's thighs provides a sterile field. For the female patient in Sim's position or for the male patient, place the drape carefully to provide a sterile field beneath the perineal area.

If sterile gloves are on top, put them on first. Then, carefully take the first drape and unfold it, keeping your gloved hands at the top of the drape. Grasp two adjacent corners of the drape and turn your hands, so that the drape covers as much of the glove as possible. Then, place the drape to provide a sterile field, keeping the top sterile and not

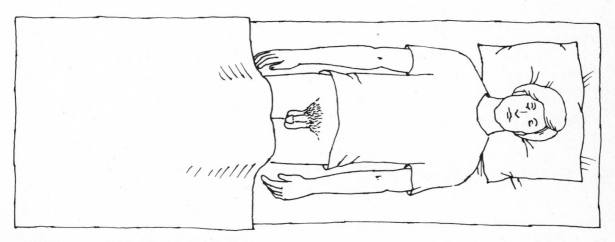

FIGURE 39.4   MALE SUPINE POSITION

touching anything but the top side of the drape with your gloved hands.

Place the second drape to secure and enlarge the sterile field. If it is fenestrated, place the opening over the penis of the male patient. The drape can be placed over the meatus of the female patient, but many nurses find that it tends to fall forward, obscuring their vision and potentially contaminating the catheter. Thus, the drape is often folded in half and placed over the pubic area.

Set up the rest of the sterile equipment. Open the cleansing solution and pour it over the swabs. Then open the lubricant and place it along the end of the catheter. If a Foley catheter is being used, attach the syringe to the balloon port; then test the balloon by inserting the fluid and withdrawing it. Leave the syringe attached. (This is not essential but can simplify later work because later you will want to hold the catheter in place with one hand, which leaves you only one hand to manipulate the syringe.)

Set up the specimen container, turned upside-down to maintain the sterility of the inside. Set the cap inside-down. Lay aside any equipment that is not needed.

6. CATHETERIZE THE PATIENT

Use your nondominant hand to expose the meatus. Remember that this hand is now contaminated and cannot be used to handle equipment again.

For a male, raise the penis at a 45-degree angle from the scrotum and retract the foreskin. For a female, separate both the labia majora and the labia minora. Retract the labia laterally and anteriorly. A common error is to place the fingers too high and too lateral to expose the meatus. If the meatus is not identifiable, move your hand for better exposure. Always identify the meatus before any other equipment is contaminated. Occasionally, when you are sure that the area of the meatus is well exposed, although you may not be positive of its exact location, cleaning will help you

to positively identify it. When the meatus is exposed and identified, begin cleaning.

Use forceps to handle the cleansing swabs, to keep your dominant gloved hand completely sterile for handling the catheter. Use each swab only once, and then discard in the prepared location where they will not contaminate your field. Do not pass the used cotton balls over the sterile field.

For a male, clean in a circular motion, starting at the meatus without retracing any area (Figure 39.5). For a female, use swabs from front to back, starting with the outside labia and moving toward the center. (See Figure 39.6.) Clean one side first and then the other. The final stroke should be vertical to clean the meatus itself.

The principle behind this pattern is to move from the area of lesser accumulation of secretions and organisms (labia) to the area of greater concentration (meatus). The stroke, if done slowly, may pull the meatus slightly open, thereby assuring identification. Some persons recommend that the first cleansing strokes be down the center across the meatus and that subsequent strokes move outward. The principle for this pattern is to move from the area you want to be the cleanest area (meatus) to the

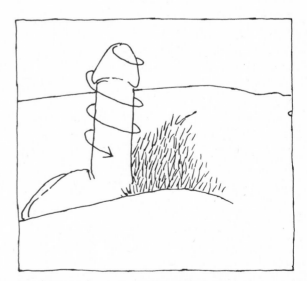

FIGURE 39.5 CLEANING THE MALE FOR CATHETERIZATION   Clean the penis with circular strokes.

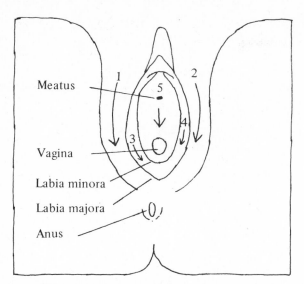

FIGURE 39.6 CLEANING THE FEMALE FOR CATHETERIZATION Clean the genitals from anterior to posterior.

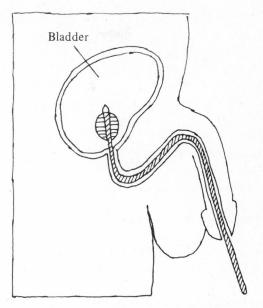

FIGURE 39.7 FOLEY CATHETER IN PLACE

area that is less critical (labia). Research has not identified which of these procedures is better. The most critical point seems to be that each swab be used only once and that the path of that swab be from anterior to posterior. For the pattern, follow your instructor's directions.

Use the sterile-gloved dominant hand to move the tray containing the catheter close to the patient (between the legs of the female patient and beside the male patient). Touch only the inside of the tray. Pick up the catheter several inches back from the tip.

Insert the lubricated catheter smoothly, approximately 2 to 3 inches into the female and 6 to 9 inches into the male. Do not use force. If you encounter an obstruction, ask the patient to breathe deeply (to relax the muscles) and gently rotate the catheter to see if it will penetrate. If it still will not enter, consult a physician before trying again. It is possible to damage the urethra and the urinary sphincters by pushing against resistant tissue.

The return of urine indicates that the catheter is in the bladder. To inflate a Foley balloon, insert the catheter 1 inch farther after urine is returned, to make sure that the

balloon does not inflate in the urethra. (See Figure 39.7.)

7. OBTAIN A SPECIMEN

If you are using a straight catheter, hold the catheter in place while you fill the specimen container.

8. DRAIN THE BLADDER AND FILL THE BALLOON

If you are using a straight catheter, drain the bladder, pinch the catheter closed, and remove the catheter quickly. Proceed to step 12.

If you are using a Foley catheter, hold it in place while you fill the Foley balloon. The catheter can continue to drain into the receptacle while this is done. Use the amount of fluid indicated on the catheter itself plus 4 or 5 ml. Because the fluid must fill the tube leading to the balloon, as well as the balloon itself, you will need this extra amount, and manufacturers indicate that balloons will not overinflate or rupture from using this amount. However, if you use too little fluid, the catheter may slip out.

Whichever type of catheter you use, never remove more than 1,000 ml from the bladder at one time, which can cause severe shock. If this large an amount is removed during the procedure, clamp the tubing for at least one hour before you resume continuous drainage.

Check for security by gently pulling the catheter until resistance is felt.

9. CONNECT THE DRAINAGE TUBING TO THE CATHETER

Be sure to maintain the sterility of the ends of the tubing at the connecting point. Place the tubing over the top of the thigh, so the leg does not occlude the tubing.

Hang the bag below the level of the bed. Make sure the bag does not touch the floor.

10. TAPE THE CATHETER TO THE PATIENT

This is done to prevent pull on the neck of the bladder as the patient moves. For a male, tape the catheter without tension to the side of the lower abdomen, to prevent the formation of a fistula at the penile scrotal angle. For a female, tape it to the thigh.

Coil excess tubing on the level of the bed, so that drainage is not impeded; urine collecting in the tube provides a medium for bacteria to multiply and ascend. Attach the tubing to the side of the bed with a plastic catheter clamp (which may be enclosed in the set) or a rubber band and a safety pin. Wrap the rubber band around the tubing and pin it to the sheet.

11. MAKE THE PATIENT COMFORTABLE

Remove the supplies. Assist the patient to a comfortable position, straighten the bed, and open the curtains. The patient may have further questions or concerns, and this is a good time to teach the patient about the Foley catheter. Let the patient know that the balloon will hold the catheter in place and that movement is quite all right. Stress the need for fluids (if permitted by the medical condition). Because of the pressure of the balloon, the patient with a Foley catheter usually feels as though he or she needs to void. Explain that this feeling will pass as the tissue becomes less sensitive to

the constant stimulation. Understanding this helps the patient to tolerate the discomfort.

12. CARE FOR THE EQUIPMENT

Gather disposable equipment and dispose of it properly. If you have used nondisposable equipment, follow your hospital's procedure for cleaning.

13. WASH YOUR HANDS.

14. RECORD THE INFORMATION

On the patient's chart, indicate the time of catheterization, the amount of urine obtained, a description of the urine, and the patient's response to the procedure. Also record the type and size of catheter inserted. If a specimen was obtained and sent to the lab, note this as well. If necessary, record the amount of urine obtained on the intake and output worksheet.

Caring for a Patient with an Indwelling Catheter

TO MAINTAIN STERILITY

The urinary tract is usually sterile. The introduction of organisms via the catheter is a common cause of urinary-tract infection. A variety of measures are used to decrease the risk of infection.

1. Place the patient on intake and output recording. This will assist you to assess the functioning of the catheter.
2. Encourage the patient to consume increased quantities of fluid. Large intake causes a constant flow of urine out of the kidneys and bladder, which tends to inhibit the upward movement of microbes. By increasing fluid intake, you are "internally" irrigating the system. Up to 4,000 ml fluids per day (for the patient without circulatory problems and with no fluid restriction) is best. This quantity may be unrealistic for an elderly patient, but encourage any increase.
3. Maintain the *closed* system. Every time

the system is opened, microorganisms can enter. Carry out all procedures so that the system is uninterrupted if at all possible. (See Module 18, Collecting Specimens, page 279, for a method of obtaining urine specimens without interrupting the system.)

4. Maintain external cleanliness around the catheter. Secretions that build up are an optimum location for bacterial growth, which could ascend the outside of the catheter. The basic necessity is thorough washing with soap and water. As an additional measure, some facilities clean the meatal area and the first several inches of exposed catheter with an antibacterial solution (providone iodine) and then apply an iodine ointment at the meatus around the catheter. Be sure to ask the patient about allergy to iodine before using the ointment.

5. Keep the catheter drainage bag below the level of the bladder at all times. This prevents potentially contaminated urine from draining back into the bladder.

6. Keep the tubing coiled by the patient's side. Tubing that hangs off the bed in loops allows urine to sit in the tubing, creating a possible reservoir for microbes, which could then ascend.

7. Keep the drainage bag off the floor. If it touches the floor, the outside picks up microbes that can then move up the outside of the bag and the catheter.

FOR PATIENT COMFORT

Other care measures are needed to prevent trauma and discomfort to the patient.

1. Tape the catheter in a way that avoids pulling it. Pull irritates the patient and can actually pull the catheter out, balloon and all. For a female patient, tape the catheter to her thigh; for a male patient, tape it to the side of his abdomen. (See Figure 39.8 for ways to tape a catheter.)

2. Take extra care when moving or ambulating a patient. You must watch the position of the tubing and bag at all times to prevent pulling.

3. Empty the bag at regular intervals (usually every eight hours), so that it does not overfill and cause urine backup in the tubing. Empty more frequently if large amounts of urine are being excreted.

4. Observe for irritation at the meatal area. If found, report it to the physician.

Removing a Foley Catheter

1. Verify the orders.
2. Wash your hands.
3. Obtain the necessary equipment.
   a. Several paper towels for wrapping the soiled catheter after removal.
   b. A means of removing the fluid from the balloon (a 10-ml syringe or scissors, which must be cleaned

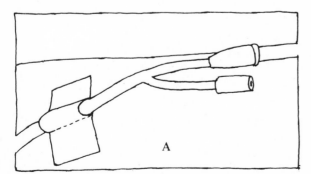 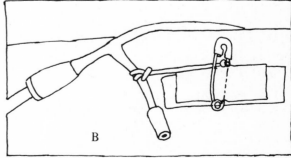

FIGURE 39.8 TAPING A CATHETER A: To decrease the chance of the tape pulling loose, the catheter is secured in a loop of tape before the ends are taped to the patient; B: alternatively, the catheter may be attached by using tape, a safety pin, and a rubber band.

      before and after use, to cut the
      balloon)
   c. Padding or a small container (a
      paper cup will work) to catch the
      fluid

4. Explain to the patient that the catheter is to be removed and that the procedure is not painful. Instruct the patient that the first voidings may burn slightly, but this is normal and is caused by catheter irritation. If it persists it should be reported. (It can indicate infection.) Also, voiding may be more frequent in small amounts at first. Usually intake and output are continued for at least 24 hours to facilitate assessment. Explain how this will be carried out if the patient is able to go to the bathroom. Encourage the patient to continue with high intake.

5. Prepare the patient, draping the covers back to expose the catheter.

6. Discontinue the catheter.
   a. Place paper towels under the catheter.
   b. Use the syringe or cut with scissors to remove fluid from the balloon.
   c. Pinch the catheter and pull it out smoothly. This should not cause discomfort but will be felt.
   d. Wrap the end of the catheter in paper towel with your free hand, while you keep the catheter itself pinched closed.
   e. Hold the catheter up to allow urine to drain from the tubing into the bag.

7. Make the patient comfortable and replace the covers.

8. Measure the output.

9. Dispose of the equipment.

10. Wash your hands.

11. Chart.
    a. Time
    b. Procedure
    c. Output
    d. Patient's response

PERFORMANCE CHECKLIST

Inserting a catheter	Unsatisfactory	Needs more practice	Satisfactory	Comments
1. Check orders.				
2. Gather equipment. a. Catheterization set				
b. Blanket for drape				
c. Light				
3. Wash your hands.				
4. Prepare patient. a. Explain procedure and rationale.				
b. Allow time for patient's questions and concerns.				
c. Provide privacy.				
d. Position patient.				
e. Drape patient.				
f. Arrange lighting.				
5. Set up equipment. a. Open pack.				
b. Put on gloves.				
c. Arrange sterile drapes.				
d. Prepare equipment. (1) Open and pour cleansing solution over swabs.				
(2) Open lubricant and apply to catheter.				
(3) Open specimen bottle or set aside.				
(4) Attach syringe to catheter and test balloon.				
6. Catheterize patient. a. Expose meatus.				
b. Clean, using swabs or cotton balls with forceps. (1) Female: Using downstrokes only, clean each side. Apply last stroke over meatus. (2) Male: Use circular motions, starting at meatus.				
c. Discard each cotton ball after use in area where it will not contaminate other equipment and without bringing soiled cotton ball over sterile field.				

	Unsatisfactory	Needs more practice	Satisfactory	Comments
d. Insert catheter. Do not touch any area with the catheter except meatus itself. Insert until urine is returned; then insert 1 inch farther: (1) Female: 2 to 3 inches				
(2) Male: 6 to 9 inches				
7. Hold catheter in place while obtaining specimen.				
8. Drain bladder and/or fill balloon.				
9. Set up drainage bag. a. Connect bag.				
b. Hang bag below level of bed, off floor.				
10. Tape catheter to patient (female: to inner aspect of thigh; male: to side of lower abdomen).				
a. Attach tubing to bed with rubber band and safety pin.				
b. Keep all coils on bed.				
11. Make patient comfortable. a. Position comfortably.				
b. Answer further questions.				
12. Care for equipment.				
13. Wash your hands.				
14. Record procedure: a. Type and size of catheter used				
b. Time of procedure				
c. Amount of urine obtained				
d. Description of urine				
e. Patient's response				
f. Disposition of specimen if taken				
Removing a Foley catheter				
1. Verify orders.				
2. Wash your hands.				
3. Obtain equipment. a. For removing fluid				
b. For wrapping soiled catheter				
4. Explain to patient. a. Procedure				
b. Nature of first voiding				

	Unsatisfactory	Needs more practice	Satisfactory	Comments
c. Need for reporting prolonged discomfort				
d. Measurement				
e. Possibility of frequency				
f. Need for high intake				
5. Prepare patient.				
6. Discontinue catheter. a. Place paper towels.				
b. Remove fluid from balloon.				
c. Pinch catheter and pull out smoothly.				
d. Wrap end of catheter in paper towel while pinched.				
e. Drain tubing.				
7. Make patient comfortable.				
8. Measure output.				
9. Dispose of equipment.				
10. Wash your hands.				
11. Chart. a. Time				
b. Procedure				
c. Output				
d. Patient's response				

QUIZ

Short-Answer Questions

1. Give three common concerns of patients being catheterized.

    a. _____

    b. _____

    c. _____

2. Mrs. Tigerson was to have a catheter inserted preoperatively. The nurse explained to Mrs. Tigerson what the procedure was, why it was being done, and what the patient should expect. The nurse then carried out the catheterization. What step in dealing with the patient's concerns did the nurse

    omit? _____

Multiple-Choice Questions

_____ 3. The length of the male urethra is approximately

    a. 4 to 5 inches.
    b. 6 to 9 inches.
    c. 7 to 8 inches.
    d. 8 to 10 inches.

_____ 4. The length of the female urethra is approximately

    a. ½ to 1 inch.
    b. 1½ to 2 inches.
    c. 2 to 3 inches.
    d. 3 to 4 inches.

_____ 5. When you are catheterizing a female patient, the catheter touches the meatus but then slides downward on the perineum and does not enter the urethra. Your next action should be to

    a. get better lighting.
    b. clean the area again.
    c. obtain a sterile catheter.
    d. clean the catheter with the remaining cleansing solution.

_____ 6. The most essential point of cleaning the female perineum for catheterization is to

    a. clean in a circular motion.
    b. clean from inner to outer areas.
    c. clean toward the anus.
    d. clean in any manner so long as you do it thoroughly.

_____ 7. Which of the following items are usually part of a catheterization set?
(1) drapes; (2) gloves; (3) catheter; (4) safety pin

    a. 1, 2, and 3
    b. 2, 3, and 4
    c. 1, 3, and 4
    d. All of the above.

_____ 8. A drape with a hole in it is called

    a. fenestrated.
    b. sequestered.
    c. windowed.
    d. no special name.

_____ 9. Which of the following must be charted after performing a catheterization?

    a. Only the name of the procedure and the time done
    b. Only those aspects that differed from a routine catheterization procedure
    c. Type and size of catheter, amount and description of urine, patient's response, and time of procedure

Module 40 Sterile Dressings

MAIN OBJECTIVE

To change sterile dressings, maintaining safety for both patients and nurse.

RATIONALE

Almost every nurse, no matter where he or she is employed, will at some time change a sterile dressing. Dressings are applied for a variety of reasons, including protection, the absorption of drainage, and the application of pressure. Second only to the nurse's responsibility to maintain rigid sterile technique is the responsibility to carefully observe and describe the wound. Is the wound healing by first intention or second intention? Is there drainage? If so, what is its color, consistency, and odor? A third responsibility is to choose the most appropriate dressing materials available and to apply them in the most secure and comfortable fashion possible.

PREREQUISITES

Successful completion of the following modules:

VOLUME 1
Assessment
Charting
Medical Asepsis

VOLUME 2
Sterile Technique

231

SPECIFIC LEARNING OBJECTIVES

	Know Facts and Principles	Apply Facts and Principles	Demonstrate Ability	Evaluate Performance
1. *Function of dressings*	State three functions of dressings	Given a patient situation, identify function of particular dressing		
2. *Dressing materials*	List dressing materials	Identify various dressing materials by name. Give rationale for use of different dressing materials in various situations.	Use various types of dressing materials appropriately	Evaluate use of dressing materials with instructor
3. *Procedure*	Explain how to change dressing	Given a patient situation, identify correct ways to perform procedure. Give rationale for correct performance of procedure.	Change dressing correctly under supervision	Evaluate own performance with instructor
4. *Observations*	State observations to be made during dressing change	Given a patient situation, describe observations accurately, using correct terminology	Make pertinent observations during dressing change	Evaluate own performance with instructor using Performance Checklist
5. *Charting*	State items to be included on note regarding dressing change	Given a patient situation, write note descriptive of dressing change. Give rationale for items to be included in note regarding dressing change.	In the clinical situation, chart complete and accurate note regarding dressing change	Provide copy to instructor for evaluation

LEARNING ACTIVITIES

1. Review the Specific Learning Objectives.
2. Read the chapters on procedures and infection in Ellis and Nowlis, *Nursing: A Human Needs Approach,* or comparable chapters in another textbook.

3. Look up the module vocabulary terms in the glossary.
4. Read through the module.
5. In the practice setting:
   a. Identify the various types of dressing materials available by name. In what situation is each appropriate?
   b. Using a pillow (or other curved surface) as an abdomen, practice doing a dressing change with the Performance Checklist as a guide. What adaptation would you make if a drain were present?
   c. When you are satisfied with your performance, have another student evaluate your performance.
   d. Have your instructor evaluate your performance.
6. In the clinical setting:
   a. Change a sterile dressing under your instructor's or a staff nurse's supervision.

VOCABULARY

aseptic
contaminated
first-intention healing
purulent
sanguinous
second-intention healing
serosanguinous
serous
sterile

STERILE DRESSINGS

Observing and Describing the Wound

Careful observation and accurate description of the wound are integral parts of changing a sterile dressing.

Observe for drainage as you remove a soiled dressing. If there is drainage of any kind present on the dressing, note the amount (count the number of dressings saturated or stained), color, consistency, and odor. Use words that accurately describe what you see. Know the meaning of such words as *sanguinous, serous, serosanguinous,* and *purulent.* Odors are best described by comparing them to a familiar smell.

Observe the wound itself. Are the edges of the wound approximated? Does it have a smooth contour? Are inflammation and edema (swelling) present? If so, to what degree? A wound that has approximated edges and a smooth contour, and that displays minimal inflammation and swelling is healing from the outside in and is said to be healing by *primary (first) intention.* There is minimal scarring with this type of healing. If the wound opens or if the edges *never were* closely approximated, the wound heals from the inside out, and the gap fills with granulation tissue. This type of healing is called healing by *secondary (second) intention.* It takes longer and leaves a larger scar.

Dressing Materials

All facilities have different dressing materials available, but there are some that are common to most facilities, although they may be called different names.

1. *4 × 4s*   These are sterile or nonsterile folded gauze pads, 4 inches by 4 inches in size. (See Figure 40.1.) In most facilities 2 × 2s and 3 × 3s are also available.
2. *Fluffs*   Fluffs are large pieces of sterile or nonsterile gauze that are loosely folded to absorb drainage (Figure 40.2). They are also used to pack wounds.
3. *ABDs (combines, combination pads)*   These are large absorbent pads (usually a coarse gauze covered by a finer gauze) that come sterile and nonsterile in various sizes (Figure 40.3). They are usually used over smaller dressing materials, and most have one side that is moisture resistant.
4. *Nonadherents*   These are special sterile dressings that have one nonadhering

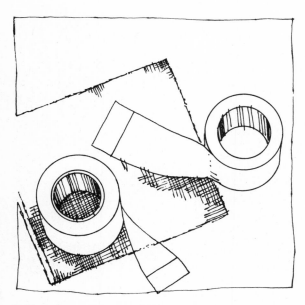

FIGURE 40.1   4 × 4s AND TAPE

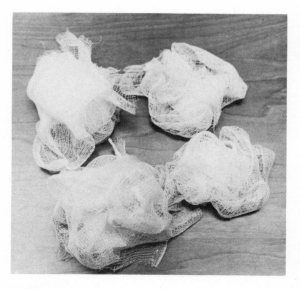

FIGURE 40.2   FLUFFS
Courtesy Ivan Ellis

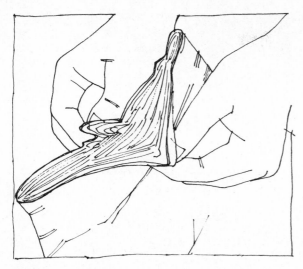

FIGURE 40.3   ABDs

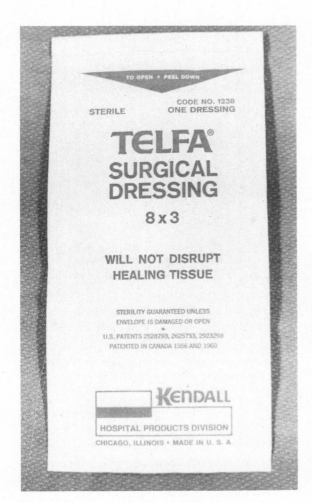

FIGURE 40.4   NONADHERENT DRESSING
TELFA® non-adherent dressing
Courtesy Kendall Co., Boston, Massachusetts

surface. (See Figure 40.4.) Nonadherents are used directly next to incisions, and often are cut to appropriate size.

5. *Roller gauze*   This is sterile gauze that comes in various widths and is used for packing as well as wrapping wounds (Figure 40.5). Roller gauze is also used to secure dressings.

6. *Tape*   Tape comes in a variety of materials (adhesive, plastic, paper) and in widths from ¼ inch to 6 inches wide. Paper tape is generally considered hypoallergenic (See Figure 40.1.)

7. *Montgomery straps or ties*   Commercially available, these straps are used to tie across large and/or bulky dressings that need frequent changing. (See Figure 40.6.) Cut to the desired width, they include one or more eyelets. Generally, twill tape or roller gauze is used to secure these straps or ties. Straps can remain on the dressing until soiled, but ties usually are changed more frequently. Montgomery straps are sometimes made from wide tape, folded back, with holes cut for eyelets.

Changing Sterile Dressings

1. Check the orders for the dressing change. In some instances, the physician

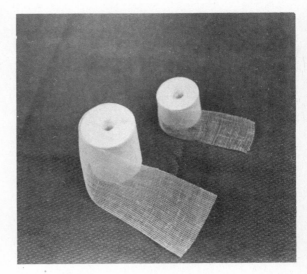

FIGURE 40.5   ROLLER GAUZE
Courtesy Ivan Ellis

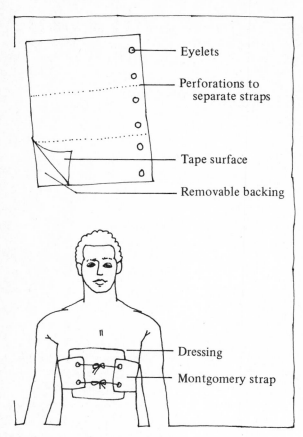

FIGURE 40.6   MONTGOMERY STRAP

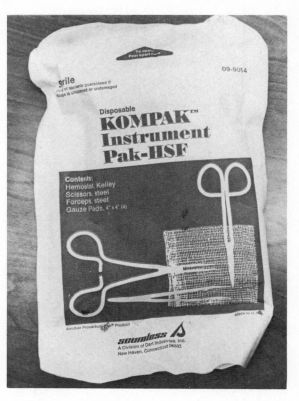

FIGURE 40.7   COMMERCIAL INSTRUMENT PACK
Courtesy Ivan Ellis

will want to do the first dressing change after surgery and then will write an order: "Change dressing prn." Or, you may be responsible for all dressing changes. In any case, a dressing may always be *reinforced;* that is, additional dressings can be applied on top of dressings already there to absorb drainage.

2. Wash your hands.

3. Gather the equipment. Some hospitals use commercially prepared packages that include all the instruments needed (Figure 40.7). Your facility may have a dressing tray partially prepared, in which case you merely add the additional sterile supplies you will need. Or you may have to gather all the sterile supplies, using a sterile towel or the individual sterile packages as a sterile field. Items you may need include scissors, thumb forceps (pickups), 4 × 4s, ABDs, tape, antiseptic solution with

cotton-tipped applicators, and sterile gloves. (See Figure 40.8.) Some facilities have special bags or paper for the disposal of soiled dressings. In others, the bedside waste bag is used. If this is done, it should be discarded and replaced immediately after the dressing is changed.

4. Identify the patient and explain what you intend to do. Allow the patient to ask questions to help ensure his or her cooperation. There is usually little, if any, pain associated with a dressing change, but, if some is to be expected, be certain to prepare the patient for it. Ask the patient to keep his or her hands away from the dressing area and to avoid talking during the procedure to limit the number of microorganisms moving in the air. Limit your own conversation to essential information. In some situations, it may be necessary for both patient and

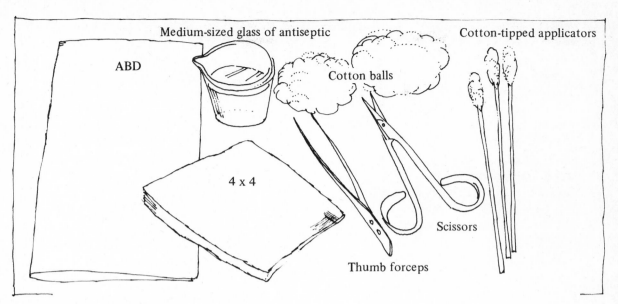

Medium-sized glass of antiseptic

ABD

Cotton-tipped applicators

Cotton balls

4 x 4

Scissors

Thumb forceps

FIGURE 40.8   DRESSING TRAY

nurse to wear masks during a dressing change. At this point, take a look at the present dressing to be certain you have sufficient and appropriate dressing materials.

5. Prepare the environment. Close windows and doors to eliminate drafts that might chill the patient and/or carry microorganisms into the open wound. Pull the drapes and draw the curtains around the bed to allow for the patient's privacy. The patient should be flat or in low-Fowler's position. Clear a working space—the overbed table serves this purpose well. Place a bag or paper for soiled dressings in easy reach. The bag edges can be taped to the mattress edge for convenience.

6. Tear strips of tape if tape is to be used. (If Montgomery straps are in use, you will not need tape unless the straps themselves are going to be changed.) Determine whether the patient has an allergy to adhesive tape, in which case you should use paper or plastic tape. Tear the tape in correct lengths and place them on the edge of an easily reached surface.

7. Expose the area to be dressed and drape the patient, if necessary, for privacy. A bath blanket can be used for this purpose.

8. Prepare to remove the present dressing. Loosen tapes from the outside toward the dressing. If body hair makes this activity uncomfortable for the patient, you may want to shave the area before applying more tape. Some dressings are covered with an elastic or cloth binder, in which case you must unhook or unpin the binder.

9. Remove the outer dressings. There are many ways this can be done. Your facility may have a preferred procedure, so be sure to consult your facility's procedure book. If the outer dressings appear dry, you can take them off with your bare hands, grasping them at the center (without applying pressure) and removing them to the side. Avoid passing dressings over any sterile area. If the outer dressings are not dry, or if you prefer, you can use forceps or wear gloves. Inner dressings are often moist or soaked and should be removed by forceps or with sterile gloves. Notice how many of what type of dressings are soiled to indicate the amount of drainage when you chart. Place the soiled dressings in the bag or on the

paper designated for that use. If forceps
or gloves were used, discard them.
10. Wash your hands.
11. Observe the wound, noting the approxi-
mation of the wound's edges, the presence of inflammation and/or edema,
and the presence, appearance, and odor
of drainage, if any.
12. Open all packages and arrange the
sterile equipment conveniently.
13. Pour the antiseptic solution if one is
being used. Use the solution of the
physician's choice or the one currently
in use at your facility. In some facilities,
the solution comes in small bottles for
individual use and does not have to be
poured. In any case, if a container is
needed for the solution, it must be
sterile and you should be careful not to
drip solution around the basin, especially on the cloth drapes.
14. Put on sterile gloves. (See Module 36,
Sterile Technique, page 168.) In some
facilities, you will also be required to
wear a mask.
15. Clean the wound with antiseptic solution if indicated or ordered by the
physician. Using cotton balls or prepared swabs, clean around the
wound and in ever-widening circles
away from the wound, moving from
clean to dirty. Discard the swab.
Use each swab only once. Clean
two or three times as indicated.
16. Redress the wound, placing dressing
materials carefully so they do not
slide off. Use materials in the order
they were in when the old dressing
was removed if that seemed effective.
If not, redress for greater effectiveness.
If a drain is present, the bulk of the
dressing should be placed over the drain
area, usually in a dependent position.
To prevent excoriation of the skin
around the drain site, partially split a
4 × 4 with sterile scissors and place it
snugly around the drain (Figure 40.9).
17. Remove your gloves and place them in
the bag of used dressing materials.

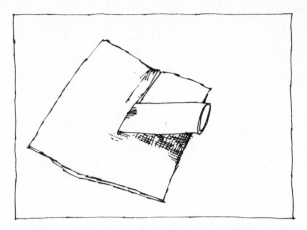

FIGURE 40.9   SPLIT GAUZE SURROUNDING
A DRAIN

18. Secure the dressing with tape, Montgomery tapes, or a binder as indicated.
Use sufficient tape to hold the dressing
in place, but do not use too much.
19. Assist the patient to a position of
comfort.
20. Care for the equipment. Remove the
bag used for soiled dressings and other
materials and put it in the appropriate
place. Rinse any glass or metal materials used to remove protein substances before sending them to central
supply.
21. Wash your hands.
22. Chart the procedure, including the time,
observations made, dressing materials
and antiseptic solution used, and any
reactions of the patient.

PERFORMANCE CHECKLIST

	Unsatisfactory	Needs more practice	Satisfactory	Comments
1. Check orders.				
2. Wash your hands.				
3. Gather necessary equipment.				
4. Identify patient and explain procedure.				
5. Prepare environment.				
6. Tear tape.				
7. Expose dressing, draping patient if necessary.				
8. Loosen old tapes.				
9. Remove old dressing and place in waste bag.				
10. Wash your hands.				
11. Observe wound.				
12. Open sterile packages and arrange equipment.				
13. Pour solution (if used).				
14. Put on sterile gloves.				
15. Clean wound with antiseptic solution if appropriate, using each swab only once.				
16. Apply dressing.				
17. Remove gloves and place in waste bag.				
18. Secure dressing.				
19. Assist patient to position of comfort.				
20. Care for equipment.				
21. Wash your hands.				
22. Chart.				

QUIZ

Short-Answer Questions

1. List three reasons for the application of dressings.

   a. _____

   b. _____

   c. _____

2. List three of the nurse's responsibilities with regard to dressing changes.

   a. _____

   b. _____

   c. _____

3. List four characteristics of drainage that must be noted when a dressing is changed.

   a. _____

   b. _____

   c. _____

   d. _____

4. List three characteristics of a wound that is healing by *primary intention*.

   a. _____

   b. _____

   c. _____

5. A special sterile dressing with a nonstick surface that is used directly next to an incision is called a _____ dressing.

6. What type of tape is generally considered to be hypoallergenic?

   _____

Module 41 Oral and Nasopharyngeal Suctioning

MAIN OBJECTIVE

To safely and effectively suction patients using either the oral or nasopharyngeal route.

RATIONALE

A variety of conditions can cause an abnormal increase in respiratory secretions. Lung and bronchial infections, central nervous system depression, and exposure to anesthetic gases are among the more frequent causes. In the newborn, saliva and amniotic fluid can be present in the mouth and throat in amounts the infant cannot expectorate. The premature newborn has an absent or decreased cough reflex and is often unable to raise secretions. In each of these situations, the secretions must be mechanically removed to facilitate breathing.

In the conscious, alert adult, the cough reflex is activated when respirations are compromised, and secretions are then expectorated. However, newborn, unconscious, or very ill patients are incapable of coughing, and must rely on the nurse and the nurse's

familiarity with the equipment and varying techniques for suctioning to carry out this function for them.

PREREQUISITES

Successful completion of the following modules:

VOLUME 1
Assessment
Charting
Medical Asepsis
Basic Infant Care

VOLUME 2
Sterile technique

SPECIFIC LEARNING OBJECTIVES

	Know Facts and Principles	Apply Facts and Principles	Demonstrate Ability	Evaluate Performance
1. Patient explanation	State information included in explaining suctioning to alert patient	Given a situation involving an alert patient, give adequate explanation	In the clinical area, explain procedure to alert patient	Evaluate effectiveness with instructor
2. Equipment	Know variety of equipment available for suctioning adults and infants	Given a patient situation, select appropriate equipment	In the clinical setting, select appropriate equipment for suctioning patient	
3. Routes for suctioning	Name common routes for suctioning	Given a patient situation, assess need for procedure and determine appropriate route	In the clinical setting, determine appropriate route for suctioning	Validate choice with instructor
4. Procedure a. Sterile technique b. Patient position c. Inserting catheter d. Applying suction e. Safety	Describe correct patient position and method to safely suction patient	Given a patient situation, describe patient position and correct procedure for suctioning, using sterile technique and observing safety precautions	In the clinical area, carry out procedure safely on alert or comatose adult or infant	Evaluate performance with instructor using Performance Checklist

5. *Assessment*	List assessments made before, during, and after suctioning	Given a patient situation, identify specific assessment needed	Clinically identify significant observations	Evaluate own performance with clinical instructor
6. *Charting*	State information to be recorded	Given a patient situation, record procedure and results correctly	In the clinical area, record data on patient's chart	Evaluate charting with clinical instructor

LEARNING ACTIVITIES

1. Review the Specific Learning Objectives.
2. Read the section on respiration in Ellis and Nowlis, *Nursing: A Human Needs Approach,* or comparable material in another textbook.
3. Look up the module vocabulary terms in the glossary.
4. Read through the module.
5. Review the Performance Checklist.
6. In the practice setting:
   a. Familiarize yourself with the suctioning equipment available.
   b. Using the available equipment and a mannequin, simulate oral and nasopharyngeal suctioning.
   c. Again, with available equipment and an infant mannequin, perform the bulb method as used on an infant.
   d. Have your partner evaluate your performance using the Performance Checklist.
   e. Compare your own evaluation with that of your partner's.
   f. Reverse roles, and repeat steps b–e.
   g. Practice assessing and recording the suctioning procedure.
   h. When you feel you have practiced the procedure adequately, have your instructor evaluate your performance.
7. In the clinical setting:
   a. Consult with your clinical instructor regarding an opportunity to suction both an alert and a comatose patient, as well as an infant.

VOCABULARY

aspiration
bronchial
cough reflex
cyanotic
hypoxia
inspiration
mucus
pharynx
saliva
secretions
trachea

ORAL AND NASOPHARYNGEAL SUCTIONING

Always carefully assess the patient before you proceed with suctioning. This is often done by listening to chest sounds and to sounds of the higher respiratory tract. Frequently, you can hear gurgling sounds from the back of the throat. A patient with severely compromised respirations from the presence of copious secretions may appear cyanotic and have labored breathing. It is important that you weigh the decision to suction a patient because the irritation of the catheter itself may only intensify the buildup of secretions. Also, during suctioning, the patient is unable to breathe in oxygen. Suctioning performed too frequently can *increase* the accumulation of secretions and cause a degree of hypoxia.

Explaining the Procedure

Suctioning can be very threatening to the alert patient. It is natural to resist foreign objects that enter the respiratory tract. This is, in fact, the basis for our protective cough reflex. You can reduce the patient's fear and attain his or her cooperation by adequately explaining the procedure and the reasons for it.

Tell the patient that you will insert the catheter gently, and ask the patient to relax as much as possible. Inform the patient that he or she may cough when the catheter is inserted or withdrawn, but explain that this may help raise the secretions to where they can be suctioned.

Equipment

If a suction catheter kit (Figure 41.1) is not available, you will need the following:

1. A clean towel to protect the patient's gown
2. A sterile catheter
   a. Adult sizes: 10–18 French, 22 inches long
   b. Child sizes: 5–8 French, 15 inches long
3. A sterile glove
4. A sterile container or basin
5. Sterile water or sterile normal saline

These items, excluding the sterile water, are all contained in the kit, although a soft drape may be substituted for the towel.

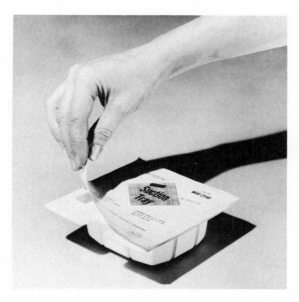 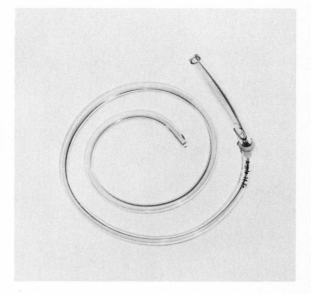

FIGURE 41.1   SUCTION CATHETER KIT
Courtesy Sherwood Medical, St. Louis, Missouri

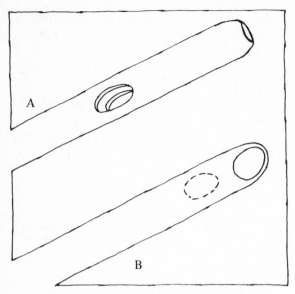

FIGURE 41.2　SUCTION CATHETERS　*A:* Open-ended catheter; *B:* whistle-tip catheter.

SUCTION CATHETERS

Suction catheters are available with several types of tips (Figure 41.2), each with special advantages. The *open-ended catheter* has a large opening at the end of the catheter and two opposite eyes. This type is effective when large plugs of mucus are present, but it does have a tendency to pull at tissue

unless it is used carefully. The *whistle-tip catheter* has a large oblique opening in the end, which has less of a tendency to grab or pull tissue than does a side eye.

With any catheter, the system must be closed in order to obtain suction, or pull. You can control this easily by using a Y-tube and placing your thumb over the open end of the Y to close the system. A button-type connector is also available. To use it, place your thumb over the opening in the protruding button. (See Figure 41.3.)

SUCTION SOURCE

Many hospitals have a suction outlet on the wall of each room. In this case, you will need only a length of clean tubing and an adapter to connect to the outlet. If wall suction is not available, obtain a portable suction machine (Figure 41.4) from the central supply department.

Always test equipment *before* the procedure. Suction tubing must be tightly fastened to the outlet to be effective; that is, to maintain a closed system. Inspect all plugs and cords on portable units: they should be in good repair to prevent sparks. Remember that sparks can be very hazardous when oxygen is in use and very often,

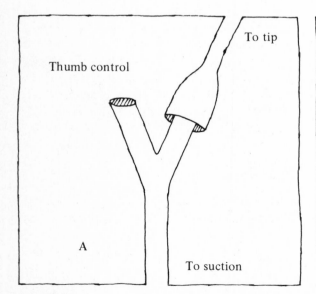

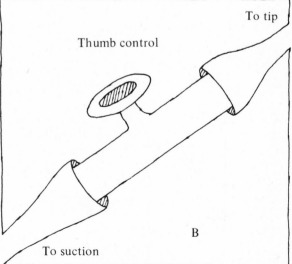

FIGURE 41.3　CONNECTORS　*A:* Y-tube connector; *B:* button-type connector.

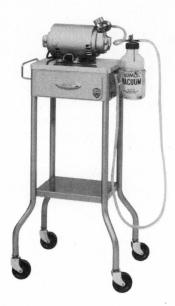

FIGURE 41.4 GOMCO PORTABLE ASPIRATOR (Suction machine)
Courtesy Chemetron Medical Products, division of Allegheny Ludlum Industries

the patient ill enough to require suctioning also is receiving oxygen.

Sterile Technique

Because the respiratory tract is continuous and moist, pathogens can readily move downward from the area being suctioned. The bronchi and lungs of an ill person are particularly susceptible to infection, so sterile technique should be used for suctioning, whether orally or nasopharyngeally. If you have to change the suctioning route for any reason (an obstruction), you must obtain a new sterile catheter.

One sterile glove is usually sufficient. Your gloved hand holds the portion of the catheter (which is sterile) in contact with the patient, while your other (clean) hand operates the machine or clean pieces of equipment.

You will use the sterile water, poured into a sterile container, to flush the catheter and tubing. Tap water contains microorganisms that are not harmful to the well person but may cause infection of the respiratory tract in the ill person.

In some settings, clean technique is used for oral suctioning. Be aware that this is not the best procedure, and make every effort to maintain an exceptional level of cleanliness.

The bulb-syringe method, for infants, is usually performed using medical asepsis only.

Routes for Suctioning

The catheter can be inserted *orally* (through the mouth to the back of the throat) or *nasopharyngeally* (through one of the nares). For an infant, the tip of the bulb is introduced into the mouth.

You should be able to see the back of the throat (pharynx), so that determining the length of insertion is usually not a problem. (See Figure 41.5.) When using the nasopharyngeal route, the length is generally that from the tip of the nose to the tip of the earlobe, or about 5 inches.

If tracheal, or deep, suctioning is necessary, it is performed by a respiratory therapist, a critical-care nurse, or a very experienced and skilled staff nurse. For tracheal suctioning, the catheter is introduced past the glottis deep into the trachea. This is done when a patient is unable to raise deep secretions to the point where they can be suctioned out.

The cough reflex can be stimulated using either route. Although unpleasant for the conscious patient, coughing raises deeper secretions, which can then be removed by suctioning.

Suctioning Procedure

1. Wash your hands.
2. Gather the necessary equipment.
   a. Suction catheter kit
   b. A sterile catheter in the appropriate size
   c. A sterile glove
   d. A sterile container or basin

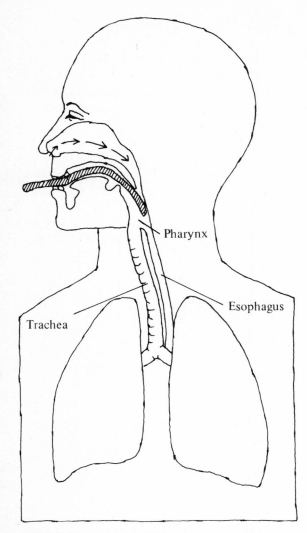

FIGURE 41.5   LOCATION OF CATHETER IN PHARYNX

e. Sterile water
f. Wall suction connector
g. Portable suction machine (if wall suction is not available)
h. A tongue depressor (for oral suctioning)
3. Explain the procedure to the patient.
4. Use adequate lighting. Have an assistant hold a gooseneck lamp or flashlight for you if the wall lighting is not sufficient.
5. Position the patient in low-Fowler's position, with the head turned slightly toward you.
6. Place the drape (from the catheter kit)

or a clean towel across the patient's chest, to protect the gown.
7. Open the catheter kit, maintaining the sterile field.
8. Glove your dominant hand.
9. Pick up the catheter with your gloved hand and attach the connector end to the suction tubing, which is held in your clean hand. Take care not to touch the tubing with the gloved hand.
10. With your ungloved hand, pour the sterile water into the basin.
11. Turn on the machine.
12. Test the machine by suctioning water once through the tubing and catheter. (The water also serves to lubricate the catheter.)
13. Insert the catheter.
    a. Through the mouth, using a tongue blade if necessary to hold the tongue aside for visibility
    b. Through the nares. (If an obstruction is met in one nostril, try the other side.)
    Never apply suction while you are inserting the catheter. You could damage the mucous membranes. Use a catheter only for a single route: if you must change the route, obtain a new sterile catheter. For example, if you have just attempted to suction a patient orally and have met with resistance, and then decide to proceed with the nasopharyngeal approach, you must discard the first catheter and obtain a second. If you are not using a kit, open separate sterile packs and proceed.
14. Holding your thumb over the opening in the catheter, apply suction for no longer than 15 seconds. In fact, it is good practice as you begin to hold your breath during the suction period, to remind you that the patient is not receiving oxygen nor inspiring while you suction.
15. When suctioning orally, suction carefully in the cheeks where secretions tend to pool.
16. Withdraw the catheter under suction

with a rotating motion. This aspirates the secretions protruding from the catheter's tip.

17. Flush the catheter.
18. Briefly turn off the suction to listen to the patient's breath sounds, to assess the need for repeated suctioning.
19. If the patient's breathing is not clear, repeat steps 14–18.
20. When the patient's breathing sounds clear, stop. You should never apply suction more than three times. Sometimes you will stop because you have not been successful in reaching the secretions. At other times, you may be forced to stop because the patient is actively fighting the procedure. Knowing when to stop suctioning requires good nursing judgment. Remember that this procedure can be very tiring, as well as frightening, for the patient.
21. With your nonsterile hand, grasp the cuff of the sterile glove and pull it downward over the used catheter in your gloved hand. This method neatly encloses the used catheter in the glove, making disposal more sanitary.
22. Detach the catheter from the tubing and dispose of it safely in a receptacle.
23. Reposition the patient.
24. Wash your hands.
25. Record the procedure on the patient's chart. Include the results and the patient's response. For example:

> 4:20 a.m. Unresponsive to painful stimuli. Nasopharyngeal suctioning performed. Mod. am't thick green mucus obtained.   J. Jones, RN

Bulb Suctioning the Infant

Most infants have minimal secretions and are able to cough, which effectively clears their air passages. However, when amniotic fluid in the passages of the newborn or increased production of mucus in the infant causes breathing to become labored, suctioning must be done to maintain a patent airway.

PROCEDURE

1. Wash your hands. Good medical asepsis is all that is necessary in this procedure because you are only suctioning in the mouth. Deeper suctioning is usually performed in the nursery by specially trained nurses.
2. Gather the necessary equipment.
   a. A sterile bulb syringe. (You should begin with a sterile syringe. However, if frequent suctioning is needed, the bulb can be rinsed well and placed in a clean towel at the side of the crib or at the foot of the crib for further use. This is often done as a prophylactic measure.)
   b. Clean diaper or towel to place under the infant's chin
   c. Kidney basin as a waste receptacle for secretions
3. Wrap the baby in a warm blanket, to prevent chilling.
4. Position the infant. You can swaddle, or wrap the baby with a small sheet if necessary. (See Module 9, Basic Infant Care, page 126.) The head should be flat on the surface of the crib. A newborn can be held "football" fashion, with the head slightly downward. Gravity will help secretions move from the back of the throat to the mouth, where they can be suctioned more readily. If held, swaddling for restraint is usually not necessary.
5. Compress the bulb before inserting it into the infant's mouth. Any compression with the tip in the mouth may force secretions deep into the respiratory tract.
6. Insert the tip into the mouth and release to aspirate.
7. Remove the syringe and compress, expressing the contents into the basin.
8. Repeat steps 5–7 until the infant's cheeks and mouth are clear.
9. Carefully suction the nares. You can use the same syringe.
10. Place the infant on his or her side after suctioning.

11. Listen for clear breath sounds.
12. Care for the equipment. Rinse and dispose as necessary.
13. Wash your hands.
14. Record. This is usually done on a check-list for the infant. Enter "bulb" in the method column. Any significant observations (unusual color, unusual amount of secretions) should be entered in the nurses' notes. For example:

> 9 a.m. Suctioned with bulb. Mod.
> am't frothy, white mucus obtained.
> J. Jones, RN

PERFORMANCE CHECKLIST

General procedure for suctioning	Unsatisfactory	Needs more practice	Satisfactory	Comments
1. Use sterile technique.				
2. Wash your hands.				
3. Gather necessary equipment. a. Suction catheter kit				
b. Catheter				
c. Glove				
d. Container				
e. Sterile water				
f. Wall suction connector				
g. Portable suction machine if necessary				
h. Tongue depressor if necessary				
4. Explain procedure to patient.				
5. Provide adequate lighting.				
6. Position patient.				
7. Place drape across patient.				
8. Open kit, maintaining sterile field.				
9. Glove your dominant hand.				
10. Keeping gloved hand sterile, attach end of catheter to tubing.				
11. With clean hand, pour water into basin.				
12. Turn on machine.				
13. Test by flushing with water.				
14. Insert catheter. Do not apply suction until catheter is in place. a. Orally: Without placing thumb over control, insert catheter directly downward toward back of throat, only as far as you can see tip of catheter.				
b. Nasopharyngeally: Insert catheter about 5 inches into nares.				
15. Place finger over control when in position and apply suction for not more than 15 seconds.				
16. If using the oral route, suction carefully in cheeks.				
17. Slowly remove catheter using a rotating motion.				

	Unsatisfactory	Needs more practice	Satisfactory	Comments
18. Flush tubing and catheter with water.				
19. Briefly turn off suction and listen to patient's breathing sounds.				
20. Repeat procedure if necessary. (Avoid repeating more than three times.)				
21. Stop when breathing is clear or other conditions indicate.				
22. Remove glove, enclosing catheter in glove.				
23. Detach catheter and discard.				
24. Reposition patient.				
25. Wash your hands.				
26. Record.				
Bulb method				
1. Wash your hands.				
2. Gather necessary equipment. a. Bulb syringe				
b. Clean diaper or towel				
c. Kidney basin				
3. Wrap infant to prevent chilling.				
4. Position infant, using swaddling restraint if necessary.				
5. Compress bulb with palm of your hand.				
6. Place tip carefully in infant's mouth and release bulb.				
7. Remove bulb and dispose of secretions.				
8. Repeat procedure if necessary.				
9. Using same syringe, suction infant's nares.				
10. Reposition infant on side.				
11. Listen for clear breathing.				
12. Rinse and dispose of equipment.				
13. Wash your hands.				
14. Chart.				

QUIZ

Short-Answer Questions

1. List two reasons why the patient must be given an adequate explanation of the suctioning procedure.

   a. _____

   b. _____

2. When using a suction catheter, why must sterility be maintained?

   _____

3. Why does a newborn or infant usually need to be suctioned?

   _____

4. When operating the equipment, why must the system be closed?

   _____

5. What is the maximum length of time you should suction on each insertion of the catheter? _____

6. Ideally, what is the maximum number of times you should suction a patient? _____

Module 42 Tracheostomy Care and Suctioning

MAIN OBJECTIVE

To care for patients with a tracheostomy correctly, and to perform suctioning through the tracheostomy in a safe effective manner.

RATIONALE

Patients with tracheostomies are frequently cared for on the general hospital unit. In view of this, the nurse must be familiar with the special care required and the variations needed for suctioning these patients. Normally, the upper respiratory passages protect the trachea, filtering out foreign material and providing some protection from micro-organisms. The trachea normally remains sterile. Because the tracheostomy opens directly into the trachea, a thorough knowledge of sterile technique is required. In addition, safety involves the constant maintenance of a patent airway.

PREREQUISITES

Successful completion of the following modules:

VOLUME 1
Assessment
Charting
Medical Asepsis
Hygiene

VOLUME 2
Sterile Technique
Sterile Dressings
Oral and Nasopharyngeal Suctioning

257

SPECIFIC LEARNING OBJECTIVES

	Know Facts and Principles	Apply Facts and Principles	Demonstrate Ability	Evaluate Performance
1. General considerations				
a. Definition	Define *tracheostomy*			
b. Indications for tracheostomy	State two reasons for tracheostomy	Given a patient situation, give rationale for tracheostomy		
c. Types of tracheostomy tubes	Name three types of tracheostomy tubes and advantages and disadvantages of each	Identify type of tube in use for particular patient		
d. Safety factors	State three important safety measures and rationale for each	Given a patient situation, state safety measures appropriate to that situation	In the clinical area, carry out measures safely with patient	
2. Tracheostomy suctioning				
a. Equipment	Describe equipment used in tracheal suctioning	In a given situation, select and adapt equipment correctly	In the clinical area, use appropriate equipment in manner described	Evaluate selection with instructor
b. Procedure	State information to be given to patient	Given a patient situation, plan appropriate patient teaching and nurse-patient interaction	In the clinical area, carry out appropriate nurse-patient interaction and patient teaching	Evaluate interaction with instructor

	Given a patient situation. plan suctioning procedure	In the clinical area, correctly suction tracheostomy patient	Evaluate own performance with instructor using Performance Checklist
Know correct positioning. Explain use of sterile technique. State distance catheter is inserted for shallow or deep suctioning. Describe method and how long to apply pressure.			
c. Charting State what needs to be recorded	Given a patient situation, list pertinent information to be charted	In the clinical setting, record accurately on patient's chart	Evaluate charting format and content with instructor
3. Cleaning and dressing a. Equipment Name equipment needed for cleaning and dressing tracheostomy	Given a specific situation, select and assemble equipment correctly	In the clinical area, correctly use equipment and materials	Evaluate use with instructor
b. Procedure State explanation to be given to patient. Know correct positioning. Explain use of sterile equipment. List steps in cleaning and dressing procedure.	Given a patient situation, state plan to clean and dress tracheostomy	In the clinical setting, carry out cleaning and dressing procedure	Evaluate own performance with instructor using Performance Checklist
c. Charting State items to be recorded			

LEARNING ACTIVITIES

1. Review the Specific Learning Objectives.
2. Read the section on the respiratory system (in the chapter on basic vital functions) in Ellis and Nowlis, *Nursing: A Human Needs Approach,* or comparable material in another textbook.
3. Look up the module vocabulary terms in the glossary.
4. Read through the module.
5. Review the Performance Checklist.
6. In the practice setting:
   a. Examine the various tracheostomy tubes available.
   b. Select and gather the equipment for suctioning a tracheostomy.
   c. If a tube can be attached to a mannequin, use the Performance Checklist as a guide and practice suctioning the tracheostomy.
   d. Gather the equipment for cleaning a tube and changing a dressing.
   e. Follow the Performance Checklist and practice cleaning the tube and changing the dressing.
   f. When you think you have mastered these skills, ask your instructor to evaluate your performance.
7. In the clinical setting:
   a. Consult with your instructor for an opportunity to give care and to suction a patient with a tracheostomy.

VOCABULARY

asphyxiation
aspirate
bronchi
button
cannula
catheter
clockwise
counterclockwise
dead air space
hydrogen peroxide
hypoxia
inflatable cuff
lumen
mucus
necrosis
obturator
prophylactic
respirator
suction
trachea
tracheal ring
tracheostomy

TRACHEOSTOMY CARE AND SUCTIONING

Tracheostomies

A tracheostomy is a surgical incision into the trachea for the purpose of inserting a tube. At one time, the procedure was performed only as an emergency measure, to allow a critically ill patient to breathe through a surgical incision and tube in the trachea when life was imminently threatened by respiratory obstruction.

In current practice, tracheostomies are performed more commonly as a prophylactic procedure, so that secretions in the respiratory tract can be removed more effectively *before* a patient's breathing is severely compromised. Tracheostomies may also be performed to decrease the amount of dead air space in the airway; and thus to reduce the effort of breathing. In some instances, a tracheostomy is done so that a respirator can be employed to breathe for the patient.

The procedure is performed by a physician usually in the critical-care unit or the operating room. A small horizontal incision is made just below the first tracheal ring, and one of a variety of tubes is inserted. Most tracheostomies are temporary. Once the patient can tolerate temporary closure (buttoning) from brief to more prolonged periods of time, the tracheostomy tube is removed and the incision then heals over. (See Figure 42.1.)

Tracheostomy Tubes

Tracheostomy care varies with the type of tube used. Several varieties are available. For many years, metal tubes were the most widely used, followed by rubber tubes. More recently, plastic tubes are used almost exclusively in acute-care settings.

The size of the tube is usually the choice of the physician who performs the procedure and inserts the tube. Most tubes, regardless of type, come in standard sizes: 0–12 or French 24–44, from smaller to larger.

PLASTIC TUBES

Most commonly used today are plastic tubes (Figure 42.2). Like rubber tubes, these usually have inflatable cuffs. The plastic tube has many advantages over metal: it has a larger lumen and softer consistency; it attaches easily to ventilating equipment; it molds more easily to the trachea; it is less irritating; and it is more comfortable for the patient. Also, it is relatively inexpensive. One disadvantage of plastic tubes is that they cannot be sterilized with ordinary methods, so they are one-use items.

METAL TUBES

Metal tracheostomy tubes consist of three parts: an outer cannula (tube), which is in

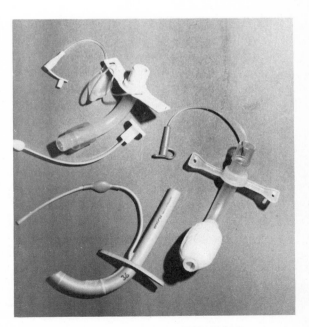

FIGURE 42.2   PLASTIC CUFFED TUBE
Courtesy Ivan Ellis

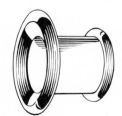

FIGURE 42.1   TRACHEOSTOMY BUTTON
Courtesy Pilling Company, Fort Washington, Pennsylvania

contact with the trachea; an inner cannula (tube), which fits snugly into the outer and is removed for cleaning; and a bulb-type obturator, which fits the outer tube but is slightly longer in length. All are made of silver. (See Figure 42.3.) The obturator is placed inside the outer tube when it is initially inserted to facilitate smooth passage and to prevent tissue from being torn. Once the tube is in place, the obturator is removed, the outer metal tube is secured with a cloth tape, and the inner cannula is inserted. The metal tube has the advantage of withstanding repeated sterilization. Disadvantages are its cost, its comparative rigidity and heaviness, its smaller lumen, and its tendency to cause excessive tracheal irritation. Also, it does not easily adapt to respirators with special equipment.

RUBBER TUBES

Rubber tubes are used infrequently. They have larger lumen than do metal tubes, and they do not have an inner cannula. They usually have an inflatable cuff, which when inflated, completely occludes the trachea, so that the only air passage is through the tube. The advantages of rubber tubing include its moderate cost, its ability to be resterilized, and its increased comfort over metal tubing, due in part to its lighter weight. Most rubber tubes can be attached to ventilating equipment with few adaptations.

Assessing the Patient

Assessing the needs of a patient with a tracheostomy for suctioning and cleaning is an important function for the nurse. This is especially critical because many of these patients are comatose, and conscious patients cannot talk because of the tracheal opening.

Assessments should be made frequently because the opening can become obstructed by the build-up of crusts and secretions. Never allow the patient to reach the point of laborious breathing. Clean by necessity, not by a definite schedule. Some patients have more secretions than others. Cleaning and dressing the tracheostomy once per shift may be adequate with some patients, while others may need care two and three times per shift.

To assess the patient; listen to the breath sounds. They should be quiet, not labored. If the respirations are labored and you hear the movement of secretions (a gurgling sound), the patient needs suctioning. You can also observe the condition of the tubes. If suctioning, cleaning, and dressing are all needed, suction first. If the secretions are removed by suctioning first, the cleaned tube and dressing will stay cleaner longer. While giving care, always observe the incision for redness and swelling, which can be symptoms of infection or irritation. Remember that suctioning removes oxygen, causes tissue irritation, and increases secretions, so the procedure should be used with discretion. Also, for tracheostomies, suctioning should not exceed ten seconds at any one time.

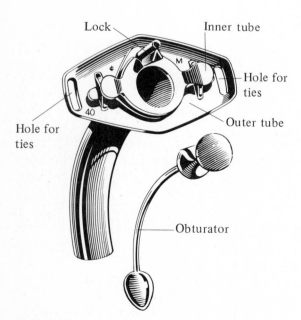

FIGURE 42.3   METAL TUBE
Courtesy Pilling Company, Fort Washington, Pennsylvania

Safety Measures

Crucial to the care of a tracheostomy is the prevention of infection, not only to the wound, but to the bronchi and lungs as well. If a patient has a new or recent tracheostomy, use sterile technique when cleaning or dressing. In many facilities, good handwashing and clean technique are used when cleaning or dressing a tracheostomy of long standing. But, regardless of how long a patient has had the tracheostomy, always use sterile technique when suctioning.

Keep emergency equipment at the bedside to prevent accidental asphyxiation. It is procedure in some facilities to keep an extra tracheostomy set at the bedside, which contains a clamp that the nurse can quickly insert into the opening to maintain patency in case the tube becomes dislodged or is coughed out, allowing the opening to close. A new sterile tube is then inserted. If a complete set is not available, always keep a sterile clamp and a tube of the correct size and type at the bedside.

If cloth material or gauze is used in care, it must be lint-free, to prevent the aspiration of particles into the respiratory tract. Avoid cutting cloth materials for this reason.

A patient who has a tube with an inflatable cuff should have the cuff deflated at regular intervals, so that pressure necrosis or erosion of the tracheal lining does not occur. The cuff is usually deflated for ten minutes out of each hour, or as the physician orders. Suction any accumulated oral secretions before deflating the cuff. During the time the cuff is deflated, take special precautions to ensure that the tapes are secure and that the tracheostomy tube is in good position, so it is not coughed out. This is not a problem if the tube has a double cuff because one cuff remains inflated while the other is deflated, providing alternating pressure areas and preventing necrosis. Some tubes are made with soft pliable cuffs that can be left inflated. Check the procedure for the type of cuff in use.

Any patient with a tracheostomy needs constant careful watching. It is also a matter of safety to provide a call bell within reach of the alert patient at all times, so that help can be summoned if respiratory difficulty occurs.

Tracheostomy Suctioning

The tracheal suctioning procedure is similar to that described in Module 41, for nasopharyngeal suctioning. If the patient with a tracheostomy is on a respirator, the procedure is much more complex and requires advanced skills that are not included in this module.

1. Wash your hands.
2. Explain the procedure. If the patient is responsive, it is imperative that the procedure be carefully explained. Without proper psychological preparation, the patient may fear choking or bleeding to death. A brief explanation should also be given to the unresponsive patient because the patient may understand even though he or she is unable to respond. The responsive patient should be asked to cough to raise secretions so they are more easily suctioned.
3. Position the patient in mid-Fowler's position. Turn the patient's head slightly toward you.
4. Provide a slate or pencil and paper to the alert patient for purposes of communicating. Tell the patient that the tracheal opening prevents air from reaching the vocal cords, so speech will not be possible. Later, a button or finger over the opening will allow the patient to speak. If the patient cannot write, establish a yes or no signal system with him or her.
5. Obtain a sterile suctioning set or similar equipment. You will need the following:
   a. A sterile glove
   b. A sterile suction catheter
   c. A sterile basin
   d. Sterile water or sterile normal saline
   e. A sterile syringe and normal saline if saline is to be instilled
   f. Sterile gauze squares

g. A portable suction machine if wall suction is not available

6. Test the suction apparatus.
   a. Turn on either the wall suction or the portable machine.
   b. Place your thumb over the end of the unsterile tubing that is attached to the suction equipment and test for "pull."
   c. Keep the suction set to a range of efficiency, usually low to medium.

7. Open the pack and put a sterile glove on your dominant hand; a second glove is not necessary. You will use the gloved (sterile) hand to handle the proximal end of the catheter, which comes in contact with the patient. You will use your ungloved hand to operate the equipment and to control the suction.

8. Draw up 1 to 5 ml sterile saline, if it is being used, into the syringe. The properties of normal saline help to liquefy thickened respiratory secretions. You must be prepared to suction quickly after instillation, so that the saline is removed without compromising alveolar exchange.

9. Pour sterile water or saline into the basin.

10. Pick up the sterile catheter in your gloved hand, and carefully insert the connector end into the suction tubing, which you are holding in your ungloved hand.

11. Turn off oxygen in use. You can hear breath sounds more clearly without the distraction of the noise of oxygen flow. Most patients can tolerate a brief interruption in oxygen administration. To allow maximum inspiration of oxygen, however, do not discontinue oxygen until just before you are ready to suction. Remember that during the actual suctioning period the patient is unable to breathe. In critically ill patients, even this relatively brief period of time can produce mild to moderate hypoxia. To offset this, an Ambu bag is sometimes employed to manually breathe the patient three deep inspirations just before and after the suctioning. Refer to a critical-care manual for the particulars of this technique.

12. Turn on the suction.

13. Instill saline if ordered.

14. Insert the catheter 4 to 5 inches into the tracheostomy, keeping the suction off.

15. Apply suction by closing the system. This is usually done by placing your thumb over a side opening at the base of the catheter. The patient will often cough in response to the irritation caused by the catheter. This helps to raise secretions. If persistent coughing occurs, however, it can indicate tracheal spasm, and the procedure should be stopped.

16. Apply suction for only ten seconds (per entry). Remember that the patient is unable to breathe during the procedure. (You can hold your own breath while suctioning to help you time the procedure.)

17. Observe the patient for dyspnea and color changes.

18. Withdraw the catheter, rotating it gently while you continue suctioning, so that higher secretions are removed and are not tracked through the lumen of the tracheostomy.

19. Rinse the catheter with either sterile water or normal saline.

20. Turn off the suction and listen for clear breath sounds.

21. If breathing is not clear, repeat the procedure.

22. If the breathing sounds clear, detach the catheter.

23. Check the patient's pulse and respiration.

24. Grasp the top of the sterile glove and pull it down over the used catheter. This provides a handy method for discarding the equipment.

25. Discard all disposable equipment.

26. Reassure the patient.

27. Check the position of the tube.

28. Wash your hands.

29. Chart the procedure and your observations. The entry should include the amount and description of secretions, as well as the patient's tolerance of the procedure. For example:

> 9:15 a.m. Tracheal suctioning performed. 2 ml normal saline instilled; mod. am't thick white mucus obtained. VS stable. Skin appears slightly reddened around tube.
>
> B. Cook, RN

Deep (Bronchial) Suctioning

Bronchial suctioning should be done only by a very skilled nurse. In this procedure, both bronchi, right and left, are suctioned, often to a depth of 10 inches. To enter the right bronchus, the patient's head is turned to the left. For easier access to the left bronchus, the patient's head is turned to the right. (See Figure 42.4.)

The suctioning procedure is basically the same as for tracheal suctioning. After any suctioning, but particularly deep bronchial

suctioning, the patient must rest before being given additional care.

Cleaning and Dressing the Tracheostomy

You would again reassure the patient, as you did when preparing to suction, and provide a means of communication before you begin to clean and dress the tracheostomy.

CLEANING PROCEDURE

1. Assess the patient. Depending on the amount and character of secretions, patients will vary in their need for cleaning and dressing.
2. Wash your hands.
3. Obtain a tracheostomy care kit or the following supplies:
   a. Sterile gloves if the tracheostomy has recently been performed
   b. 4 x 4 gauze squares
   c. A cleansing solution (often a hydrogen peroxide mixture, alcohol, or saline)
   d. A basin

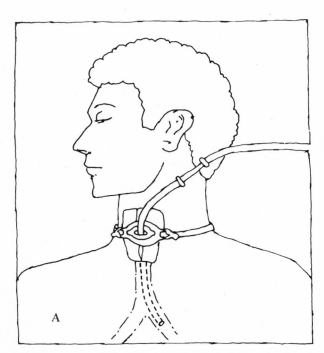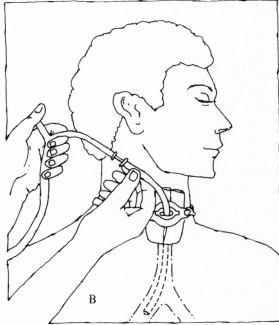

FIGURE 42.4   POSITIONS FOR BRONCHIAL SUCTIONING   *A:* Suctioning left bronchus; *B:* suctioning right bronchus.

e. A tracheostomy brush, pipe cleaners, or swabs, to clean the cannula surfaces

f. Sterile water

4. Explain what you are going to do. Many patients are afraid that the tube may become dislodged during care. By demonstrating competency you can reassure the patient.

5. Provide a slate or pencil and paper to the alert patient for communication.

6. Position the patient in mid-Fowler's position.

7. Set up the supplies.

8. Put on sterile gloves, if necessary.

9. To clean a cannula-type tracheostomy tube:

a. Hold the outer tube carefully in place with one hand as you turn the lock clockwise with your other hand to unfasten the inner cannula.

b. Slide the inner cannula out by curving it toward you.

c. Place the cannula in the basin.

d. Immerse it in the cleansing solution for a few minutes.

e. Apply friction with brush, pipe cleaners, or swabs to remove mucus and crusts.

f. Rinse well in cold sterile water.

g. Dry thoroughly with sterile, lint-free gauze or towel.

h. Inspect and remove any particles of lint.

i. If the patient's secretions are copious, or if he or she coughs while you are cleaning the inner cannula (so that these secretions come in contact with the inside surface of the outer tube), remove the secretions and thoroughly dry the inner surfaces as described below, to prevent the surfaces of the two tubes from adhering.

j. Hold the outer tube and replace the clean inner cannula.

k. Turn the lock counterclockwise to secure.

l. Test to make sure that the inner cannula is secure.

If a rubber or plastic tube with no inner cannula is being used, carefully clean the inner surfaces with pipe cleaners or swabs dampened (not saturated) with normal saline.

10. Dispose of the equipment.

11. Wash your hands.

12. Record the procedure.

DRESSING PROCEDURE

Ideally, this is a two-person procedure, although a single person can carry it out carefully.

1. Assess the patient.

2. Wash your hands.

3. Gather the necessary equipment.

a. 4 × 4 gauze squares

b. Twill tape ties

c. Scissors

d. Swabs

e. A cleansing solution

f. Oral-care equipment

4. Remove the old dressing and discard.

a. *Two persons* Have your assistant hold the tube while you remove the old dressing.

b. *One person* Place one hand gently around the tube to keep it secure as you carefully remove the soiled gauze.

5. With swabs moistened in saline or hydrogen peroxide solution, clean around the edges of the tracheostomy opening.

6. Notice any redness or swelling of the wound margins.

7. Prepare the dressing.

a. Open the first fold of a 4 × 4 gauze square.

b. Fold it in half lengthwise.

c. Fold each end toward the center (Figure 42.5).

d. Place it around the tube with the ends up.

This type of dressing eliminates the need to cut the material, which could free lint that could be inhaled.

8. Remove the holding tape.

a. *Two persons* Have your assistant

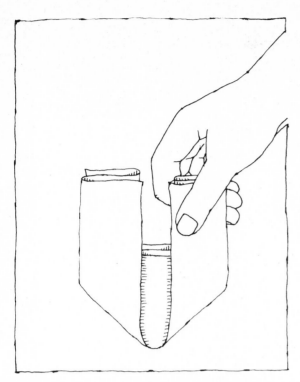

FIGURE 42.5   TRACHEOSTOMY DRESSING

apply light pressure to the tube, to prevent dislodging it, while you cut the tape, remove it, and discard.

b. *One person*   Leave the twill tapes in place while the old dressing is removed and the new one is placed. Cut and prepare both ties. Thread the new ties through the slits above the old ties, and tie the new ties. Then, cut and remove the old ties. Or, an alert, oriented patient can be asked to hold the tube in place while you change the tapes.

It is possible to develop the dexterity to hold the tracheostomy tube with the nondominant hand and use the dominant hand to remove the old tape and fasten the new. Once both new tapes have been attached, the ties are held firmly while being tied around the back of the neck.

9. Carefully slip the prepared dressing, ends extending up, around the tube.
10. With the tube held in place, tape the new dressing.

a. Make a slit near the end of the twill tape.
b. Thread the tape through the flange on one side of the tube.
c. Pass the end through the tape slot and pull until it is snug.
d. Bring the tape around the back of patient's neck (Figure 42.6).
e. Thread the loose end through the remaining flange.
   Tie at the side of the neck tightly enough so the tube is held securely, but loosely enough so that there is not undue pressure on tissues. It is helpful if the assisting nurse holds a finger under the tape as it is tied to allow for slack.
11. Check the position of the tube.
12. Perform oral care following the guidelines in Module 8, Hygiene, page 106. Because a patient with a tracheostomy has a changed breathing pattern (without air moving freely though the mouth), the oral cavity becomes dry and there is a build-up of sores and crusts. This can lead to odor, which is distressing to both the patient and those caring for

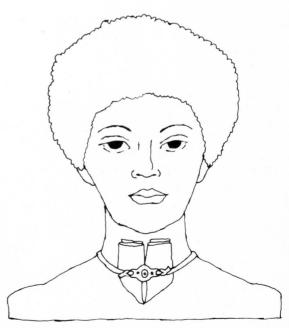

FIGURE 42.6   TAPES HOLDING THE TRACHEOSTOMY TUBE

him or her. Because the patient needs
meticulous and frequent oral care,
make this a part of the general tracheostomy care, so that it is neither for-
gotten nor neglected.
13. Dispose of the equipment.
14. Wash your hands.
15. Record the procedure and your observations. For example:

> 2:15 p.m. Tracheostomy dressing
> changed. Skin in good condition. No
> exudate present around tube.
>   B. Cook, RN

PERFORMANCE CHECKLIST

Tracheal suctioning	Unsatisfactory	Needs more practice	Satisfactory	Comments
1. Use sterile technique.				
2. Wash your hands.				
3. Explain procedure to patient.				
4. Position patient in mid-Fowler's.				
5. Provide means of communication.				
6. Obtain sterile suctioning set or assemble equipment. a. Sterile glove				
b. Sterile suction catheter				
c. Sterile basin				
d. Sterile water				
e. Sterile syringe and saline if saline is to be injected				
f. Sterile gauze squares				
g. Portable suction machine if necessary				
7. Test suction machine or wall suction.				
8. Open pack and glove dominant hand.				
9. Draw up saline into syringe if necessary.				
10. Pour sterile water or saline into basin.				
11. Holding catheter in gloved hand, attach to suction tubing without contaminating proximal portion of catheter.				
12. Turn off oxygen if in use.				
13. Turn on suction.				
14. Instill saline if ordered.				
15. Insert catheter 4 to 5 inches.				
16. Apply suction.				
17. Suction for approximately ten seconds.				
18. Observe patient closely.				
19. Withdraw catheter, rotating it gently, while continuing to suction.				
20. Rinse catheter with sterile water.				
21. Turn off suction and listen to breath sounds.				
22. Repeat procedure if necessary.				

	Unsatisfactory	Needs more practice	Satisfactory	Comments
23. If breathing sounds clear, detach catheter.				
24. Check patient's pulse and respiration.				
25. Grasp cuff of sterile glove and pull downward over catheter.				
26. Discard disposable equipment.				
27. Reassure patient.				
28. Check position of tube.				
29. Wash your hands.				
30. Chart procedure and observations.				
Deep (bronchial) suctioning Follow the steps for tracheal suctioning with these adaptations:				
1. Raise patient's shoulder on side you plan to suction in order to provide better access to bronchus.				
2. Turn head in opposite direction.				
3. Insert catheter 8 to 10 inches.				
4. Suction as directed for tracheal suctioning.				
5. Allow patient to rest before continuing with care.				
Cleaning the tracheostomy tube				
1. Assess patient.				
2. Wash your hands.				
3. Obtain tracheostomy care kit or gather following supplies: a. Sterile gloves (if new tracheostomy)				
b. Sterile gauze squares				
c. Cleansing solution				
d. Basin				
e. Tracheostomy brush, pipe cleaners, or swabs				
f. Sterile water				
4. Explain procedure to patient.				
5. Provide means of communication.				
6. Position patient in mid-Fowler's.				
7. Set up supplies.				

	Unsatisfactory	Needs more practice	Satisfactory	Comments
8. Put on sterile gloves if necessary.				
9. To clean:				
a. Cannula-type tracheostomy tube				
(1) Holding outer tube firmly in place, turn lock clockwise to release.				
(2) Remove inner cannula by moving it toward you.				
(3) Place cannula in basin.				
(4) Immerse in cleansing solution.				
(5) Remove remaining crustations on inner lumen with brush, pipe cleaners, or swabs.				
(6) Rinse thoroughly in cold sterile water.				
(7) Dry with sterile gauze or towel.				
(8) Remove any lint.				
(9) Remove any mucus from inside outer tube with swab.				
(10) Hold outer tube and replace clean inner cannula.				
(11) Fasten lock.				
(12) Test to make sure inner cannula is secure.				
b. Plastic or rubber-type tracheostomy tube				
(1) Clean inner surface of tube with pipe cleaner or lintless swabs moistened with sterile normal saline.				
(2) Remove any moisture with dry swabs.				
10. Dispose of equipment.				
11. Wash your hands.				
12. Record procedure.				

Dressing the tracheostomy	Unsatisfactory	Needs more practice	Satisfactory	Comments
1. Assess patient.				
2. Wash your hands.				
3. Gather necessary equipment. a. Gauze squares				
b. Twill tape ties				
c. Scissors				
d. Swabs				
e. Cleansing solution.				
f. Oral-care equipment				
4. Remove old dressing and discard.				
5. With moistened swabs, clean around incision.				
6. Observe for redness or irritation.				
7. Prepare dressing.				
8. With assistant holding tube (if possible), cut holding tape, remove, and discard.				
9. Still holding tube in place, slip new dressing around underlip of tube.				
10. Thread twill tape through flanges of tube and tie to side.				
11. Check position of tube and tautness of tape.				
12. Perform oral care.				
13. Dispose of equipment.				
14. Wash your hands.				
15. Record procedure and observations.				

QUIZ

Multiple-Choice Questions

_____ 1. The patient with a tracheostomy cannot talk because

    a. he or she is too ill.
    b. air does not reach the vocal cords.
    c. there is swelling of the trachea.
    d. of the presence of secretions.

_____ 2. Emergency equipment that should always be kept at the bedside of a tracheostomy patient includes: (1) tape; (2) clamp; (3) tracheostomy tube; (4) oxygen.

    a. 2 and 3
    b. 1, 2, and 3
    c. 2, 3, and 4
    d. All of the above

_____ 3. The primary reason for periodically deflating a cuffed tracheostomy tube is to

    a. promote the patient's comfort.
    b. adjust the position of the tube.
    c. remove and clean the tube.
    d. prevent tissue necrosis.

_____ 4. When performing shallow tracheal suctioning, how far should the catheter be inserted?

    a. 1 inch
    b. 3 inches
    c. 5 inches
    d. 8 inches

_____ 5. To suction the right bronchus, to which side should the patient's head be turned?

    a. Same
    b. Opposite
    c. First one side, then the other
    d. It doesn't matter.

_____ 6. When performing bronchial suctioning, the catheter may be inserted as deeply as

    a. 3 inches.
    b. 5 inches.
    c. 10 inches.
    d. 15 inches.

_____ 7. Which of the following solutions might be used to clean a tracheostomy
              tube? (1) alcohol; (2) hydrogen peroxide; (3) Betadine; (4) normal saline

              a. 3 and 4
              b. 2 and 4
              c. 1, 2, and 4
              d. All of the above

_____ 8. The primary reason for tying the tapes holding the tracheostomy in place
              loosely enough is to prevent

              a. undue pressure that could cause respiratory obstruction.
              b. skin irritation.
              c. circulatory impairment.
              d. discomfort.

_____ 9. The greatest threat to the patient with a tracheostomy is the danger of

              a. hemorrhaging.
              b. pneumonia.
              c. infection.
              d. asphyxiation.

Module 43 Administering Oral Medications

MAIN OBJECTIVE

To prepare and administer oral medications safely to patients.

RATIONALE

One of the nurse's most routine and yet most critical responsibilities is the preparation and administration of medications; and oral medications comprise the bulk of medications administered. The basic procedures used can be applied not only to the administration of oral medications, but to the administration of medications by other routes as well.

The responsibility extends beyond preparation and administration. The nurse must know how medicines act, usual dosage, desired effects, and side effects, so that he or she can evaluate the effectiveness of medication and recognize adverse effects when they occur. You will acquire this knowledge gradually as you study pharmacology and care for patients with varying problems.

PREREQUISITES

1. Successful completion of the following modules:

   VOLUME 1
   Assessment
   Charting
   Medical Asepsis

2. Before giving medications, you must have a satisfactory level of proficiency in the mathematics of dosages and solutions. A math quiz is included here, on the next page. If you are not able to answer at least 11 of the 14 items correctly, plan to complete one of the many programmed instruction units available on the mathematics of dosages and solutions. Consult your instructor for guidance.

SELF-TEST: MATHEMATICS OF DOSAGES AND SOLUTIONS

Directions: Read each problem carefully. Show your work beneath the
questions and place your answers in the right-hand column.

1. Pronestyl 500 mg is ordered q.i.d. for Mr. Jones. How many 250-mg
tablets will be needed for a 5-day supply?

   q.i.d = 4×d   4 tab/day   ×5
                        ×2 tabs/dose   ‾‾
                        ‾‾   40
                        8

   40

2. To give codeine phosphate gr 1/2 from tablets gr 1/6, how many tablets
should you use?

   1/2   3/6
   1/6   1/6

   3 tabs

3. How many grams are in 250 mg?

   $\frac{1,000 mg}{1 gm} = \frac{250 mg}{x}$ 1000√250 0.25

   1000x = 250

   0.25 gm

4. How many milliliters are in 1.5 oz?

   1.5   1 oz   1.5 oz
   30   ‾‾‾‾ = ‾‾‾‾‾   45
   45   30 ml   x

   45 ml

5. You are to prepare Streptomycin sulfate for injection. On hand is a vial
containing 1.0 gm dry drug. The label reads: "Add 9.2 ml diluent to
yield 10.0 ml solution." Each milliliter will contain how many milligrams
of the drug?

6. You are to administer 30 units of U-100 insulin at 7:30 a.m. When you
prepare the insulin, what will your dosage be in milliliters?

   $\frac{30u}{x ml} = \frac{100u}{1 ml}$ 100x = 30   100√30   0.30

   .30 ml

7. How many minims of medication should be given to administer 25 mg
of a medication marked "75 mg = 1 ml"?

8. The order for intravenous fluid reads: "1,000 ml 5% glucose in water to
run 10 hours." Determine the number of drops per minute the IV should
run if the administration set delivers 15 gtt/ml.

   ml/hr
   drops/hr
   drops/min

   $\frac{1000 ml}{10 hr}$ $\frac{100 ml}{x drops} = \frac{1 ml}{15 drops}$ 60√1500   25

   100 ml/hr   x = 1500   120
                                      ‾‾‾
                                      300

   25 gtt/min

9. If the centigrade temperature is 40° C, what is the Fahrenheit reading?

_____   _____

10. If the adult dose of a medication is 500 mg, is the pediatric dose more likely to be 200 mg or 800 mg?

_____   *200 mg*

11. Name two factors that are commonly used to calculate pediatric dosage.

_____   a. *Weight*

b. *age*

12. A patient is given 500 ml 10% glucose solution IV. How many calories does the patient receive?

_____   _____

13. How much morphine sulfate should a 6-month-old infant receive if the adult dosage of morphine sulfate is 20 mg?

_____   _____

14. How much aspirin should a 3-year-old child receive if the adult dosage of aspirin is 10 grains?

_____   _____

Key

1. 40 tabs
2. 3 tabs
3. 0.25 gm
4. 45 ml
5. 100 mg
6. 0.30 ml
7. 5 min
8. 25 gtt/min

9. 104° F
10. 200 mg
11. a. Age
    b. Weight
12. 200 calories
13. 0.8 mg
14. 2 grains

SPECIFIC LEARNING OBJECTIVES

	Know Facts and Principles	Apply Facts and Principles	Demonstrate Ability	Evaluate Performance
1. Abbreviations	Know meanings of abbreviations listed on page 281	Correctly interpret medication orders that include abbreviations	Correctly use and interpret abbreviations used in preparation and administration of medications	Evaluate own performance with instructor
2. Equivalencies	Know equivalencies listed on page 282	Given problems, work out equivalencies in apothecary, metric, and household systems	In the clinical situation, correctly work out problems involving equivalencies under supervision	Evaluate own performance with instructor
3. Administration methods	State two broad methods of administering medication. Discuss at least two different methods of administering medications using individual medication supplies.	Outline medication administration procedure used in assigned facility	Correctly carry out medication administration procedure used in assigned facility with supervision	Evaluate own performance with instructor using Performance Checklist and facility procedure
4. Safety and accuracy	State three "checks" and five "rights"		Use three checks and five rights consistently	Evaluate own performance with instructor
5. Giving oral medications	Know procedure for preparation and administration of oral medication	Adapt steps of procedures to those used in assigned facility	Prepare and administer oral medication according to procedures in assigned facility	Evaluate own performance with instructor
6. Charting	Know information to be charted regarding medications administered	Identify charting method used in assigned facility	Correctly chart medications administered according to method used in assigned facility	Evaluate own performance with instructor

LEARNING ACTIVITIES

1. Review the Specific Learning Objectives.
2. Read the section on administering medications in Ellis and Nowlis, *Nursing: A Human Needs Approach,* or comparable material in another textbook.
3. Look up the module vocabulary terms in the glossary.
4. Read through the module.
5. Study the abbreviations and equivalencies on pages 281 and 282.
6. In the practice setting:
   a. Identify
      (1) A paper soufflé cup
      (2) A calibrated medicine glass (usually made of glass or plastic, but can be made of heavy waxed paper)
      (3) A medicine tray or cart
   b. Review the medication administration method used in your facility.
   c. Go through the procedure step by step referring to the Performance Checklist as necessary. Use the appropriate method for your facility.
   d. When you feel you can remember the procedure, ask your instructor to check your performance.
7. In the clinical setting:
   a. Consult with your clinical instructor for an opportunity to give medications with supervision.

VOCABULARY

capsule
dose
five rights
meniscus
route
stock drugs
tablet
three checks
unit dose

ADMINISTERING ORAL MEDICATIONS

Systems of Administration

In any health care facility, medications are administered according to a procedure defined by that facility. First, the procedure is usually based on one of two supply systems. *Stock supply* refers to drugs that are kept on the unit in fairly large containers and from which the medication orders for all patients on the unit are taken. *Individual patient supplies* are currently used more commonly. These consist of enough medication for a single occasion, for one shift, for an entire day, or for an undefined period of time. Second, the procedure is based on a recording system, which is a way of keeping track of the medications ordered and those that have or have not been given.

MEDICATION CARDS

Perhaps the oldest and still most widely used procedural method is that of using a small card on which are recorded the patient's name, room number, medication, dose, and route. The nurse administering the medications checks the card against a permanent record of all medications ordered, such as the Kardex. Then, using the cards as a guide, the nurse prepares and administers the medications. Recording is done on the patient's chart.

CENTRAL MEDICATION RECORDS

In some health care facilities, a large notebook, or Kardex, containing sheets listing the medications for each patient is used, both as a permanent record and as a guide as the medications are prepared and administered. It is often used for recording the administration as well. In these cases, the physician's order sheet is used as a safety check.

COMMERCIAL MEDICATION SYSTEMS

Commercially produced systems are also available to assist in the safe administration of medications. One is the Brewer system,

which consists of a large machine that contains medications commonly used on a given unit; a cart, including individual drawers for the medications of each patient; and a special recording form.

PHARMACY SYSTEMS

In recent years, pharmacy personnel have begun to play a larger role in the administration of medications to patients. This system is quite widely used, especially in large health care facilities, and is known as the *unit-dose system.* Although it can vary substantially in procedure from one facility to another, basically it consists of the provision by pharmacy personnel of prepackaged and prelabeled individual doses of medications for patients. The medications are administered by nursing personnel on the nursing unit or by nursing or pharmacy personnel from the pharmacy. Studies have shown that the unit-dose system provides for greater accuracy and convenience (especially in terms of time saved).

Safety and Accuracy

THE THREE CHECKS

Whatever system is used, there are certain basic considerations that always apply. The first of these is the *three checks:* the name and the dosage of the medication are checked (from the label) against that ordered (1) as the medication is taken off the shelf or out of the drawer, (2) before it is opened, and (3) before it is replaced. In the case of the unit-dose system, the three checks can be accomplished by reading the label as the individual prepackaged medication is taken from a drawer, before it is opened, and from the empty package after it has been poured.

THE FIVE RIGHTS

Another of the considerations basic to the administration of medication is the *five rights.* They serve as a guide for remembering (1) the right drug, (2) in the right dose, (3) by the right route, (4) to the right patient, and (5) at the right time. This is certainly not *all* the nurse has to know, but fewer medication errors would be made if the five rights were consistently considered.

The right drug, the right dose, the right route, and the right time are ensured by following the three checks. To ensure that you have the right patient, the patient must be carefully identified. This is usually accomplished by checking the identification band given the patient on admission and/or by asking his or her name prior to giving the medication. In the case of confused or unconscious patients, obviously the former method is necessary.

Stay with the patient until all medications have been swallowed. It is *not* appropriate to leave medications at the bedside for patients to take on their own unless so ordered by the physician. Among the medications commonly left at the bedside are antacids and nitroglycerin, although medications that patients have been taking regularly at home may also be their responsibility.

The nurse who prepares a given medication should administer it. Stated another way, you should administer *only* those drugs that you prepared. Only the person who prepared the drug actually knows what it is and what strength or dosage it is, unless it is still in the unit-dose packaging.

Measuring Dosage

The measurement of liquid medications is somewhat of a special procedure. The medicine glass or cup must be read at eye level, with the thumbnail placed at the bottom of the meniscus at the correct level on the medicine glass, to ensure accuracy.

Oral Medication Procedure

1. Obtain cards, Kardex, notebook, or other source of list of medications a patient is to receive. This will vary with the facility.
2. Check the medications listed against the physician's or nurse's orders (in some facilities nurses can write orders for certain medications, such as laxatives). The procedure in your facility

COMMON ABBREVIATIONS

PO	by mouth
a.c.	before meals
p.c.	after meals
q.d.	every day
q.o.d.	every other day
b.i.d.	twice a day
t.i.d.	three times a day
q.i.d.	four times a day
stat	immediately
$\bar{c}$	with
$\bar{s}$	without
$\bar{ss}$	one half
h.s.	at bedtime
p.r.n.	as needed
q.h.	every hour
q.2h.	every two hours

Also see the Table of Equivalencies, page 281.

may include a double-check system, in which case it may not always be necessary to check against the order sheet. In this procedure, as well as in all others, know the policy at *your facility.* Check the patient's name and room number, the name of the medication, the dosage, the route of administration, and the time(s) to be given.
3. Wash your hands.
4. Gather the equipment. You will need soufflé cups for tablets and capsules and medicine cups (calibrated) for liquids.
5. Read the name of the medication to be given from the record.
6. Check the label on the medication and take that medication from the shelf or drawer.
7. Check the label again, before pouring.
8. Remove the correct amount of medication for the individual dose to be given at this time.
   a. For a tablet or capsule (not prepackaged):
      (1) Pour from the bottle into the bottle cap until you have the correct dosage.
      (2) Transfer to the soufflé cup.

TABLE OF EQUIVALENCIES

1. Metric doses and apothecaries' equivalents

Liquid

Metric	Approximate apothecaries' equivalents
1,000 ml	1 quart
500 ml	1 pint
250 ml	8 fluidounces
30 ml	1 fluidounce
15 ml	4 fluidrams
5 ml	1 fluidrams
1 ml	15 minims
0.06 ml	1 minim

Solid

Metric	Approximate apothecaries' equivalents
30 gm	1 ounce
15 gm	4 drams
4 gm	60 grains (1 dram)
1 gm	15 grains
0.5 gm	7½ grains
60 mg	1 grain
30 mg	1/2 grain
15 mg	1/4 grain
10 mg	1/6 grain
8 mg	1/8 grain
1 mg	1/60 grain
0.6 mg	1/100 grain
0.4 mg	1/150 grain
0.3 mg	1/200 grain
0.2 mg	1/300 grain
0.1 mg	1/600 grain

2. Approximate household measures

1 teaspoonful	1 fl dr	4–5 ml
1 tablespoonful	½ fl oz	15 or 16 ml
1 jigger	1½ fl oz	45 ml
1 cup	8 fl oz	240 ml

3. Prescription abbreviations

gr	grain or grains
gtt*	drops
ʒ	dram
℥	ounce
a̅a̅	equal parts
s̅s̅	one half
cc**	cubic centimeter
gm	gram
mg	milligram
mcg	microgram
ml	milliliter
mEq	millequivalent
min	minim

*Gutta(e)
**Although technically not exactly equivalent, ml and cc are often used interchangeably.

b. For a liquid:
(1) Place the cap upside-down on the countertop, so as not to contaminate it.
(2) With the medicine cup at eye level, pour the liquid to the desired level in the cup, using the bottom of the concave meniscus as your guide.

Generally all pills to be given to the same patient at the same time can be placed in one container. However, if the administration of a medication is contingent on a pulse or blood pressure measurement, keep that medication separate from the others, and make the measurement immediately after identifying the patient.

9. Return the bottle to the shelf. Check the label one last time, being sure to read it carefully.
10. Place the medication on the tray or cart.
11. Place a medication card or label on the poured medication for identification.
12. Approach and identify the patient.

13. Explain what you are going to do and, if appropriate, what the medication is for and how it works. The information should be simple and presented in language easily understood by the patient. Explain any specific needs related to the drug, such as increased fluid intake.

14. Give the patient a glass of fresh water. (You may have to change the water in the bedside pitcher.) If the medication has an unpleasant flavor, you can give juice with it instead of water, so long as this is not contrary to the patient's diet order or the drug manufacturer's directions. If the patient has a favorite juice, indicate it on his or her record, so that the next nurse to administer the medication will know and will not have to ask the patient again.

15. Watch the patient take the medication. If you are not certain it has been swallowed, or if there seems to be a problem with swallowing, have the patient open his or her mouth and look inside to see if the medication is still there. If the patient is unable to swallow a tablet or capsule, give it in a vehicle, such as applesauce or jelly. It is common practice to crush tablets (except those with enteric coating) and to empty the contents from capsules to mix with the vehicle. Whole pills or capsules are sometimes given in a teaspoon of jelly.

16. Leave the patient in a comfortable position.

17. Discard the medication container if it is disposable. If not, rinse it out and replace it on the tray or cart for reprocessing.

18. Wash your hands.

19. Indicate on the medication record that the medication was given. Again, the exact method for doing this will vary with the facility. Usually, the name of the medication, the dosage, the route of administration, the time, and your signature (with abbreviation indicating your position) are included. Initials are often used to indicate that an individual medication has been given, but a full signature is usually required on the medication record at least once during each shift.

If for some reason the medication is *not* given (for example, it may be held at the nurse's discretion or refused by the patient), indicate this on the medication record. In many facilities, this is indicated by a circle around the time that it should have been given along with an explanation in the nurses' notes. When the physician is notified regarding a medication not given, this should also be noted on the chart.

20. Go on to the next patient or, if you are finished, return to the medication area.

21. Replace any extra supplies and tidy the area.

22. Return to the patient 20 to 30 minutes after administering the medication to check its effects.

PERFORMANCE CHECKLIST

	Unsatisfactory	Needs more practice	Satisfactory	Comments
1. Obtain list of medications for patient.				
2. Check against order sheet.				
3. Wash your hands.				
4. Gather necessary equipment.				
5. Read name of medication from record.				
6. Check label and take medication from shelf or drawer.				
7. Check label a second time.				
8. a. For tablets or capsules, pour into bottle cap and transfer to soufflé cup unless prepackaged.				
b. For liquid, place cap upside-down on counter and pour medication at eye level.				
9. Return bottle to shelf and check label a third time.				
10. Place medication on tray.				
11. Label medication.				
12. Take to bedside and identify patient.				
13. Explain to patient as appropriate.				
14. Give medication to patient, along with water or juice, and assist as appropriate.				
15. Watch to be sure patient has swallowed medication.				
16. Leave patient in comfortable position.				
17. Discard medication container.				
18. Wash your hands.				
19. Chart whether medication was taken, according to facility's procedure.				
20. Go on to next patient or return to medication area.				
21. Replace extra supplies and tidy area.				
22. Return to patient 20 to 30 minutes later to check for effect.				

QUIZ

Short-Answer Questions

1. Medication procedures are usually based on the use of one or two general supply methods. Name these two methods.

    a. _____

    b. _____

2. At what times does the nurse check the name and dosages of the medication against that ordered when using the three checks?

    a. _____

    b. _____

    c. _____

3. List the five rights.

    a. _____

    b. _____

    c. _____

    d. _____

    e. _____

4. Name two methods of identifying the patient prior to giving medications.

    a. _____

    b. _____

5. 1 mg = _____ grains

6. 1 ℥ = _____ ml

7. 1 ml = _____ min

8. 5 ml = _____ ℥

9. The medication ordered is gr v; the tablets available are marked in milligrams. How many milligrams are equivalent to 5 grains? _____

10. The order is 10 ml liquid medication. The patient must take this medication at home. How many teaspoons will this be? _____

Multiple-Choice Questions

_____ 11. Mrs. Brown is to receive a medication PO q.i.d. This means

        a. by mouth every other day.
        b. before meals every day.
        c. after meals every day.
        d. by mouth four times a day.

_____ 12. Mr. Green is to receive medication c̄ meals. This means

        a. before meals.
        b. after meals.
        c. with meals.
        d. none of the above.

_____ 13. When pouring a liquid medication, you should measure from

        a. the top edge of the meniscus.
        b. the bottom of the meniscus.
        c. neither of these.
        d. It makes no difference.

Module 44 Administering Topical Medications

MAIN OBJECTIVE

To prepare and correctly administer topical medications using ophthalmic, otic, nasal, dermatological, vaginal, and rectal routes.

RATIONALE

Drugs can be administered by a variety of routes, depending on the patient's condition, the drug itself, and the desired effect. The nurse must be able to prepare and administer drugs correctly using these various routes, keeping in mind the basic concepts of safe administration as well as those related to these special routes. The nurse's knowledge of the anatomy and physiology related to the particular organ being treated, and of the actions, usual dosage, desired effects, and side effects of the particular drug being administered, is imperative for safe practice.

PREREQUISITES

1. Successful completion of the following modules:

    VOLUME 1
    Assessment
    Charting

    VOLUME 2
    Medical Asepsis
    Sterile Technique
    Irrigations
    Administering Oral Medications

2. A review of the anatomy and physiology of the eye, ear, nose, skin, vagina, and rectum

SPECIFIC LEARNING OBJECTIVES

	Know Facts and Principles	Apply Facts and Principles	Demonstrate Ability	Evaluate Performance
1. Ophthalmic medications *a. Technique*	State whether sterile technique or medical asepsis is used	Given a patient situation and medication order, determine whether sterile technique is required.	Use sterile technique or medical asepsis when administering eye medication.	Evaluate own performance with instructor
b. Rationale	Describe four reasons why patient might be receiving eye medication	Given a patient situation, identify why patient might be receiving eye medication.	In the clinical setting, identify reason for eye medication.	Evaluate own performance with instructor
c. Positioning	Describe positioning of patient for instillation of eye medication.		In the clinical setting, correctly position patient.	Evaluate own performance with instructor
d. Procedure	Describe how to administer eyedrops and ointments.		Correctly instill eyedrops and ointments.	Evaluate with instructor using Performance Checklist
2. Otic medications *a. Technique*	State when sterile technique is used and when medical asepsis is appropriate.	Given a patient situation, identify whether to use sterile technique or medical asepsis.	Use correct technique when administering otic medications	Evaluate own performance with instructor
b. Positioning	Describe positioning of adult and pediatric patient for instillation of eardrops, including position of auricle.	Given a patient situation, select appropriate positioning for patient.	In the clinical setting, correctly position adult and pediatric patients to receive eardrops.	Evaluate own performance with instructor
c. Procedure	Describe how to administer eardrops. State how long patient should remain on his or her side after administration of eardrops.		Correctly instill eardrops. Instruct patients to remain on side five to ten minutes after administration of eardrops.	Evaluate with instructor using Performance Checklist

3. Nasal medications a. Technique	State whether sterile technique or medical asepsis is used	Given a patient situation and medication order, determine whether sterile technique is required	In the clinical setting, use careful asepsis when administering nasal medications	Evaluate own performance with instructor
b. Rationale	Know most common reason for administration of nasal medication. State rationale for administration of water-soluble nasal medications.		In the clinical setting, check to be sure nasal medications are water-soluble	
c. Positioning	Describe positioning of patients to receive nasal medications, including Proetz and Parkinson positions.	Given a patient situation, identify appropriate position for patient	In the clinical setting, correctly position patient	Evaluate own performance with instructor
d. Procedure	Describe how to administer nosedrops and nasal sprays. State how long patient should remain in position after nosedrops have been instilled.		Correctly administer nosedrops and nasal sprays. In the clinical setting, instruct patients to remain as positioned for five minutes after administration of nosedrops	Evaluate with instructor using Performance Checklist
4. Dermatological medications a. Rationale	State rationale for use of lotions, ointments, liniments, and powders.	Given a patient situation, state preparation that might be used.		
b. Procedure	State how to apply medications to skin.	Given a patient situation, describe method of applying medication to skin.	Correctly apply medication to patient's skin	Evaluate own performance with instructor

	Know Facts and Principles	Apply Facts and Principles	Demonstrate Ability	Evaluate Performance
5. *Vaginal medications* a. *Positioning* b. *Procedures*	List methods of instilling vaginal medications State how long patient should remain quiet after medicated douche		Correctly administer vaginal medications Instruct patient to remain quiet for 20 minutes following douche	Evaluate with instructor using Performance Checklist
6. *Rectal medications* a. *Positioning* b. *Rationale*	State most common form of rectal medication. State rationale for administration of retention enema after bowel movement.			Evaluate with instructor using Performance Checklist
c. *Procedures*	Describe how to administer rectal suppository. State how long patient should remain quiet after suppository insertion.		Correctly administer rectal medication by suppository. Instruct patient to remain quiet for 20 minutes following administration of suppository. Administer retention enema after patient has had bowel movement.	Evaluate own performance with instructor
7. *Charting*	State items to be included in charting for each route discussed	Given a patient situation, do sample charting for medication discussed	In the clinical setting, correctly chart ophthalmic, otic, nasal, dermatological, vaginal, and rectal medications	Evaluate own performance with instructor

LEARNING ACTIVITIES

1. Review the Specific Learning Objectives.
2. Read the section on administering drug therapy in Ellis and Nowlis, *Nursing: A Human Needs Approach,* or comparable material in another textbook.
3. Look up the module vocabulary terms in the glossary.
4. Read through the module.
5. Using a partner for a patient, in the practice setting:
   a. Simulate the instillation of eyedrops. If they are available, your instructor may want you to use Lytears or a similar solution.
   b. Simulate the instillation of eardrops in the ear of an adult. Do not use any actual drops.
   c. Simulate the instillation of nosedrops and nasal sprays. Do not use any actual drops or sprays. Position your partner appropriately for the administration of a nasal spray and in the three positions described for nose-drops.
   d. Practice the explanation and positioning for administration of a vaginal cream. Teach your "patient" self-administration.
   e. Practice the explanation and positioning for administration of a rectal suppository.
   f. Change roles with your partner and repeat steps a–e.
   g. Evaluate one another's performance.
6. In the clinical setting:
   a. Seek out opportunities to administer topical medication with supervision.

VOCABULARY

aspiration pneumonia
auricle
canthus
conjunctival sac
dermatological
dorsal recumbent position
douche
ethmoid sinus
instillation
liniment
local
lotion
ocular
ointment
ophthalmic
otic
rectal
Sim's position
sphenoid sinus
suppository
systemic
topical
tympanic membrane
vaginal

ADMINISTERING TOPICAL MEDICATIONS

All of the topical medications discussed in this module will be administered using the first 13 steps of the Oral Medication Procedure (Module 43). Equipment needed and exact method of administration will vary according to the medication. Directions will usually be given by the physician or be found in a package insert.

Ophthalmic Medications

The administration of eyedrops or ocular ointments is a sterile procedure, which is done to soothe irritated tissue, to dilate or constrict the pupil, to treat eye disease, or to provide anesthesia. In addition to the five rights discussed in Module 43, you must be certain that you have the "right" (correct) eye.

1. Wash your hands immediately before administering the eye medication.
2. Explain to the patient what you plan to do and what he or she can do to help.
3. Clean the eyelid(s) and lashes. Use a sterile cotton ball soaked in sterile normal saline. Move from inner canthus to outer canthus, using each cotton ball for only one wipe.
4. Have the patient turn his or her head slightly to the side (away from the eye being medicated), and tip it slightly backward. This can be done with the patient lying in bed or sitting in a chair.
5. Have the patient look up.
6. Rest your dominant hand (holding the medication) on the patient's forehead, to avoid poking the patient in the eye. Use your other hand to pull down on the lower lid of the eye to be medicated, exposing the lower conjunctival sac. Exert gentle pressure with the hand resting on the patient's face, holding a cotton ball or 2 x 2 gauze to catch any excess medication. (See Figure 44.1.)

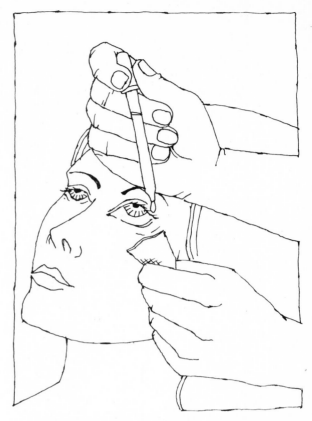

FIGURE 44.1   ADMINISTERING EYEDROPS

7. Administer medication.
   a. Eyedrops:
      (1) Draw only as much solution into the dropper as you will need because unused solution is never returned to the medication bottle.
      (2) Once you have the medication in the dropper, hold the bulb end up, so the medication cannot run up into the bulb. It is possible for the solution to become contaminated with particulate matter from the rubber bulb. In fact, many eye medications are now packaged in a flexible plastic container with an opening designed to deliver the drops.
      (3) Holding the eyedropper close to but not touching the eye, drop the designated number of drops into the middle of the exposed conjunctival sac.

b. Ointment:
   (1) Squeeze out a ribbon of medication long enough for the entire lower conjunctival sac, moving from inner canthus to outer canthus.
   (2) Discontinue the ribbon by twisting the tube.
   (3) Wipe any excess ointment from the tube with sterile gauze.

8. Ask the patient to close the eye gently. If the eye is squeezed tightly shut, the ointment or drops are pushed out. If eyedrops were instilled, have the patient move the eyeball around while it is closed to help disperse the medication. If ointment was used, have the patient keep the eye closed a full minute following the instillation to allow the medication to melt.

9. Some medications (among them Atropine) have systemic effects if allowed to pass into the lacrimal system and from there be absorbed into the general circulatory system. To prevent this, gently press the inner angle of the eye against the nose.

10. Make the patient comfortable.

11. Dispose of the equipment.

12. Wash your hands.

13. Record as you would for oral medication, step 19, page 283, including which eye was treated.

Otic Medications

The administration of medication to the ear is a clean procedure, except when the tympanic membrane is not intact, in which case sterile technique is used. Medication can be introduced into the ear to soften wax, to relieve pain, or to treat disease. It is imperative that you have the correct ear in addition to the other five rights.

1. Wash your hands.
2. Explain to the patient what you plan to do and what he or she can do to help.
3. Warm the medication to be instilled to body temperature by holding the container in your hand for a short time or by placing the container in warm water.

4. If you are using a glass dropper, check to be sure it is not rough on the end. In the case of an uncooperative adult patient or a pediatric patient, you may want to attach a flexible rubber tip to prevent injury to the patient in the event of sudden movement. Fill the dropper.

5. Have the patient lie on the opposite side of the ear being medicated.

6. Pull gently upward and backward on the top of the ear auricle (Figure 44.2) in order to straighten the canal. This allows the medication to reach all parts of the canal. In the infant and small child (under three), the canal is almost straight,

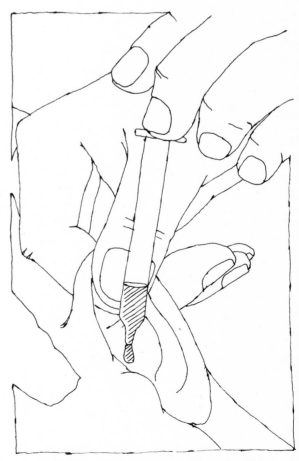

FIGURE 44.2   ADMINISTERING EARDROPS TO AN ADULT

so pull the top of the ear downward and backward.

7. Instill the correct number of drops, directing them toward the side of the ear canal.
8. Have the patient remain on his or her side for five to ten minutes after the drops have been instilled, to allow maximum contact with the canal.
9. Insert cotton loosely into the canal *only* if ordered. (This is occasionally ordered to keep the medication in contact with the canal and to prevent its running out.) Never pack the ear tightly.
10. Make the patient comfortable.
11. Dispose of the equipment.
12. Wash your hands.
13. Record as you would for oral medication, step 19, page 283, including which ear was treated.

Nasal Medications

Nasal medication is often given in the form of nosedrops and is usually ordered to relieve nasal congestion. Nosedrops and nasal sprays are usually water-soluble because of the danger of aspiration pneumonia with oil-based solutions. The administration of nasal medication is not a sterile procedure, but careful medical asepsis should be practiced because of the close and direct connection between the nose and the sinuses.

1. Wash your hands.
2. Explain to the patient what you plan to do and what he or she can do to help.
3. Have the patient clear his or her nasal passages, using a tissue and blowing gently.
4. Position the patient according to the area you want to medicate.
   a. Dropper:
      (1) *The opening of the eustachian tube* The patient should lie flat on his or her back.
      (2) *The ethmoid and sphenoid sinuses* The patient should be in the Proetz position, with head hanging straight back over the edge of the bed (Figure 44.3).

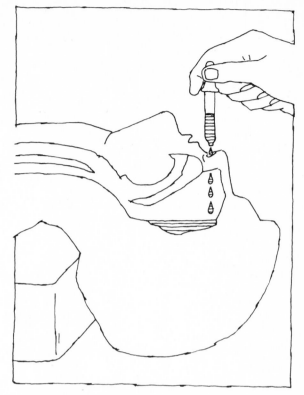

FIGURE 44.3   PROETZ POSITION FOR ADMINISTERING NOSEDROPS

      (3) *The frontal and maxillary sinuses* The patient should be in the Parkinson position, with head slightly over the edge of the bed and turned toward the affected side (Figure 44.4).
   When the patient is positioned with the head hanging over the side of the bed, you should help support the head with one hand to prevent strain on the neck muscles.
   b. Nasal spray: Position patient in chair with head tilted back.
5. Administer medication.
   a. Dropper:
      (1) Draw in sufficient medication for both nostrils.
      (2) With the tip of the dropper about 1/3 inch inside the nostril, instill the number of drops ordered into each side. Be careful not to touch the side of the nostrils, which could cause the patient to sneeze.

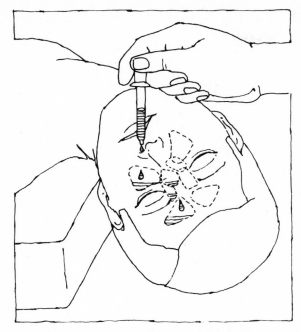

FIGURE 44.4   PARKINSON POSITION FOR
ADMINISTERING NOSEDROPS

    (3) Have the patient remain as po-
        sitioned for five minutes after
        the medication has been in-
        stilled.
  b. Nasal spray:
    (1) As you spray the medication
        into one nostril, have the patient
        hold the other one shut.
    (2) Ask the patient to inhale as the
        spray is being administered.
    (3) Repeat on the other nostril.
    (4) Keep the patient's head back for
        one or two minutes.
    Patients often administer their own
    nasal sprays.
6. Make the patient comfortable.
7. Dispose of the equipment.
8. Wash your hands.
9. Record as you would for oral medica-
    tion, step 19, page 283.

Dermatological Medications

Medications applied to the skin are often in
the form of lotions, ointments, or liniments,
and occasionally powders. *Lotions* protect,
soften, soothe, and/or provide relief from
itching. *Ointments* have an oil base, and
body heat causes them to melt after application. Medications that fight infection or
soothe inflamed tissues often come in ointment form. If obtained from a stock jar,
remove the ointment with a sterile tongue
blade. Discard any excess; do not return it
to the jar. *Liniments,* which are applied by
rubbing, are used to provide relief from
tight aching muscles. *Powders* are used for
their soothing drying action. The procedure
requires sterile technique if the application
is on an open or infected area.

1. Wash your hands.
2. Explain to the patient what you plan to
    do and what he or she can do to help.
    In some situations, the patient can be
    taught to apply the medication to his or
    her own skin, especially when the area
    to be treated is in easy view and reach.
3. Provide for the patient's privacy if
    necessary.
4. Provide for adequate lighting.
5. Position the patient so that the area to
    be treated is accessible. In some cases
    you may need assistance, for example,
    with the support of a limb.
6. Be sure the area to be treated is clean.
    Skin medications are often applied im-
    mediately after a bath or shower.
7. Apply the medication to the area to be
    treated. Using gloves wastes less medi-
    cation and is less irritating than using
    gauze. Clean gloves should be worn to
    apply any topical medication that can
    be absorbed through the skin, like a
    steroid cream. In situations in which
    sterile technique must be maintained,
    wear sterile gloves or apply the ma-
    terial with a sterile tongue blade or
    applicator. Apply the medication in
    thin even layers unless otherwise or-
    dered. To apply powder, spread it
    lightly and evenly, taking care not to
    let it accumulate between skin folds.
    Avoid shaking the powder directly
    over the patient; put it in your own
    hand first, and then apply it to the
    patient. Instruct the patient to turn his
    or her head away to prevent inhalation.

8. Use a light dressing to cover the area *only* if ordered by the physician. Some medications should not be covered.
9. Return the patient to a position of comfort.
10. Dispose of equipment.
11. Wash your hands.
12. Record as you would for oral medication, step 19, page 283, including the area treated and the appearance of the area before treatment.

Vaginal Medications

Several vehicles are used for the instillation of vaginal medications. These include creams, suppositories, and douche. Medical asepsis is used. Be especially alert to the patient's feelings of embarrassment.

1. Wash your hands.
2. Explain to the patient what you plan to do and what she can do to help.
3. Provide for the patient's privacy. Close the bed curtains.
4. Provide for lighting.
5. Position the patient in the dorsal recumbent position with knees elevated and spread as for catheterization (see Module 39). Sim's position can also be used.
6. Drape the patient.
7. Instill the medication.
   a. Vaginal creams: introduce creams with a narrow tubular *applicator* that has a plunger attached.
   b. Suppositories: introduce suppositories with a *gloved* and *lubricated* finger.
   c. Douche:
      (1) Obtain the equipment and follow the procedure for vaginal irrigation in Module 38, page 202.
      (2) Have the patient remain quiet for 20 minutes following the douche to allow the medication to reach all surfaces.

In some instances, a hospitalized patient can be taught to give vaginal medications to herself.

8. Return the patient to a position of comfort.
9. Care for the equipment.
10. Wash your hands.
11. Record as you would for oral medications, step 19, page 283.

Rectal Medications

Rectal medications are usually given for their local effect, but some—for example, aspirin suppositories— are given for systemic effect. Suppositories are the most commonly used rectal medication, although creams and retention enemas can also be used. Medical asepsis is appropriate for all.

1. Wash your hands.
2. Explain to the patient what you plan to do and what he or she can do to help.
3. Provide for the patient's privacy.
4. Provide adequate lighting.
5. Position the patient. Most commonly, the patient should be in the side-lying position. If for some reason this is difficult for the patient, have him or her assume the dorsal recumbent position, with the knees flexed.
6. Drape the patient.
7. Instill the medication.
   a. Suppository:
      (1) Using a *gloved lubricated* finger, insert the *suppository* beyond the internal sphincter.
      (2) Ask the patient to breathe in and out through the mouth while you are inserting the suppository. This helps relax the sphincter muscles.
      (3) Have the patient remain quiet for 20 minutes following the insertion of a suppository.
   b. Rectal cream
      (1) Introduce the cream with the special tip, which is attached directly to the *tube of cream*.
      (2) Remove the tip and clean after each use.
   c. Retention enema: Administer the enema after a bowel movement for

maximum absorption of the medication. See Module 19, Administering Enemas, page 289, for the necessary equipment and the procedure.

8. Clean the anal area with tissue to remove the lubricant.
9. Return the patient to a position of comfort.
10. Care for the equipment.
11. Wash your hands.
12. Record as you would for oral medications, step 19, page 283.

PERFORMANCE CHECKLIST

Ophthalmic medications	Unsatisfactory	Needs more practice	Satisfactory	Comments
1. Wash your hands.				
2. Explain procedure to patient.				
3. Clean eyelid(s) and lashes.				
4. Position patient with head to side and tipped back.				
5. Have patient look up.				
6. Rest dominant hand on patient's forehead.				
7. Pull down on lower lid to open eye wide with other hand.				

8. Administer medication.
  a. Eyedrops:
    (1) Draw solution into eyedropper.				

(2) Hold bulb end up.				
(3) Without touching eye, instill drops.				
b. Ointment: (1) Squeeze out medication.				
(2) Discontinue by twisting tube.				
(3) Wipe excess off tube.				
9. Have patient close the eye gently.				
10. Have patient move eyeball or keep eye closed as appropriate.				
11. Press inner angle of eye against nose if necessary.				
12. Make patient comfortable.				
13. Dispose of equipment.				
14. Wash your hands.				
15. Record.				
Otic medications				
1. Wash your hands.				
2. Explain procedure to patient.				
3. Warm medication to body temperature.				
4. Examine and fill glass dropper.				
5. Position the patient on opposite side of ear being medicated.				
6. Pull auricle of ear to straighten canal.				

	Unsatisfactory	Needs more practice	Satisfactory	Comments
7. Instill drops.				
8. Have patient remain as positioned for five to ten minutes.				
9. Insert cotton loosely if ordered.				
10. Make patient comfortable				
11. Dispose of equipment.				
12. Wash your hands.				
13. Record.				
Nasal medications				
1. Wash your hands.				
2. Explain procedure to patient.				
3. Have patient clear nasal passages.				
4. Position patient. a. Dropper: according to area you want to reach				
b. Nasal spray: in chair with head tilted back				

5. Administer medication.
  a. Dropper:
    (1) Draw sufficient medication for both nostrils.				

(2) Insert tip and instill drops.				
(3) Have patient remain in position for five minutes.				
b. Nasal spray: (1) Spray medication into nostril with patient holding other closed.				
(2) Have patient inhale.				
(3) Repeat on other nostril.				
(4) Keep patient's head back for one or two minutes.				
6. Make patient comfortable.				
7. Dispose of equipment.				
8. Wash your hands.				
9. Record.				

	Unsatisfactory	Needs more practice	Satisfactory	Comments
Dermatological medications				
1. Wash your hands.				
2. Explain procedure to patient.				
3. Provide for patient's privacy.				
4. Provide adequate lighting.				
5. Position patient appropriately.				
6. Be sure area being treated is clean.				
7. Apply medication appropriately.				
8. Use light dressing if ordered.				
9. Make patient comfortable.				
10. Dispose of equipment.				
11. Wash your hands.				
12. Record.				
Vaginal medications				
1. Wash your hands.				
2. Explain procedure to patient.				
3. Provide for patient's privacy.				
4. Provide adequate lighting.				
5. Position patient in dorsal recumbent position with knees elevated. (Sim's position can also be used.)				
6. Drape patient.				
7. Instill medication.				
8. Return patient to position of comfort.				
9. Care for equipment.				
10. Wash your hands.				
11. Record.				

Rectal medications	Unsatisfactory	Needs more practice	Satisfactory	Comments
1. Wash your hands.				
2. Explain procedure to patient.				
3. Provide for patient's privacy.				
4. Provide adequate lighting.				
5. Position patient in side-lying position.				
6. Drape patient.				
7. Instill medication.				
8. Clean anal area.				
9. Return patient to position of comfort.				
10. Care for equipment.				
11. Wash your hands.				
12. Record.				

QUIZ

Multiple-Choice Questions

_____ 1. Administration of which of the following requires the use of sterile technique? (1) ophthalmic medications; (2) nasal medications; (3) vaginal medications; (4) rectal medications

    a. 1 only
    b. 1, 2, and 3
    c. 1 and 3
    d. 2, 3, and 4

_____ 2. Eyedrops are instilled into what part of the eye?

    a. Cornea
    b. Inner canthus
    c. Conjunctival sac
    d. Outer canthus

_____ 3. When administering eardrops to an infant, how is the ear canal straightened?

    a. By pulling the auricle upward and backward
    b. By pulling the auricle downward and backward
    c. By pulling the auricle upward and forward
    d. By pulling the auricle downward and forward

Short-Answer Questions

4. Why are nosedrops and nasal sprays usually water-soluble?

_____

5. The Proetz position is used to reach which sinuses?

_____

6. List three reasons for the administration of lotions.

    a. _____

    b. _____

    c. _____

7. List two patient positions that can be used for the insertion of vaginal medication.

    a. _____

    b. _____

8. How long should the patient remain in bed after the administration of a medicated douche?_____

9. How far should a rectal suppository be inserted? _____

10. Why is it helpful to have the patient breathe in and out through the mouth when you are inserting a rectal suppository?

_____

Module 45 Giving Injections

MAIN OBJECTIVE

To prepare and administer subcutaneous, intramuscular, and intradermal medications safely to patients.

RATIONALE

The safe preparation and administration of subcutaneous, intramuscular, and intradermal medications is a routine nursing responsibility that requires dexterity; sterile technique; a knowledge of the actions, usual dosage, desired effects, and side effects of the drug being given; as well as a knowledge of how and where to give the drug. In addition, this last requires a knowledge of human anatomy. Because drugs given by these routes not only are absorbed more quickly than by mouth, but are irretrievable once injected, a firm mathematics foundation and routine practice of the three checks and the five rights are mandatory.

PREREQUISITES

1. Successful completion of the following modules:

   VOLUME 1
   Assessment
   Charting
   Medical Asepsis

   VOLUME 2
   Sterile Technique
   Administering Oral Medications

2. Satisfactory completion of the self-test on mathematics of dosages and solutions on pages 276–277. If you cannot meet this level of proficiency, you need additional practice in the mathematics of dosages and solutions. There are many programmed texts available for independent study.
3. A review of anatomy as it relates to site selection for subcutaneous, intramuscular, and intradermal injections.

SPECIFIC LEARNING OBJECTIVES

	Know Facts and Principles	Apply Facts and Principles	Demonstrate Ability	Evaluate Performance
1. *Equipment* *a. Syringes*	Name five types of syringes available. Identify parts of syringe.	Given a patient situation, identify type of syringe appropriate for use. State which parts of syringe are kept sterile.	In the clinical situation, use correct type of syringe for injection. Handle syringe without contaminating sterile parts.	
b. Needles	Identify two methods used to size needles. Identify parts of needle.	Explain system used to size gauge of needle. State which parts of needle are kept sterile for injection.	Select needle appropriate to viscosity of medication to be injected. Handle needle without contaminating sterile parts.	Evaluate own performance with instructor
c. Medication containers	Name two types of containers commonly used for injectable medications	Differentiate between vial and ampule.	Correctly demonstrate removal of solution from vial and ampule	Evaluate own performance using Performance Checklist
2. *Subcutaneous administration* *a. Advantages and disadvantages*	Name three advantages of subcutaneous medication administration over oral medication administration. Name primary disadvantage of subcutaneous medication administration.	Given a patient situation, identify advantage of giving medication subcutaneously. State implications for nurse based on disadvantage.	In the clinical setting, identify advantages of giving medication subcutaneously	
b. Equipment selection	State needle and syringe size most commonly used for subcutaneous injections.	Given a patient description, select needle and syringe appropriate for subcutaneous injection.	In the clinical setting, select needle and syringe appropriate for patient.	Evaluate own performance with instructor
c. Site selection	State angle at which needle is inserted for subcutaneous injections. State three areas acceptable for subcutaneous injections.	Given patient description, identify appropriate angle for injection. Given a patient situation, describe which site(s) is appropriate for subcutaneous injection.	In the clinical setting, select appropriate angle for injection for patient. In the clinical setting, select appropriate site for injection.	

d. Injection technique	List steps in preparation and injection of subcutaneous medications	Adapt steps to procedures in assigned clinical facility	Prepare and inject saline in practice setting under supervision. Prepare and inject medication under supervision.	Evaluate own performance with instructor using Performance Checklist
3. Intramuscular administration a. Advantages and disadvantages	Describe speed of absorption of medication given intramuscularly versus subcutaneous administration. Name five disadvantages of intramuscular injections.	Given a patient situation, select type of injection to be given in terms of absorption speed	In the clinical setting, identify absorption speed of injection to be given	
b. Equipment selection	State needle and syringe size most commonly used for intramuscular injections.	Given a patient situation, select needle and syringe appropriate for intramuscular injection.	In the clinical setting, select needle and syringe appropriate for patient.	Evaluate selection with instructor
c. Site selection	State angle at which needle is usually inserted for intramuscular injections. State four sites acceptable for intramuscular injections.	Given a patient description, identify appropriate angle for injection. Given a patient situation, describe which site(s) is appropriate for intramuscular injection.	In the clinical setting, select appropriate angle for injection for patient. In the clinical setting, select appropriate site for injection.	Evaluate own performance with instructor. Evaluate selection with instructor
d. Injection technique	List steps in preparation and injection of medications intramuscularly, including Z-track technique	Identify critical way in which procedure differs from subcutaneous injection.	Prepare and inject saline in one or more sites in practice setting under supervision. Prepare and inject medication under supervision.	Evaluate own performance with instructor using Performance Checklist

	Know Facts and Principles	Apply Facts and Principles	Demonstrate Ability	Evaluate Performance
4. *Intradermal administration* *a. Uses*	State two reasons for use of intradermal injection technique	Given patient situations, identify appropriate situation for use of intradermal technique	In the clinical setting, correctly identify situation for which intradermal injection would be used.	Evaluate with instructor
b. Equipment selection	State needle and syringe size most commonly used for intradermal injections		In the clinical setting, select appropriate needle and syringe for intradermal injection.	Evaluate own performance with instructor
c. Site selection	State angle at which needle is inserted for intradermal injection. State two commonly used sites for intradermal injections.	Given a patient situation, select area appropriate for intradermal injection	In the clinical setting, select site appropriate for intradermal injection.	Evaluate own performance with instructor
d. Injection technique	List steps in preparation and injection of intradermal medications.	Adapt steps to procedure in assigned clinical facility	In the practice setting, prepare and inject saline intradermally under supervision. In the clinical area, prepare and inject intradermal medication under supervision.	Evaluate own performance with instructor using Performance Checklist
5. *Charting*	Know information to be charted	Identify charting method used in assigned facility	Correctly chart injections given according to method used in assigned facility	Evaluate own performance with instructor

GIVING INJECTIONS

LEARNING ACTIVITIES

1. Review the Specific Learning Objectives.
2. Read the chapter on medication administration in Ellis and Nowlis, *Nursing: A Human Needs Approach,* or a comparable chapter in another textbook.
3. Look up the module vocabulary terms in the glossary.
4. Read through the module.
5. In the practice setting:
   a. Observe and handle the assortment of needles and syringes available at your school and in your facility.
      (1) Using a 2- or 3-ml syringe and a 1½-inch needle, draw 1 ml solution from a multiple-dose vial.
      (2) Using the same equipment, draw *all* the solution from an ampule containing 1 or 2 ml solution.
      (3) Demonstrate changing a needle as you would if the first one had been contaminated.
      (4) Demonstrate drawing up the equivalent of 65 units of U-100 insulin in an insulin syringe. Draw up the equivalent of 40 units U-100 insulin in a regular 2-ml syringe or a tuberculin syringe.
   b. Read the procedures.
      (1) Using the Performance Checklist as a guide, give 1 ml solution to an orange as though it were being given subcutaneously.
      (2) Using the Performance Checklist as a guide, give 1 ml solution to an orange as though it were being given intramuscularly.
      (3) Using the Performance Checklist as a guide, give a subcutaneous injection (1 ml normal saline) to your partner under supervision.
      (4) Using the Performance Checklist as a guide, give an intramuscular injection to your partner under supervision, first using the dorsogluteal site and then the ventrogluteal site.
      (5) Using the Performance Checklist as a guide, give an intramuscular injection to your partner under supervision, using the Z-track technique.
      (6) Using the Performance Checklist as a guide, give an intradermal injection to your partner under supervision.
6. In the clinical setting, when your instructor approves your practice performance, give subcutaneous, intramuscular, and intradermal injections in your facility under supervision.

VOCABULARY

ampule
aspirate
barrel
bevel
gauge
hub
intradermal
intramuscular
Luer-Lok
lumen
needle
plunger
point
shaft
subcutaneous
syringe
vial
viscosity
wheal
Z-track

GIVING INJECTIONS

Equipment

To give any injection, you will need a
syringe, a needle, a swab and disinfectant
to clean the skin, and, of course, a medication.

Syringes come in a variety of sizes, shapes,
and materials. There are also several commercially made syringes designed for use
with specific prefilled cartridges.

SYRINGES

Glass and Luer-Lok Syringes   Once the
mainstay of every hospital's syringe supply,
the glass syringe (Figure 45.1) is less widely
used now that plastic disposable syringes
are available. However, because they can be
sterilized and included in surgical, obstet-
rical, and treatment setups, and because
they adapt to the special tips (Luer-Lok)
that are necessary for attachment to some
irrigation devices, they are still quite popular.

Glass and Luer-Lok syringes are available
in 2-ml, 5-ml, 10-ml, 20-ml, and 50-ml sizes.
They can be secured with special control
handles which are sometimes used to administer local and regional anesthesia. The Luer-
Lok attaches the needle to the syringe by a
threaded seal, which makes the connection
more secure than the friction connection of
a standard syringe.

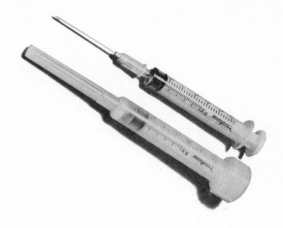

FIGURE 45.2   DISPOSABLE PLASTIC SYRINGE
Courtesy Monoject Division of Sherwood Medical

Disposable Plastic Syringes   Plastic disposable syringes (Figure 45.2) are widely used
and are available in a variety of sizes, with
or without needles attached. They usually
come packaged either in a paper or cello-
phane wrapper or in a rigid plastic container.

Syringes that come with a needle attached are convenient and time saving if the
needle happens to be the correct size and
length. The needle fits on the syringe by
simple friction. It is designed to be secure so
long as it is pushed straight on and its cover
is pulled straight off. When the hub of the
needle is twisted, it releases and comes off
the syringe.

Prefilled Syringes and Cartridges   A variety
of prefilled syringes and cartridges are available. The syringes usually come with appropriate needles attached and with directions
for use. Especially helpful are syringes prefilled with those drugs needed for emergency
use. Prefilled syringes are disposable.

Prefilled cartridges contain medication
and have an appropriate needle attached.
The disposable cartridge and needle are
designed to fit into a nondisposable metal
or plastic syringe. Although drawing up the
medication is eliminated, which does make
the procedure less difficult, mixing medications can be *more* difficult.

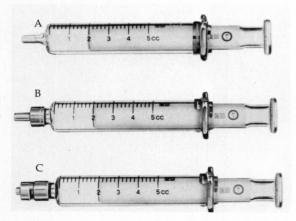

FIGURE 45.1   GLASS SYRINGES   *A:* Glass Luer;
B: metal Luer; *C:* Luer-Lok.
Courtesy American Hospital Supply Corp.,
McGaw Park, Illinois

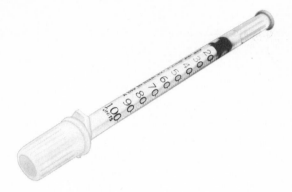

FIGURE 45.3 DISPOSABLE INSULIN SYRINGE
Courtesy Becton Dickenson & Co.

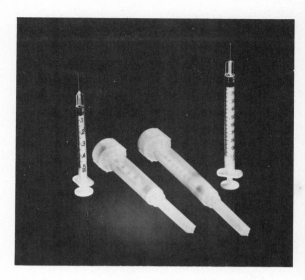

FIGURE 45.4 DISPOSABLE TUBERCULIN SYRINGE
Courtesy Monoject Division of Sherwood Medical

Insulin Syringes Insulin syringes are used specifically to measure dosages of insulin. They are available in both plastic (disposable) and glass (reusable) versions. (See Figure 45.3.) Although U-40 and U-80 insulin and insulin syringes are still in use, U-100 insulin is rapidly becoming the only insulin used in many health care facilities. Once U-100 insulin is the only insulin in circulation, dosage errors should be rare.

Tuberculin Syringes Tuberculin syringes are usually chosen for the administration of very small amounts of medication because they are marked in 0.01-ml increments. They are often marked in minims as well, which makes them ideal for infant and pediatric use. These syringes are also available in disposable plastic (Figure 45.4) and reusable glass forms.

Although an insulin syringe is the safest to use when administering insulin, insulin can also be measured accurately in a tuberculin syringe if an insulin syringe is not available.

NEEDLES

Needles for use with syringes come in standardized lengths (3/8 to 5 inches) and gauges (13 to 27). The needles you will use most frequently will be from ½ to 2 inches in length and from 25 to 18 gauge. Needles are also available in both disposable and reusable versions. The reusable ones have metal

hubs as well as a metal shaft and generally have the lumen size indicated on the hub. (Figure 45.5 shows the parts of a needle.) Disposable needles have a plastic hub and a metal shaft, and the length and gauge are indicated on the outside of the package. Sometimes color coding is used to indicate a needle's size, but this is not standardized from one company to another. Therefore,

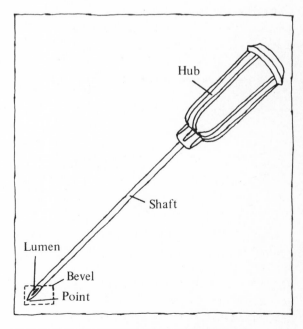

FIGURE 45.5 THE PARTS OF A NEEDLE

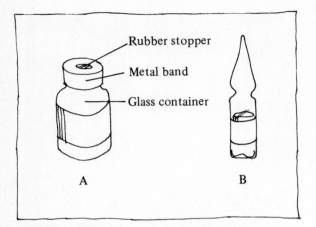

FIGURE 45.6   MEDICATION CONTAINERS
A: Vial; *B:* ampule.

use extra caution as you move from one
facility to another: be familiar with the type
of needle in use.

Reusable needles are sharpened periodically before resterilization. Occasionally, the
points are damaged, causing burrs on the
tips. If you find a burr, do not use the
needle.

The larger the gauge number of a needle,
the smaller the lumen. A needle with a small
lumen is less painful to the patient when it
is inserted. Base your choice of needle on
the relative viscosity or thickness of the
medication. For example, most clear fluid
solutions can be given intramuscularly with
a 22- or 23-gauge needle. Subcutaneous injections of these kinds of fluids can be given
with a 25- or 26-gauge needle. However,
thicker opaque medications given intra-

muscularly may require a 20- or 21-gauge
needle. Larger needles are used primarily for
giving blood or for injecting special intravenous fluids.

MEDICATION CONTAINERS

The two types of containers for injectable
medications that you will encounter most
frequently are the *vial* (either multiple dose
or single dose) and the *ampule* (Figure 45.6).
The procedures below give directions on how
to withdraw solution from each of these.

Withdrawing Solution from Containers

VIALS

1. Wash your hands.
2. Using an alcohol or other type of antiseptic swab, clean the rubber top of the
   vial with a firm circular motion.
3. Discard the swab.
4. Prepare the syringe and needle, selecting
   the type of syringe used in your facility,
   being careful to keep the needle, the
   syringe tip, the inside of the barrel,
   and the side of the plunger sterile.
   (See Figure 45.7.)
5. Draw as much air into the syringe as
   you have calculated you will need volume of solution.
6. With the vial resting on the countertop,
   remove the needle guard and insert the
   needle through the rubber tip of the
   vial.

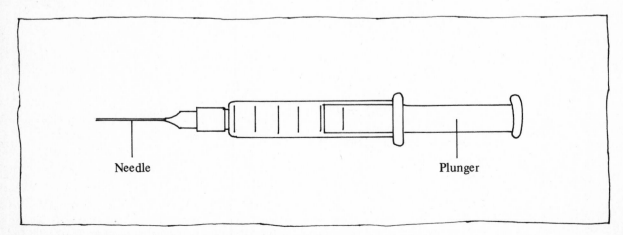

FIGURE 45.7   THE PARTS OF A SYRINGE TO BE KEPT STERILE

7. Push the air into the vial by pushing the plunger of the syringe into the barrel. This will prevent a vacuum when you withdraw the medication.

8. Pick the vial up in your nondominant hand and hold it upside-down at eye level. Many persons find it easiest to do this between the index and middle fingers. (Practice various techniques until you feel comfortable with one.) Pull the plunger down to withdraw the necessary amount of medication. Make sure the tip of the needle is beneath the level of the fluid in the inverted vial.

9. If air bubbles are present in the syringe, flick your index finger against the barrel of the syringe to move them near the top, so that they can be expelled. Keeping the syringe vertical will enable the air to collect under the needle opening.

10. When you have drawn just slightly more than the amount of solution wanted, remove the needle from the vial.

11. With the needle pointing vertically, pull back slightly to aspirate the fluid from the needle into the syringe.

12. Push the plunger gently into the barrel until 1 drop of medication appears at the point of the needle. This drop can be removed with a gentle shake of the syringe and needle. (This prevents the medication from being on the outside of the needle and irritating the tissues as the needle is injected.) If extra fluid must be ejected, the syringe can now be pointed downward over a sink or receptacle, so that excess medication does not flow back over the needle.

13. Replace the needle guard, being careful to touch the needle to the inside of the needle guard only. If the outside of the guard is touched, the needle has been contaminated and must be replaced.

AMPULES

1. Wash your hands.

2. If there is medication in the upper part of the ampule, move it down into the

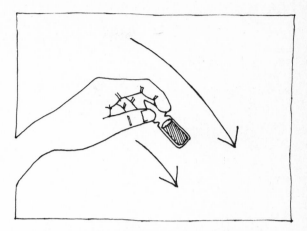

FIGURE 45.8 SHAKING FLUID TO THE BOTTOM OF AN AMPULE Grasp the ampule by the tip and shake it firmly downward, as you would a thermometer.

lower part of the ampule by flicking the tip of the ampule with your index finger. Another method is to grasp the ampule by the tip and shake it firmly downward, as you would shake down a thermometer (Figure 45.8).

3. Using an alcohol or other type of antiseptic swab, clean the narrowest part of the ampule with a firm circular (twisting) motion.

4. Prepare the syringe and needle, using the procedure appropriate to the type of syringe used in your facility, being careful to keep the appropriate parts sterile.

5. Using a swab or gauze square to protect your hand from cuts, break off the top of the ampule away from yourself. To do this, hold the base of the ampule in one hand, grasp the top firmly with the other hand, and exert pressure (Figure 45.9).

6. Remove the needle guard.

7. Hold the ampule firmly in your nondominant hand, either resting on the counter or supported in your hand, between your index and middle fingers. Insert the needle into the open end of the ampule, being careful to touch the ampule on the inside only. (See Figure 45.10.) Many facilities now provide

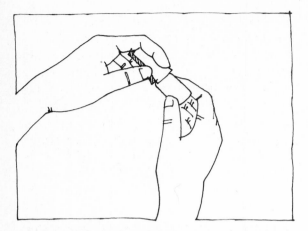

FIGURE 45.9   BREAKING THE NECK OF AN
AMPULE   Cover the neck of the ampule to protect
yourself from cuts. Then hold the ampule away
from yourself with one hand and break the top off
with the other.

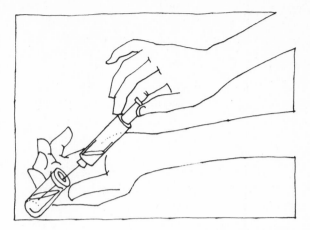

FIGURE 45.10   ASPIRATING FLUID FROM AN
AMPULE   Hold the ampule in your nondominant
hand and insert the needle in the ampule. Pull back
the plunger, keeping the needle in the solution, and
withdraw the needle when you have drawn slightly
more solution than you need.

special filter needles to withdraw medication from ampules. These filters prevent the aspiration of particulate matter
into the syringe. They are not designed
to be used for injection and must be
replaced with an appropriate needle
after the medication has been drawn up.
8. Pull the plunger of the syringe back,
   being careful to keep the needle in the
   solution to avoid drawing air into the
   syringe.
9. Withdraw the needle from the ampule
   when you have drawn just slightly more
   than the amount of solution needed.
10. Proceed with steps 11–13 of the proce-
    dure for removing fluid from vials.

Ensuring Accurate Dosages

When the *exact* measurement of a medication is critical—for example, a dosage of
insulin or heparin—it is common practice to
have two qualified individuals check the
dosage together. Present the order and the
filled syringe, still attached to the medication container if possible, to the person
with whom you are checking.

Subcutaneous Administration

ADVANTAGES AND DISADVANTAGES

Subcutaneous (SC) injections of medication
have several advantages over the oral method
of administration. First, if the patient has
adequate circulatory status, you can depend
on rapid, almost complete absorption of the
medication. Second, gastric disturbances do
not effect the medication given subcutaneously. And third, the patient does not have
to be conscious or rational to receive the
medication.

The greatest disadvantage in this method
of administration is that it penetrates the
body's first line of defense, the skin. Thus,
it is imperative that sterile technique be
used for the safety of the patient. Another
disadvantage is the amount of patient teaching that is necessary for the patient who
must continue subcutaneous administration
at home.

SELECTING THE EQUIPMENT

In most instances, a 25-gauge, 5/8-inch
needle is used for subcutaneous injections.
You should remember, however, that an

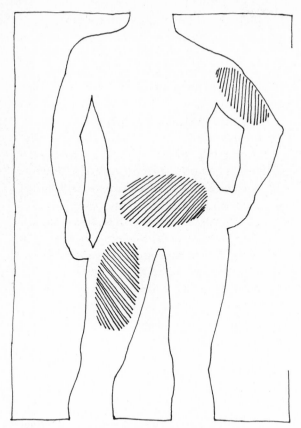

FIGURE 45.11   COMMON SITES FOR SUBCU-
TANEOUS INJECTION

extremely thin or especially obese patient
may need individual consideration.

Because the maximum amount of solution
that can be comfortably given subcutaneously is from 1½ ml to 2 ml, generally nothing larger than a 2-ml syringe is necessary,
although in some facilities the smallest
regular syringe available is 2½ ml. Certainly
insulin and tuberculin syringes could also be
used for lesser amounts.

SELECTING THE SITE

Subcutaneous tissue lies directly below the
skin. Thus, it is generally recommended that
the needle be inserted at a 45- to 60-degree
angle, but again individual consideration must
be given to very thin or extremely obese
patients. In obese patients, you may have
to use a 90-degree angle to reach subcutaneous tissue.

The site you select will vary with individual patients and circumstances. Generally,
areas in the upper arms, anterior aspects of
the thighs, and the lower abdominal wall
are acceptable (Figure 45.11). The upper
back can also be used for patients who receive frequent subcutaneous injections. (See
Figure 45.12.)

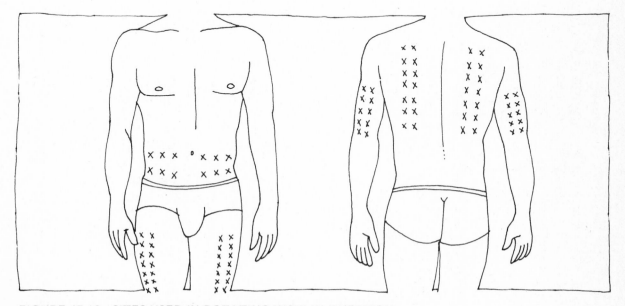

FIGURE 45.12   SITES USED IN ROTATING INSULIN INJECTION

INJECTION PROCEDURE

1. Check the injection orders according to the routine at your facility.
2. Wash your hands.
3. Calculate the volume of medication you will need.
4. Select the appropriate equipment.
5. Remove the medication from the vial or ampule. Use the three checks to ensure that the correct dose of the correct medication has been drawn up.
6. Carry the medication card, syringe, and needle (with needle guard in place), along with an alcohol or other antiseptic swab, to the bedside. Use a tray so that you have a clean area on which to keep the syringe in case you have to position the patient. When giving an injection to a child, you can conceal the syringe in your hand to avoid frightening the child as you enter the room. In all cases, a child who is old enough to understand should be verbally prepared prior to the injection.
7. Identify the patient by identification band, by asking his or her name, or by both methods.
8. Explain what you are going to do, including what the medication is for and how it works if appropriate. Explanations for children should be brief and general, and *truthful*.
9. Pull the bed curtains around the patient to provide privacy.
10. Provide adequate lighting.
11. Choose the site for the injection.
12. Expose the area.
13. Clean the site with a swab, using a circular motion and moving from the middle of the site outward.
14. Give the skin time to dry.
15. Place the swab between the third and fourth fingers of your nondominant hand.
16. Remove the needle guard, being careful to pull it straight off and away from the needle. Again, the needle should touch only the *inside* of the guard.
17. Using your nondominant hand, pinch the skin at the site selected between the thumb and index finger to elevate the subcutaneous tissue. If the patient is obese, you may have to spread the skin firmly apart to make the skin taut. An injection is less painful to a patient if the skin is taut when pierced; also, tautness allows the needle to enter the skin more easily.
18. Hold the syringe like a dart (the barrel between the thumb and index finger of your dominant hand) and insert the needle through the skin with a quick dartlike thrust. The needle should be at an angle appropriate for the patient. (See Selecting the Site, page 315.)
19. As soon as the needle is inserted, transfer your nondominant hand to the barrel of the syringe to steady it, and transfer your dominant hand to the plunger.
20. Pull back gently on the plunger (aspiration), to be sure the needle is not in a blood vessel. Injection of a medication into a blood vessel can injure the vessel (the medication may not be appropriate for intravenous administration) and can produce a more immediate and considerably stronger effect than desired, possibly leading to serious complications. If blood appears in the syringe, the needle is in a blood vessel. Withdraw the needle; discard the medication, needle, and syringe; and start over. You would not use the blood-tinged medication because it would almost certainly lead to a discolored and sore area.
21. If no blood appears in the syringe, inject the medication by pushing the plunger into the barrel with slow and even pressure. Slow infusion allows the medication to move into intracellular spaces, making room for additional fluid and reducing pain from pressure on the tissue.
22. Using your nondominant hand, steady the tissue immediately adjacent to the puncture site and quickly remove the needle. This prevents the skin from

dragging on the needle as it is removed and causing pain.

23. Gently massage the injection site with the alcohol swab and discard it.
24. Replace the needle guard.
25. Provide for the patient's comfort.
26. Return the supplies to the area designated for their storage or disposal. Follow your facility's procedure for cleaning or disposing of syringes and needles. This will usually include breaking or cutting off the needle, and placing both needle and syringe in a special container.
27. Wash your hands.
28. Using the medication card, record the administration of the medication on the patient's medication record. In some facilities, the site used is also recorded in the nurses' narrative notes.

Intramuscular Administration

ADVANTAGES AND DISADVANTAGES

Some of the advantages in the use of the intramuscular (IM) route for medications are the same as for the subcutaneous route: (1) medication is almost completely absorbed, (2) gastric disturbances do not affect the medication, and (3) the patient does not need to be conscious or rational to receive the medication. Also, absorption occurs even more rapidly than with the subcutaneous route because of the greater vascularity of muscle tissue. Irritating drugs are often given intramuscularly because there are very few nerve endings in deep muscle tissue.

Disadvantages include the penetration of the skin, the possibility of nerve damage, pain that lingers on long after the injection, and abscesses. There is also more involved patient teaching for the individual being discharged on an IM medication.

SELECTING THE EQUIPMENT

A 19- to 22-gauge needle is used for intramuscular injections. Your choice should depend on the viscosity of the medication. Also, the length of the needle depends again on the size of the patient, but will usually be 1 to 2 inches long. The most commonly used is a 22-gauge, 1½-inch needle.

Syringe size varies, but generally either a 2-ml or 5-ml syringe is used. In most facilities, no more than 5 ml medication is given into any one intramuscular injection site at a time.

SELECTING THE SITE

Dorsogluteal Site   This is perhaps the most common of the four intramuscular injection sites for adults. The injection is given in the gluteus medius muscle.

The patient should be lying prone with his or her toes pointed inward. This position helps you to accurately locate the site and relaxes the muscle, but can be difficult or impossible for many patients to assume. The area should be adequately exposed (that is, all clothing must be completely away), again to aid you in identifying the site.

There are two methods for locating this site. The first and most traditional is to divide the buttock into quadrants, and then give the injection in the upper outer quadrant (Figure 45.13).

The landmarks are the upper iliac crest, the inner crease of the buttocks, the outer lateral edge of the patient's body, and the lower edge of the buttock (inferior gluteal fold). The landmarks should be palpated, not merely located by sight. Errors can easily be made, particularly in the location of the iliac crest.

Once the location of the upper outer quadrant has been established, give the injection 2 to 3 inches below the crest of the ilium. By observing these precautions, you avoid injecting into large blood vessels or the sciatic nerve.

The second method for locating the same site (some use it as a check) is to draw an imaginary line between the posterior superior iliac spine and the greater trochanter of the femur (see Figure 45.13). An injection given laterally and superiorly to this

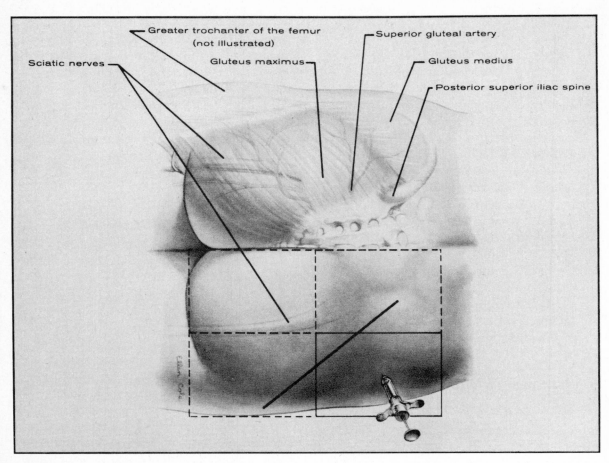

FIGURE 45.13   DORSOGLUTEAL SITE FOR INTRAMUSCULAR INJECTION   The quadrant outlined in solid lines surrounds the dorsogluteal site. The solid diagonal line can also be used to locate the site. *Courtesy of Wyeth Laboratories, Philadelphia, Pennsylvania*

line will be away from the sciatic nerve because the line runs lateral to the nerve.

Ventrogluteal Site   The ventrogluteal site has several advantages over the dorsogluteal site. There are no large nerves or blood vessels in the area, it is generally less fatty, and it is cleaner because there is less danger of fecal contamination. In addition, because the gluteal muscle is not completely developed in small children, the ventrogluteal site, rather than the dorsogluteal site, is preferred for them, at least until a child is walking.

The patient can be in one of several positions: prone, side lying, standing, or with the feet up in stirrups.

The anatomical landmarks of the ventro-gluteal site are the greater trochanter, the crest of the ilium, and the anterior superior iliac spine. To identify the site, first locate these landmarks on the patient. Then, place the heel of your hand on the greater trochanter and point one finger toward the anterior superior iliac spine and an adjacent finger toward the crest of the ilium, forming a triangle with the iliac bone. (The size of your hand and the patient's bone structure may require small adjustments in your hand position to form this triangle.) The injection site is the middle or lower aspect of this triangle, approximately 1 inch below the iliac bone (Figure 45.14).

Once the site is located, proceed with the injection as you would for a dorsogluteal

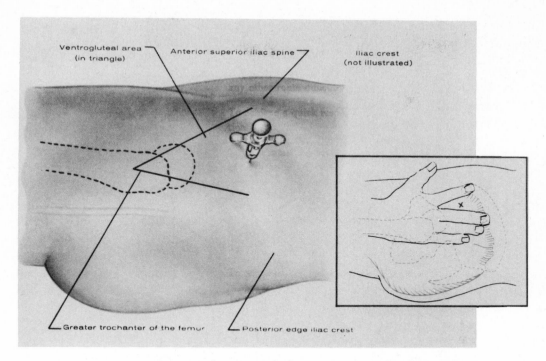

FIGURE 45.14 VENTROGLUTEAL SITE FOR INTRAMUSCULAR INJECTION
Courtesy of Wyeth Laboratories, Philadelphia, Pennsylvania

injection, *except* point the needle slightly toward the iliac bone as you insert it.

Vastus Lateralis Site The lateral thigh is relatively free from major nerves and blood vessels and is accessible in the dorsal recumbent or sitting position. This site is recommended particularly for infants and small children, whose gluteal muscle is still poorly developed.

In adults, the superior boundary is a hand-breadth below the greater trochanter; the inferior boundary is a hand-breadth above the knee. On the front of the leg, the midanterior thigh serves as a boundary; on the side of the leg, the midlateral thigh is the boundary. The result is a narrow band (approximately 3 inches wide) that is suitable for intramuscular injection. (See Figure 45.15.)

Insert the needle only to a depth of 1 inch and hold it parallel to the surface of the bed. This site is particularly well suited for large or obese patients. Small or slender people seem to have considerable pain when this site is used.

The anterior surface of the midlateral

thigh is suitable for intramuscular injections in infants and small children. Again, insert the needle to a depth of just 1 inch. To concentrate the muscle mass and make the injection easier, compress the muscle tissue between your fingers.

Deltoid Site The deltoid muscle of the arm can also be used as a site for intramuscular injection. Although it is easily accessible, its use is limited because the smaller muscle is not capable of absorbing large amounts of medication. Another, possibly more critical, limitation on the use of this site is the danger of injury to the radial nerve.

The deltoid site is rectangularly shaped. The upper boundary is 2 to 3 finger-breadths down from the acromion process on the outer aspect of the arm. The lower boundary is roughly opposite the axilla. Lines parallel to the arm, one third and two thirds of the way around the outer lateral aspect of the arm, form the side boundaries. (See Figure 45.16.)

Although the size of the muscle varies somewhat with the size of the person, the amount of medication injected at this site should be limited to a maximum of 2 ml, preferably of nonirritating medication.

INJECTION PROCEDURE

1. Proceed according to steps 1–16 of the subcutaneous injection procedure on page 316.
2. Using your nondominant hand, spread the skin at the site selected between your thumb and index finger, making it taut. If the patient is very small or emaciated, you may have to pinch the skin between the thumb and index finger to ensure sufficient muscle tissue.
3. Holding the syringe like a dart (the barrel between the thumb and index finger of your dominant hand), insert the needle through the skin with a quick dartlike thrust. The needle should usually be at a 90-degree angle, and the

length of the needle should be appropriate to the size of the patient.

4. Continue according to steps 19–27 of the subcutaneous injection procedure on page 316.

Z-TRACK TECHNIQUE

The Z-track technique of intramuscular injection is used when a drug either stains the tissues (Imferon) or is extremely irritating (Vistaril). The correct use of the Z-track technique prevents a drug's leaking back up through the needle track and staining or causing irritation.

Select equipment following the procedure for routine intramuscular injections, generally using a 2-inch needle. When a 2-inch needle is not available, a 1½-inch needle can be used.

The dorsogluteal area is the best site to use for injection, if possible.

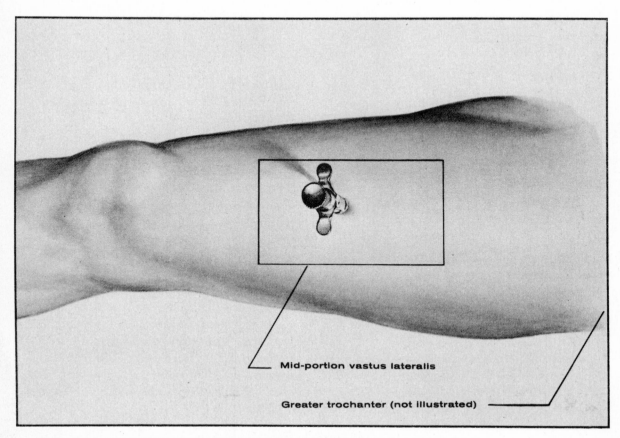

Mid-portion vastus lateralis

Greater trochanter (not illustrated)

FIGURE 45.15   VASTUS LATERALIS SITE FOR INTRAMUSCULAR INJECTION
Courtesy of Wyeth Laboratories, Philadelphia, Pennsylvania

1. Proceed according to steps 1–16 of the subcutaneous injection procedure on page 316.
2. Using the side of your nondominant hand, pull the skin laterally until it is taut.
3. Holding the syringe like a dart, insert the needle at a 90-degree angle.
4. As soon as the needle is inserted, use the thumb and index finger of your nondominant hand to steady the syringe, using your dominant hand to aspirate.
5. Inject the medication slowly and wait several seconds.
6. Remove the needle quickly, and im-

mediately release the skin being held taut by your nondominant hand. The skin will cover the needle opening, preventing leakage.
7. Do *not* massage the injection site.
8. Continue according to steps 24–27 of the subcutaneous injection procedure on page 317.

Intradermal Administration

USES

The intradermal route is commonly used for diagnostic purposes, usually for diagnosing allergies and sensitivities, and for the admin-

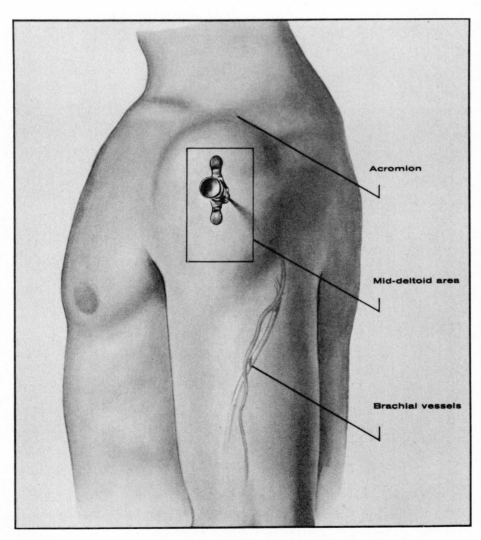

Acromion

Mid-deltoid area

Brachial vessels

FIGURE 45.16   DELTOID SITE FOR INTRAMUSCULAR INJECTION
Courtesy of Wyeth Laboratories, Philadelphia, Pennsylvania

istration of the tuberculin test. It has the longest absorption time of all of the parenteral routes.

SELECTING THE EQUIPMENT

Because a very small amount of drug is used, a 1-ml, or tuberculin, syringe is used, along with a short (1/4 to 5/8 inch), fine-gauge (25–27) needle.

SELECTING THE SITE

Intradermal literally means "between the skin layers," and the injection is administered just under the epidermis. The inner surface of the forearm is most commonly used, although the subscapular region of the back can be used as well.

INJECTION PROCEDURE

Because intradermal injections are frequently given in out-patient settings, you may have to adapt this procedure accordingly.

1. Proceed according to steps 1–16 of the subcutaneous injection procedure on page 316.
2. Using your nondominant hand, stretch the skin at the selected site, making it taut.
3. Hold the syringe at a 10- to 15-degree angle with the bevel of the needle up.
4. Insert the needle just until the bevel is no longer visible.
5. Aspirate gently.
6. Inject the medication slowly.
7. Remove the needle.
8. Do *not* massage. A small wheal (raised area) is left at the point of injection.
9. Provide for the comfort of the patient.
10. Do any patient teaching that is necessary. Usually, this includes what the patient should watch for over what time period (for example, redness or induration for 24 to 48 hours).
11. Return the supplies to the area designated for their storage or disposal. Follow your facility's procedure for cleaning or disposing of the syringes and needles.
12. Wash your hands.
13. Chart.

PERFORMANCE CHECKLIST

Subcutaneous injections	Unsatisfactory	Needs more practice	Satisfactory	Comments
1. Check orders.				
2. Wash your hands.				
3. Calculate volume of medication needed.				
4. Select appropriate equipment.				
5. Remove medication from vial or ampule.				
6. Carry medication card, syringe, and needle to bedside on tray.				
7. Identify patient.				
8. Explain procedure to patient.				
9. Provide for patient's privacy.				
10. Provide adequate lighting.				
11. Choose injection site.				
12. Expose area.				
13. Clean site using circular motion.				
14. Allow site to dry.				
15. Place swab between fingers of nondominant hand.				
16. Remove needle guard.				
17. Pinch or spread tissue as indicated.				
18. Insert needle at appropriate angle.				
19. Transfer nondominant hand to barrel of syringe, and dominant hand to plunger.				
20. Pull back on plunger (aspirate). If blood appears, discard and start over.				
21. Inject medication slowly.				
22. Steady tissue while removing needle.				
23. Massage injection site.				
24. Replace needle guard.				
25. Provide for patient's comfort.				
26. Return supplies, and clean and/or discard.				
27. Wash your hands.				
28. Record.				

	Unsatisfactory	Needs more practice	Satisfactory	Comments
Intramuscular injections				
1. Follow steps 1–16 of Performance Checklist for subcutaneous injections.				
2. Spread or pinch tissue as indicated.				
3. Insert needle at appropriate angle (usually 90 degrees).				
4. Follow steps 19–27 of Performance Checklist for subcutaneous injections.				
Z-track technique				
1. Follow steps 1–16 of Performance Checklist for subcutaneous injections.				
2. Pull skin laterally until taut.				
3. Insert needle at 90-degree angle.				
4. Aspirate.				
5. Inject slowly, and wait several seconds.				
6. Remove needle and *immediately* release skin.				
7. Do *not* massage injection site.				
8. Follow steps 24–27 of Performance Checklist for subcutaneous injections.				
Intradermal injections				
1. Follow steps 1–16 of Performance Checklist for subcutaneous injections.				
2. Stretch skin taut at appropriate site.				
3. Hold syringe at 10- to 15-degree angle, with bevel of needle up.				
4. Insert needle just until bevel is no longer visible.				
5. Aspirate gently.				
6. Inject slowly.				
7. Remove needle.				
8. Do *not* massage.				
9. Provide for patient's comfort.				
10. Do patient teaching indicated.				
11. Return supplies, and clean and/or discard.				
12. Wash your hands.				
13. Chart.				

QUIZ

Short-Answer Questions

1. Name five types of available syringes.

    a. _____

    b. _____

    c. _____

    d. _____

    e. _____

2. What is the most common concentration of insulin in use at the present time? _____

3. Needles are sized according to _____ and _____ .

4. Name two types of containers that are commonly used for injectable solutions.

    a. _____

    b. _____

5. Air is injected before removing the solution when which type of container is in use? _____

6. List three advantages of subcutaneous medication administration over oral medication administration.

    a. _____

    b. _____

    c. _____

7. What needle size is most commonly used for subcutaneous injections?

    _____

8. Name three areas that are acceptable for subcutaneous injections.

    a. _____

    b. _____

    c. _____

9. Absorption is most rapid in which of the three routes discussed?

    _____

10. What needle size is most commonly used for intramuscular injections?

    _____

11. Name four landmarks that are used to identify the dorsogluteal site.

    a. _____

    b. _____

    c. _____

    d. _____

12. Name three advantages of the ventrogluteal site over the dorsogluteal.

    a. _____

    b. _____

    c. _____

13. What are two disadvantages of using the deltoid site for intramuscular injection?

    a. _____

    b. _____

14. In both subcutaneous and intramuscular injection, what is done immediately following the insertion of the needle? _____

    _____

15. Why is the above action taken? _____

    _____

Multiple-Choice Questions

_____ 16. In a very slim person, which of the following angles would be most appropriate for subcutaneous injection?

    a. 45-degree angle
    b. 60-degree angle
    c. 90-degree angle

_____ 17. After which of the following injection techniques is massage *not* indicated? (1) intradermal; (2) subcutaneous; (3) intramuscular; (4) Z-track technique

    a. 1 and 2
    b. 1 and 4
    c. 2 and 3
    d. 3 and 4

Module 46 Preparing and Maintaining Intravenous Infusions

MAIN OBJECTIVE

To set up intravenous infusions correctly and to maintain infusions with comfort and safety for patients.

RATIONALE

Intravenous infusions are used when patients need fluids, electrolytes, or nutritional supplements that cannot be taken orally. They are also used when an ongoing means of giving intravenous medications is necessary.

Because the infusion provides direct access to the bloodstream, there are many hazards involved in the procedure: it provides an optimum entry for infectious organisms; it can allow foreign material, including air, to be introduced and to act as emboli; both the equipment and the solution can irritate the tissue; and it can cause bleeding. It is the nurse's responsibility to guard against these dangers. Also, the fluid's rate of flow is critical: too rapid a flow can create a fluid overload of the circulatory system, resulting in death if not corrected. The nurse must monitor and maintain the correct infusion rate. It is also the nurse's responsibility to ensure that the correct fluid is administered using the appropriate equipment.

PREREQUISITES

1. Successful completion of the following modules:

   VOLUME 1
   Assessment
   Charting
   Medical Asepsis
   Intake and Output

   VOLUME 2
   Sterile Technique
   Administering Oral Medications

2. Satisfactory completion of the self-test on mathematics of dosages and solutions on pages 276–277. If you cannot meet this level of proficiency, you need additional practice in the mathematics of dosage and solutions. There are many programmed texts available for independent study.
3. A review of the anatomy and physiology of the vascular system.

327

SPECIFIC LEARNING OBJECTIVES

	Know Facts and Principles	Apply Facts and Principles	Demonstrate Ability	Evaluate Performance
1. Equipment a. Fluid containers	List equipment needed for setting up infusion. Describe two types of fluid containers.		In the practice laboratory or clinical setting, select correct equipment to set up infusion.	Check for correct equipment
b. Administration sets	State purpose of each type of administration set	Given a patient situation, identify type of administration set needed	In the clinical area, select correct administration set.	Verify selection with instructor
2. Regulating the flow	State two methods of calculating correct drip rate	Given a patient situation, identify whether IV must be regulated	Calculate drip rate correctly. Regulate IV correctly.	Verify calculation with instructor
3. Setting up an intravenous infusion	List steps for setting up IV. State rationale for checking fluid for clarity and sterility.		In the practice setting, set up IV correctly	Check entire setup using Performance Checklist
4. Changing fluid containers and tubing	State frequency for changing fluid container and tubing. State appropriate procedure for dressing IV site.		In the practice setting, change IV tubing, fluid container, and dressing correctly	Evaluate own performance using Performance Checklist

Topic				
5. Removing and replacing gown	Describe method for removing and replacing gown with IV in place		In the practice setting or clinical area, remove and replace gown with IV in place	Check IV to be sure it is infusing properly when finished
6. Discontinuing intravenous infusion	Describe procedure for discontinuing IV		In the clinical area, discontinue IV	Check site for bleeding and inflammation. Evaluate performance with instructor.
7. Monitoring and maintaining an infusion	Describe phlebitis. Describe infiltration. List causes of obstruction of flow. List appropriate checks to be made when assessing IV.	Given a patient situation, differentiate between phlebitis and infiltration. Given a patient situation, identify problem that exists with IV.	In the clinical area, make complete assessment of IV. In the clinical area, determine correct action for problems identified. Chart assessment.	Verify adequacy of assessment with instructor. Verify decision with instructor.
8. Charting	State what should be charted regarding IV		In the clinical area, chart correctly regarding IVs	Use Performance Checklist to check charting

LEARNING ACTIVITIES

1. Review the Specific Learning Objectives.
2. Read the section on intravenous fluid in Ellis and Nowlis, *Nursing: A Human Needs Approach*, or comparable material in another textbook.
3. Look up the module vocabulary terms in the glossary.
4. Read through the module.
5. In the practice setting:
   a. Examine the IV equipment. Identify each of the following:
      (1) Regular venosets
      (2) Microdrip (pediatric sets) and macrodrip sets. Differentiate between the two.
      (3) Blood administration sets
      (4) Secondary administration sets (piggybacks)
      (5) Extension tubing
      (6) In-line filters
      (7) Controlled-volume sets (Peditrol, Soluset, Volutrol)
      (8) IV standards
      (9) Fluid containers (bottles, plastic bags)
      (10) Armboards
   b. Read the directions on the package regarding how to set up the brand of equipment you will be using.
   c. Set up an IV line as if it were to be started. Pay particular attention to maintaining sterility.
   d. Attach the end of the IV line to another fluid container, so that the fluid will run from the first container to the second. This will simulate an ongoing IV line.
   e. Regulate the drip rate:
      (1) To 32 drops per minute
      (2) To whatever rate would be needed to deliver the fluid remaining in the container in four hours. You will have to figure the drip rate. Consult the equipment container to identify the drops per ml delivered by the tubing.
   f. Change the fluid container only.

   g. Change the bottle and IV tubing and redress.
   h. Using a mannequin, remove and replace a gown with the IV in place.[1]
   i. Remove the IV from the mannequin's arm as if you were discontinuing the IV.
6. Practice charting for the following situations:
   a. You have hung an IV, 1,000 ml 5% D_5 W, to be given over eight hours from 4:00 p.m. to 12:00 midnight.
   b. You are maintaining an IV, and it is the end of your shift. On the previous shift, 1,000 ml 5% D_5 W was started. When your shift began, 100 ml had been given; 500 ml fluid remain. (Make up any observation data that would be needed.)
   c. You are carrying out an order to discontinue an IV. The entire amount, 500 ml normal saline, has been given.

VOCABULARY

embolus
fluid overload
infiltration
infusion
intravenous
phlebitis
thrombophlebitis

[1] If you do not have a mannequin, consult with your instructor on improvising a substitute.

PREPARING AND MAINTAINING INTRAVENOUS INFUSIONS

Equipment

For all types of intravenous infusions, the same basic equipment is needed.

1. Sterile intravenous solution as ordered
2. An administration set that contains tubing to deliver the fluid and a means of regulating the flow rate
3. An IV standard
4. A means of entry into the vein (needle or catheter)
5. Tape, and cleaning and dressing materials
6. Ointment (if indicated by the hospital's procedure)

We will discuss the first three items here because they are the responsibility of the person setting up and maintaining the IV. The last three are discussed in Module 48, Starting Intravenous Infusion, because they are the responsibility of the person starting the IV.

FLUID CONTAINERS

The most familiar fluid containers are *glass bottles.* In order for the fluid to flow out of the bottle, there must be some kind of mechanism for air to enter the bottle. This can be a vent incorporated into the bottle. (See Figure 46.1.) If there is no air vent in the bottle, there must be an air vent in the administration set. The air vent usually has a filter that removes contamination from the air entering the bottle. Bottles are available in a partially filled 50-ml size, and in 150-, 250-, 500-, and 1,000-ml sizes. The most common is 1,000 ml.

Many fluids are now supplied in *plastic bags* (Figure 46.2). Because the plastic bag simply collapses as fluid is removed, no air vent is needed. This prevents nonsterile air

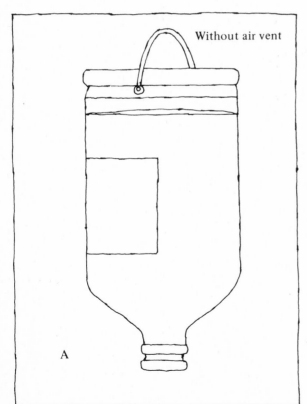
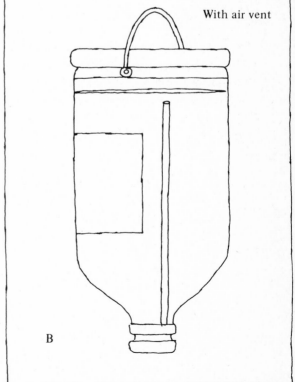

FIGURE 46.1   GLASS IV FLUID CONTAINERS   *A:* Without air vent; *B:* with air vent.

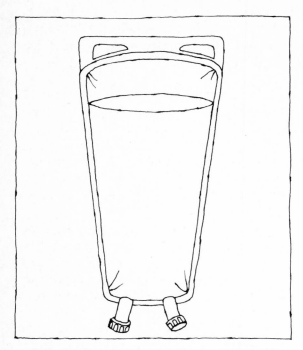

FIGURE 46.2   PLASTIC IV FLUID CONTAINER

from coming in contact with the IV fluid. The most common size is 1,000 ml, but other sizes are available.

ADMINISTRATION SETS

The conventional administration set consists of plastic tubing with a plastic spike that is inserted into the fluid container. This spike must be kept sterile. Below the spike is a drip chamber, which allows the rate of fluid administration to be monitored by counting the drops falling into the chamber. A roller valve or screw clamp is used to control the rate. The syringe tip (male adapter end of the tubing) fits into the hub of the needle in the vein. Most sets have one or more soft-rubber entry ports that reseal after puncture by a needle. These are used to inject medications into the IV line. If any

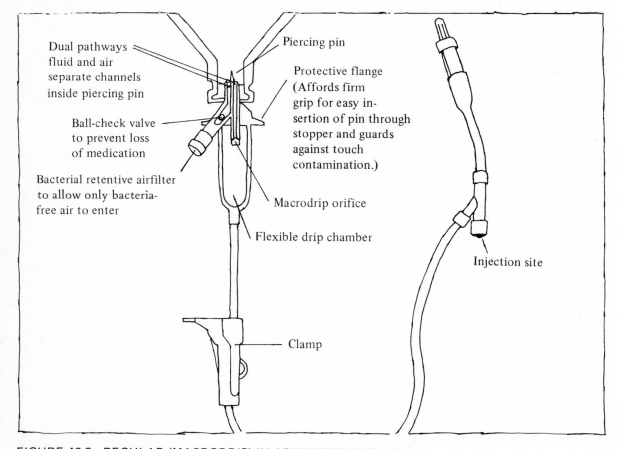

Dual pathways fluid and air separate channels inside piercing pin

Ball-check valve to prevent loss of medication

Bacterial retentive airfilter to allow only bacteria-free air to enter

Piercing pin

Protective flange (Affords firm grip for easy insertion of pin through stopper and guards against touch contamination.)

Macrodrip orifice

Flexible drip chamber

Injection site

Clamp

FIGURE 46.3   REGULAR (MACRODRIP) IV ADMINISTRATION SET   Note the airway is in the set.
Courtesy Abbott Laboratories, Chicago, Illinois

other part of the plastic is punctured with a needle, a leak will occur.

The sets are constructed so that the orifice in the drip chamber delivers a predictable number of drops for each milliliter of fluid. The most common sets are called *macrodrip sets.* These deliver 10 to 15 drops per ml (cc)[2] (See Figure 46.3.) The sets do vary, so consult the manufacturer's package for a correct figure. Remember that this figure is correct for regular, water-type fluids; when very viscous fluids, such as those containing amino acids and fats, are given, the drops per milliliter may be fewer. (The figure is usually supplied with the product.)

Most manufacturers also supply *microdrip sets* (Figure 46.4). These sets deliver 60 drops per ml and can be identified by the fine metal orifice in the drip chamber.

Blood administration sets are characterized by a larger lumen, which delivers fewer

[2]See the Table of Equivalencies on page 282.

drops per ml and a large built-in filter in the drip chamber, which removes any clots or precipitates in the blood. (See Figure 46.5.)

Secondary Sets   These sets are designed to allow more than one fluid container to be hung up at the same time, in one of three ways. Using a *tandem setup,* the second container is attached to the first by the secondary set. The fluid container on the secondary set (farthest from the patient) empties first.

The second method is the *piggyback set-up.* The secondary set is used to attach the second bottle to the primary set's tubing. Using the piggyback setup, either bottle can be made to run by shutting off the tubing to one container above the junction, keeping the tubing to the other container open. (See Figure 46.6.)

Two containers can also be hung at the same time by using a *Y-type administration set* (Figure 46.7). When both arms of the Y

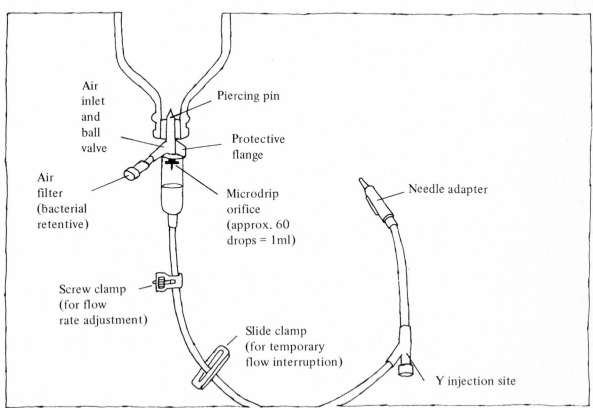

FIGURE 46.4   MICRODRIP ADMINISTRATION SET   Note the fine metal orifice in the drip chamber.
Courtesy Abbott Laboratories, Chicago, Illinois

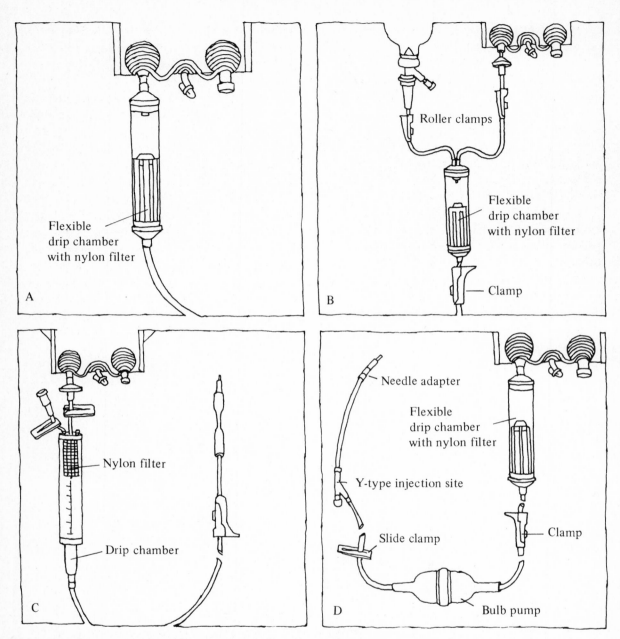

FIGURE 46.5   BLOOD ADMINISTRATION SETS *A:* Standard blood set; *B:* Y-type blood set; *C:* precision-volume blood set; *D:* blood pump set.
Courtesy Abbott Laboratories, Chicago, Illinois

are open, the container with the fluid at a higher level will empty first, and then the other container will empty. The Y set can also be used to alternate solutions.

If the tubing does not contain a special stop valve for the first emptying container, then the infusion must be monitored closely. The branch to the first emptying container must be turned off while there is still fluid

in the tube. If air is allowed to enter one arm of the Y, it will be pulled into the fluid stream coming from the second bottle and could cause a significant air embolus.

Extension Tubing   Extension tubing (Figure 46.8) is simply a length of IV tubing with a male adapter on one end and a female adapter on the other, so that it can be attached to the main set to create longer tubing. Extension tubing is often added to allow a patient greater mobility.

In-line Filters   In-line filters (Figure 46.9) are currently being used to guard against particulate matter in IV fluids and medications. They are usually inserted at the end of the tubing that connects the tubing and the needle.

Controlled-volume sets   Controlled-volume administration sets (Figure 46.10) have a 100- to 250-ml chamber, which is attached just below the fluid container. The drip chamber is below this chamber. These sets usually deliver a microdrip; that is, 60 drops per ml. They are used when careful control of fluid volume is needed, for example, with a pediatric patient, in critical-care settings, or when medication must be added to limited fluid volume. Common brands are Peditrol, Soluset, and Volutrol.

Certain controlled-volume administration sets deliver a macrodrip, or regular drip, at 15 gtt/ml. Be sure to check the package.

IV STANDARDS

IV standards (poles or stands) can be attached to a bed, placed on the floor on casters, or suspended from the ceiling with chains or hooks. (See Figure 46.11.) The height of the standard affects the flow rate: the higher the standard, the greater the pressure and the faster the rate.

EXTENSION HANGER

There are various metal wires that are used to allow one bottle on an IV standard to be hung lower than the other. The higher bottle then flows in first.

ARMBOARDS

If it is necessary to immobilize the extremity on which the IV is located, an armboard can be used. Some armboards are simply padded boards; others are commercially produced, molded plastic (Figure 46.12). Small armboards are sometimes improvised out of cardboard, using towels for padding.

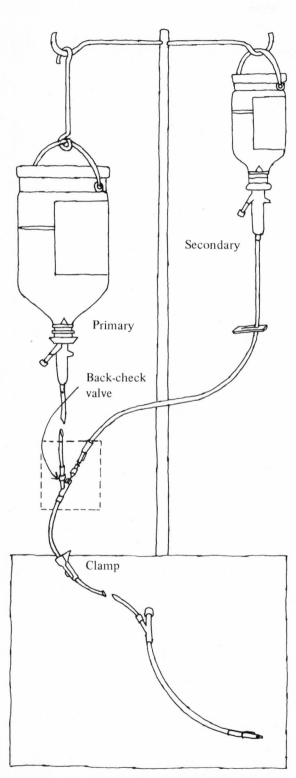

Secondary

Primary

Back-check valve

Clamp

FIGURE 46.6   SECONDARY PIGGYBACK SET
Courtesy Abbott Laboratories, Chicago, Illinois

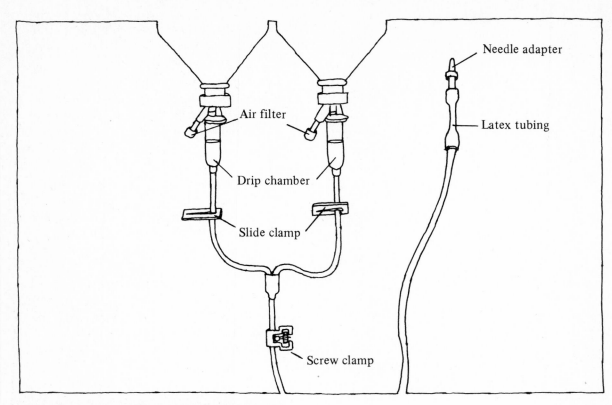

FIGURE 46.7   Y-TYPE ADMINISTRATION SET
Courtesy Abbott Laboratories, Chicago, Illinois

HYPODERMOCLYSIS SETS

Hypodermoclysis, or clysis, is the administration of fluid into the subcutaneous tissue. It is seldom used because of discomfort to the patient and problems of absorption and control. The sets look like conventional IV administration sets, except that there are two tubings attached to the drip chamber. Long, small-gauge needles are attached to the tubing (Figure 46.13), inserted subcutaneously, and taped in place. The usual sites are the anterior thighs, the subscapular areas of the back, and the subclavicular areas of the chest.

Regulating the Intravenous Infusion

The intravenous drip rate must be regulated in drops per minute to provide the ordered quantity of fluid over the ordered period of time. Many companies provide tables that give you this information, but you should know how to figure the rate when tables are not available. Here, we give two methods of calculation; try both and determine which is the easier for you.

In order to figure the rate using either method, you need three items of information:

1. The volume of fluid to be infused

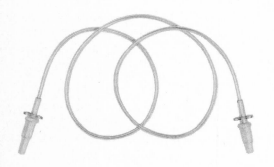

FIGURE 46.8   EXTENSION TUBING
Courtesy C. R. Bard, Inc., Murray Hill, New Jersey

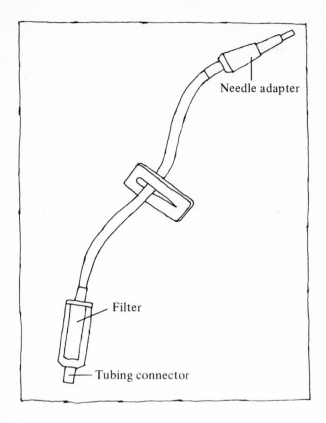

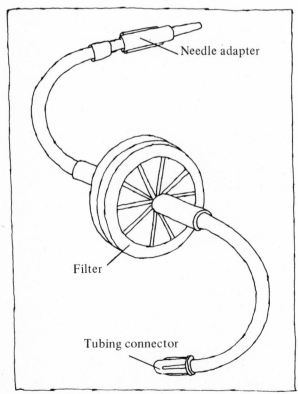

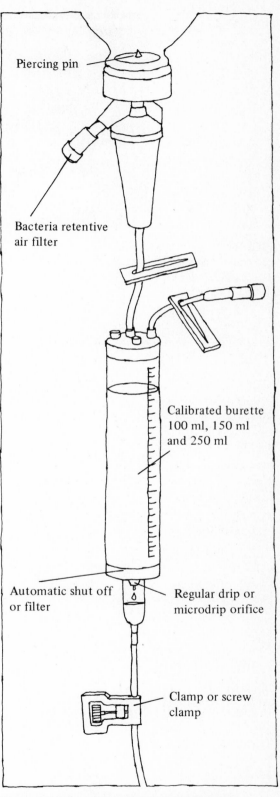

FIGURE 46.9 TWO TYPES OF IN-LINE FILTERS

FIGURE 46.10 CONTROLLED-VOLUME ADMINISTRATION SET
Courtesy Abbott Laboratories, Chicago, Illinois

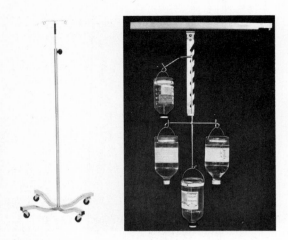

FIGURE 46.11 IV STANDARDS
Courtesy American Hospital Supply Corp.,
McGaw Park, Illinois

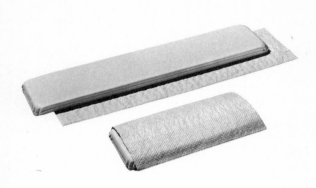

FIGURE 46.12   ARMBOARDS
Courtesy American Hospital Supply Corp.,
McGaw Park, Illinois

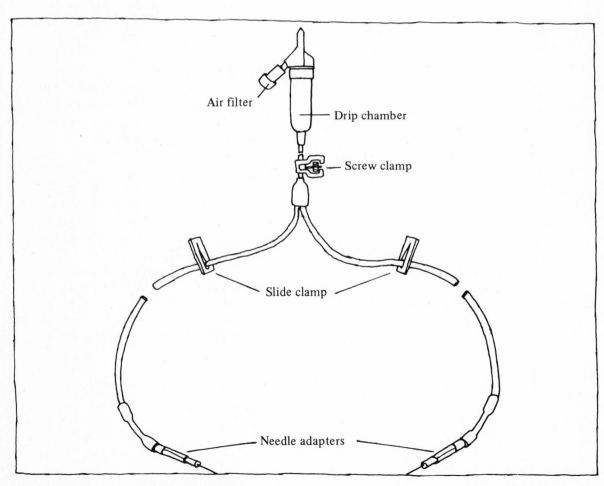

FIGURE 46.13 HYPODERMOCLYSIS SET
Courtesy Abbott Laboratories, Chicago, Illinois

2. The length of time this volume of fluid is to run

3. The "drop factor" (number of drops per ml) for the administration set, which is commonly found on the package. (Most administration sets provide 10 gtt/ml, 15 gtt/ml, or 20 gtt/ml. Microdrip sets and most controlled-volume sets provide 60 gtt/ml.)

METHOD 1

Use the following formula:

$$\frac{\text{volume (in ml) x drop factor}}{\text{time in minutes (hours x 60)}} = \frac{\text{gtt}}{\text{min}}$$

The drops per minute is the correct drip rate.

METHOD 2

1. Divide the total volume by the number of hours, to obtain the *milliliters per hour.*

$$\frac{\text{volume}}{\text{hrs}} = \text{ml/hr}$$

2. Divide the milliliters per hour by 60, to obtain the *milliliters per minute.*

$$\frac{\text{ml/hour}}{60} = \text{ml/min}$$

3. Multiply the milliliters per minute by the drop factor to obtain the *drops per minute.*

$$\text{ml/min x drop factor} = \text{gtt/min}$$

Note: The drop rate of microdrip sets, which deliver 60 gtt per ml, is always equal to the number of milliliters per hour. Try a few examples using the methods above to check this out.

Setting Up an IV

1. Check the physician's orders. Pay particular attention to the type of fluid and solution concentration, and to the infusion rate. Many abbreviations are used; three of the most common are for concentrations of dextrose and/or saline.

5% dextrose in water = D_5W

5% dextrose in normal saline = D_5N/S
half-strength normal saline = $\frac{1}{2}N/S$

If you do not understand the orders, be sure to ask.

2. Wash your hands.

3. Select the equipment. Obtain the correct fluid container using the three checks. Select an infusion set. Consider the amount of fluid to be administered and the rate. If a very slow rate is needed, a microdrip set will provide more accurate regulation. If medications are to be given, a set with multiple injection ports may be needed. For an infant or child, the use of a controlled-volume set is usually routine. If there is a great deal of equipment around the patient, an extension tubing to lengthen the IV line may be needed. Make sure that an IV standard is available. Also, have an armboard available; you often don't know whether you'll need an armboard until after the IV is in place. (A tray is usually set up with the equipment for starting the IV. This equipment is discussed in Module 48, Starting Intravenous Infusions.)

4. Check the patient's identity and prepare the patient psychologically. Do not take the equipment to the patient's bedside until the person who is going to start the IV is ready. Patients become very anxious about the procedure and possible discomfort. Just before the IV is started, verify the patient's identity and then tell the patient that an intravenous has been ordered. Do not dwell on details, but explain that once it is going, there should be relatively little discomfort. The person starting the IV should explain that procedure.

5. Prepare the patient physically. The physical preparation of the IV site is the responsibility of the person starting the IV. You can check the type of clothing the patient is wearing and make sure it can be removed over the IV.

6. Set up the equipment.
   a. Examine the fluid container against

a light to check for cloudiness, particulate matter, or other evidence of contamination. If in doubt, do not use the fluid. Select another bottle and save the potentially contaminated bottle to be returned to the pharmacy or the central supply department.

b. Open the package containing the tubing. Be sure to maintain the sterility of the connectors. If the connectors are covered with plastic caps, leave the plastic caps in place until you are ready to connect the tubing. Check the drop factor of the tubing.

c. Open the entry area of the fluid container according to the manufacturer's directions. There should be evidence that the container was sealed, which certifies sterility. Be careful that you do not contaminate the entry port.

d. Follow the manufacturer's directions about cleaning the entry port with an alcohol swab. Most fluid containers are sealed, so that the entry area is sterile and does not need to be cleaned.

e. Close the regulator on the tubing.

f. Insert the tubing into the fluid container through the correct entry port.

g. Invert the bottle with the tubing hanging down. It is convenient to be able to hang the bottle on a hook or standard at this time.

h. For a flexible-plastic drip chamber, squeeze the chamber to fill it half full with fluid. A rigid drip chamber usually fills when the container is inverted.

i. Hold the end of the tubing over a basin or a waste container. Open the regulator gradually and allow the tubing to fill. If the end of the tubing is tightly capped, that cap must be loosened to allow the tubing to fill. Replace the cap when the tubing is full. Be sure that all large bubbles are eliminated. Very tiny bubbles that do not together constitute a large

bubble are not dangerous, so don't be alarmed if a small bubble is inadvertently administered. However, it is not wise practice to knowingly administer *any* air.

Changing the Fluid Container and Tubing

The Center for Disease Control currently recommends that all IV tubings be changed every 48 hours, to decrease the incidence of phlebitis at the site (see page 342). Containers are changed every 24 hours.

1. Check the orders.
2. Wash your hands.
3. Gather the necessary equipment.
    a. Tape
    b. Dressing materials
    c. A new fluid container (verify using three checks)
    d. A new administration set
4. Set up the equipment.
5. Check the patient's identity.
6. Hang the new container on the standard beside the current container.
7. Remove the tape and dressing on the IV site to expose the hub of the needle. Be gentle and careful. Do not pull at the needle.
8. Examine the needle site for signs of swelling or inflammation.
9. When the hub is exposed, shut off the IV flow.
10. Hold the hub of the needle firmly and remove the tubing with a twisting motion.
11. Continue holding the hub of the needle with one hand while you remove the cap of the new tubing and insert it firmly into the hub with the other.
12. Immediately start the new IV infusion at a slow drip rate.
13. Redress the site according to your hospital's procedure. If your facility has no procedure, use the following:
    a. Clean the site with a water-soluble iodine pledget (Acu-dyne, Betadine).
    b. Place a small amount of water-soluble iodine ointment on the needle site.
    c. Tape the needle hub in place. Place

the center of the tape strip, sticky side up, under the hub. Cross the tape ends over the top of the hub, creating a V or chevron. Secure the tape.

   d. Place a sterile 2 × 2 gauze square over the needle.

   e. Make an occlusive, or airtight, seal over the dressing with tape.

   f. Write the date and time dressed directly on the tape to facilitate record keeping. The date and time of *starting* the IV may also be recorded on the tape each time the dressing is changed. Initial the recording.

14. Regulate the IV to the ordered infusion rate.
15. Dispose of the used equipment.
16. Wash your hands.
17. Chart.

CHANGING THE CONTAINER ONLY

1. Wash your hands.
2. Take the new fluid container to the bedside stand. Use the three checks to verify the fluid.
3. Check the patient's identity.
4. Remove the cover from the entry port, and place the container on the bedside stand.
5. Turn off the IV flow.
6. Invert the old fluid container.
7. Remove the tubing connector, being sure not to touch the tubing end.
8. Insert the tubing into the new container.
9. Invert the new container and hang it on the IV standard.
10. Turn on the flow and regulate the rate.
11. Dispose of the old container.
12. Wash your hands.
13. Chart.

Changing a Gown over an IV

TO REMOVE

1. Remove the gown from the free arm and chest.

2. Gather the sleeve on the IV arm until it forms a compact circle of fabric. Hold this circle firmly.
3. Move the sleeve down over arm, being particularly careful as you pass over the IV site. The sleeve should now be around the tubing, not around the arm.
4. Move the gown up the tubing toward the fluid container.
5. Remove the fluid container from the standard.
6. Remove the gown over the fluid container.
7. Replace the container.

TO REPLACE

Proceed in the opposite direction.

1. Gather the appropriate sleeve of the gown into a firm circle.
2. Remove the fluid container from the standard.
3. Put the gown over the fluid container (Figure 46.14).
4. Rehang the fluid container.
5. Carefully move the gown over the tubing and onto the arm.
6. Adjust the gown on the IV arm.
7. Place the patient's other arm in the gown and fasten the gown.

Discontinuing an IV

1. Check the orders. It is very upsetting to patients and staff to have an IV discontinued by mistake.
2. Wash your hands.
3. Gather the necessary equipment.
   a. A sterile cotton ball, or an alcohol swab (safe, but uncomfortable) or a 2 × 2 sterile gauze square
   b. A Band-Aid
4. Check the patient's identity.
5. Explain to the patient that the procedure will not hurt.
6. Shut off the IV flow.
7. Carefully remove the tape and dressing.
8. Hold the cotton ball or swab (according to your facility's policy) above the entry site. Be ready to exert pressure as soon

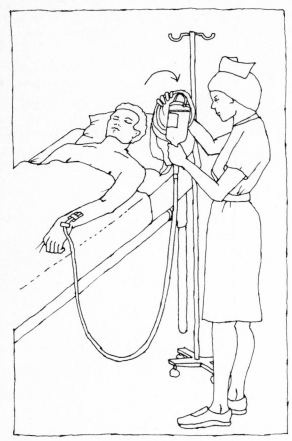

FIGURE 46.14   CHANGING A PATIENT'S
GOWN WITH AN IV IN PLACE

as the needle is out, but do not exert
pressure on the site while pulling the
needle out. This compresses the vein
wall between the needle and the swab
and can damage the vein.

9. Remove the needle by pulling straight
out in line with the vein. Check needle
or catheter to be sure it is intact.
10. Immediately put pressure on the site.
11. Raise the patient's arm above his or her
head for about one minute. Hold until
the bleeding is controlled.
12. Put a Band-Aid over the site.
13. Remove all the equipment. Be sure to
note the volume of fluid remaining in
the container, in order to accurately
record intake.
14. Wash your hands.
15. Chart, including intake.

Charting

For charting purposes, IVs can be treated
like three other categories: (1) medications,
(2) fluids, and (3) treatments.

Like medications, the charting must include the exact time started and stopped and
the exact contents in detail. Like fluids,
careful records of fluid quantities must be
recorded, often on the intake and output
worksheet, to facilitate assessing the patient's fluid balance. Like treatments, the
patient's response is noted.

Some charts contain a separate sheet on
which IVs are recorded (Figure 46.15), but
the fluid quantities are still entered on the
intake and output sheet. On other charts,
IVs are recorded with medications and
treatments. Many hospitals number each
bottle sequentially, to facilitate accuracy
in administration and record keeping.

When complete tubing is changed or when
the IV site is redressed, a notation is made.
This can be on a separate flow sheet, on the
IV sheet, or on the nurses' notes.

While an IV is in place, assessment data
must be recorded. Even if no problems are
noted, evidence that assessment has been
done is required. All items checked should
be noted.

Monitoring and Maintaining an Infusion

An important nursing responsibility is to
monitor an IV infusion and to maintain its
flow. When monitoring, you are looking for
signs and symptoms of phlebitis (or thrombophlebitis), infiltration, and obstruction of
flow.

Phlebitis—inflammation of the vein—can
be present with or without a clot in the vein.
When there is a clot, it is technically *thrombophlebitis.* In actual practice, the two
terms are used interchangeably. Phlebitis is
characterized by redness, warmth, pain, and
swelling at the IV site. It seems to occur
more rapidly when plastic rather than metal
needles are used, when electrolytes (especially potassium) are in the solution, and
when antibiotics are being administered

PARENTERAL FLUID SHEET									
DATE	TIME	NO.	SOLUTION	ADDITIVES	Amount Start	Time De'd	Amount Remaining	Total Amt. Given	Signature & Remarks
10/9/78	8⁰⁰a	1	5% D/LR	None	1000cc.	2⁰⁰p	None	1,000ml	Jo Nurse R.N.
10/9/78	2⁰⁰p	2	5% D/LR	None	1000cc	8⁰⁰p	None	1,000ml	E. Careful R.N.

BALLARD COMMUNITY HOSPITAL
Seattle, Washington

FIGURE 46.15   PARENTERAL FLUID SHEET
Courtesy Ballard Community Hospital, Seattle, Washington

through the IV. This is due to direct irritation of the vessel. Changing the dressing and tubing every 48 hours seems to decrease the incidence of phlebitis, which suggests that microorganisms also play a role in its development.

When phlebitis occurs, the best course of action is to discontinue the IV and to use warm moist packs on the site to relieve the discomfort. When an IV is critical, or when there is just a small amount of fluid left, the IV may be continued at a slow rate. Observe carefully for any increase in redness or swelling.

Infiltration is caused by the leaking of IV fluid into the surrounding tissue. Pallor, swelling, coolness, pain at the site, and usually a diminished IV flow rate are all indications of infiltration. It occurs more frequently with metal needles that have become dislodged and have penetrated a vein wall. It also can occur around a plastic needle that has been in place for a period of time. An infiltrated IV *must* be discontinued.

A decrease in flow rate or the complete cessation of fluid flow are indications of *obstruction*. Obstruction can be caused by a clot forming over the needle lumen, by particulate matter clogging the filters, by the lumen of the needle being positioned against the wall of the vein, by kinking or pressure on the tubing, or by a position of the arm that occludes the vessel proximal to the IV site. Locate the source of the obstruction, and correct it. (See the trouble-shooting chart on pages 345–347.)

Routine Assessment

Make a systematic check of the entire infusion each time you are at the patient's bedside. Most IVs are checked hourly. Pediatric and critical-care IVs are commonly checked every 30 minutes.

1. Review the entire system for obvious problems.
2. Check the bottle
   a. Note the date and time.
   b. Is it the correct solution?
   c. Which number bottle is it?
   d. What time will it be finished?
3. Check the drip chamber.
   a. Is it dripping?
   b. Is there flow?
   c. Is the rate correct?
4. Check the tubing over its entire length for kinks or obstructions.
5. Check the IV site for signs of phlebitis or infiltration:
   a. Color
   b. Skin temperature
   c. Pain
   d. Swelling
6. If an armboard is in use, remove it periodically to move the extremity, or to examine for skin irritation or circulatory impairment. Then replace.
7. Chart.

TROUBLE-SHOOTING IV PROBLEMS

Problem	Action	Reason
1. IV off schedule	Figure rate to finish IV over remaining time. If new rate is over 3 ml per minute for adult or drastically changed (from 30 ml/hr to 100 ml/hr), consider patient's condition and consult with physician before increasing rate.	a. Fluid is absorbed and utilized over time. Too rapid infusion will simply result in high urine output unless patient's cardiovascular system is inadequate, in which case fluid overload may occur. b. If fluid is behind schedule, infusing at original rate will result in inadequate fluid intake for 24-hour period. c. Figuring new rate provides adequate fluids in an evenly distributed pattern. d. Exact rate may be critical to patient, and therefore should be determined by physician.
2. Incorrect solution	Slow rate to minimum while initiating change to correct solution. Assess patient. Follow incident procedure for hospital. Notify physician.	You want to minimize amount of incorrect solution given, without losing access to vein. In some instances, type of solution is critical, and additional laboratory tests may be needed to determine action.
3. Tubing kinked	Straighten tubing and check flow rate again.	Kinked tubing slows flow rate. When kink is removed, rate may increase significantly.
4. Flow stopped	Take the following steps to reestablish flow: a. Look for obstruction of tubing and correct if present. b. Open regulator completely, move to new position, and regulate again if flow begins. c. Reposition arm. d. Place bottle lower than needle to see if blood flows back, which would indicate tubing is patent. e. Gently raise needle hub. If this starts flow, support hub with cotton pledget.	a. Pressure of arm, side rails, and other equipment can obstruct IV tubing. b. Changes in position or "fatigue" of plastic may alter flow rate. c. Flexing or twisting the forearm can obstruct vein proximal to IV site, stopping flow. d. Pressure in vein causes backflow of blood when pressure in tubing is reduced. e. Bevel of needle may be against side of vein.

Problem	Action	Reason
	f. Pinch off tubing close to arm above soft-rubber section of tube; then squeeze soft rubber firmly.	f. Slight pressure may force wall of vein away from needle. It may also release small clot. (A clot small enough to be dislodged in this manner is small enough not to be of danger as an embolus.)
	g. Obtain sterile needle and syringe. Insert into injection port closest to needle. Pinch off tubing above syringe and aspirate. Then open flow.	g. Aspiration can remove clot or clogged fluid. (Clot or clog moves into syringe and is removed; therefore, it is not hazardous to patient.)
	h. Using sterile needle and syringe, insert needle into tubing at port and aspirate IV fluid into syringe (approximately 2 to 2½ ml). Pinch off tubing above entry port and inject fluid forcefully.	h. Irrigation of IV with 2 to 2½ ml fluid would not loosen clot large enough to pose danger as embolus. (This may not be permitted by your facility. Be sure to know your facility's policy.)
5. Bubbles in tubing	a. For a few small ones, high in tubing: (1) Turn off flow. (2) Stretch tubing taut downward. (3) Flick tubing with fingernail. Bubbles will flow up to drip chamber. (4) Start flow and regulate.	a. Air is lighter than fluid, and therefore rises.
	b. For large amounts of air, high in tubing: (1) Turn off flow. (2) Insert sterile open needle into injection port close to air. (3) Open flow slowly. When air reaches needle it will bubble out. (4) Start flow and regulate.	b. Because air is lighter than fluid, when it reaches opening it rises out of tubing.
	c. For air low in tubing, below last port: (1) Turn off flow. (2) Obtain sterile needle and syringe. (3) Insert into port closest to patient.	c. Aspiration creates suction, pulling contents of tubing, including air, into syringe.

Problem	Action	Reason
	(4) Pinch tubing distal to port, to close it off.	
	(5) Aspirate. Blood will return into tubing.	
	(6) Start flow rapidly, to flush out blood.	
	(7) Regulate flow.	
6. Drip chamber completely full of fluid, so drip is not visible	For flexible drip chamber: a. Pinch off tubing. b. Invert container. c. Squeeze fluid back into container. d. Hang up bottle. e. Release tubing.	With drip chamber full, it is not possible to monitor fluid rate. When fluid is squeezed into container, air at top of bottle can enter drip chamber.

PERFORMANCE CHECKLIST

Setting up an IV	Unsatisfactory	Needs more practice	Satisfactory	Comments
1. Check physician's orders.				
2. Wash your hands.				
3. Select correct equipment.				
4. Check patient's identity and prepare patient psychologically.				
5. Prepare patient physically.				
6. Set up equipment. a. Examine fluid container.				
b. Open package of tubing.				
c. Open entry area of fluid container.				
d. Clean opening if directed by manufacturer.				
e. Close regulator on tubing.				
f. Insert tubing into container.				
g. Invert fluid container and hang if possible.				
h. Establish fluid in drip chamber.				
i. Clear air from tubing and fill with fluid.				

Changing the fluid container and tubing				
1. Check orders.				
2. Wash your hands.				
3. Gather necessary equipment, using three checks. a. Tape				
b. Dressing materials				
c. Fluid container				
4. Set up equipment.				
5. Check patient's identity.				
6. Hang new container on standard.				
7. Remove tape and dressing.				
8. Examine site.				
9. Shut off IV flow.				
10. Remove old tubing from needle hub.				
11. Remove cap of new tubing and insert into needle hub.				
12. Start IV at slow rate.				

	Unsatisfactory	Needs more practice	Satisfactory	Comments
13. Dress site. a. Clean.				
b. Place ointment on needle site.				
c. Tape needle hub.				
d. Cover with sterile gauze flat.				
e. Seal with tape.				
f. Mark date and time of dressing change, and initial.				
14. Regulate IV drip rate.				
15. Dispose of used equipment.				
16. Wash your hands.				
17. Chart.				
Changing fluid container only				
1. Wash your hands.				
2. Take new fluid container to bedside. (Use three checks to verify order.)				
3. Check patient's identity.				
4. Remove cover from entry port of new container.				
5. Turn off IV flow.				
6. Invert old fluid container.				
7. Remove tubing without contamination.				
8. Insert tubing into new container.				
9. Invert and hang new container.				
10. Start and regulate flow rate.				
11. Dispose of old container.				
12. Wash your hands.				
13. Chart.				

	Unsatisfactory	Needs more practice	Satisfactory	Comments
Removing patient's gown				
1. Remove from free arm and chest.				
2. Gather sleeve into circle.				
3. Pull circle down over arm.				
4. Pull gown over tubing.				
5. Remove fluid container from stand.				
6. Remove gown over container.				
7. Replace container.				
Replacing patient's gown				
1. Gather sleeve into circle.				
2. Remove fluid container from stand.				
3. Place gown over container.				
4. Replace container.				
5. Move gown over tubing and onto arm.				
6. Position gown on arm.				
7. Put gown on free arm and fasten.				
Discontinuing an IV				
1. Check orders.				
2. Wash your hands.				
3. Gather necessary equipment. a. Sterile cotton ball or alcohol swab				
b. Band-Aid				
4. Check patient's identity.				
5. Explain procedure to patient.				
6. Shut off IV flow.				
7. Remove tape and dressing.				
8. Hold cotton pledget ready.				
9. Remove needle.				
10. Exert pressure on site.				
11. Raise patient's arm.				
12. Apply Band-Aid.				

	Unsatisfactory	Needs more practice	Satisfactory	Comments
13. Remove all equipment.				
14. Wash your hands.				
15. Chart.				
Routine checking				
1. Review system.				
2. Check bottle: a. Date and time				
b. Correct solution				
c. Bottle number				
d. Time to be finished				
3. Check drip chamber: a. Dripping				
b. Flow				
c. Correct rate				
4. Check for kinks or obstructions.				
5. Check site: a. Color				
b. Skin temperature				
c. Pain				
d. Swelling				
6. Remove armboard and examine arm.				
7. Chart.				
Trouble-shooting problems				
1. IV off schedule: a. Calculate rate.				
b. Reset flow.				

	Unsatisfactory	Needs more practice	Satisfactory	Comments
2. Incorrect solution: a. Slow rate.				
b. Change to correct solution.				
c. Follow incident procedure.				
d. Notify physician.				
3. Tubing kinked: a. Straighten out tubing.				
4. Flow stopped: a. Look for obstruction.				
b. Correct.				
5. Bubbles in tubing. a. Remove by stretching tube or with syringe.				
6. Drip chamber full of fluid. a. Squeeze fluid back into container.				

QUIZ

Short-Answer Questions

1. List the six items of equipment that are needed for an intravenous infusion.

   a. _____

   b. _____

   c. _____

   d. _____

   e. _____

   f. _____

2. What is one advantage, in terms of sterility, of the plastic IV fluid container? _____

3. What is the proper action if the fluid in the container looks cloudy?

   _____

4. If two fluid containers are to be hung on a Y set, what are the two ways to make sure that the appropriate one drains first?

   a. _____

   b. _____

5. Figure the drop rate for each of the following problems:

   a. 1,000 ml to be given over eight hours; the drop factor is 15 gtt/ml.

   _____

   b. 650 ml to be given over four and a half hours; the drop factor is 10 gtt/ml. _____

   c. 200 ml to be given over two hours; the drop factor is 20 gtt/ml.

   _____

   d. 100 ml to be given over three hours using a microdrip set, which delivers 60 gtt/ml. _____

6. How often should the entire intravenous setup be changed?

   _____

7. Why is it important to regulate the drip rate exactly?

   _____

8. What are two measures that will stop bleeding after an IV is discontinued?

   a. _____

   b. _____

9. Give five possible causes of obstruction in the IV flow.

   a. _____

   b. _____

   c. _____

   d. _____

   e. _____

10. What are the four common symptoms of phlebitis at the IV site?

   a. _____

   b. _____

   c. _____

   d. _____

11. What are the five common symptoms of infiltration of the IV?

   a. _____

   b. _____

   c. _____

   d. _____

   e. _____

12. List six major elements that are part of a routine assessment of an IV.

   a. _____

   b. _____

   c. _____

   d. _____

   e. _____

   f. _____

Module 47 Administering Intravenous Medications

MAIN OBJECTIVE

To prepare and administer intravenous medications using an intravenous line that is in place, a controlled-volume administration set, an intermittent infusion set (heparin trap or heparin lock), and a minibottle.

RATIONALE

Intravenous medications are being used with increasing frequency when rapid effect is necessary, when medications are too irritating to be given by another route, or when the discomfort of frequent intramuscular injections is to be avoided. IV medications are also commonly used for critically ill patients.

The nurse must be aware of the many potential hazards of intravenous medications. Sterile technique must be faultless to prevent infection, and all aspects of the procedure must be done correctly. Of course, careful attention to the three checks and five rights is always necessary.

PREREQUISITES

1. Successful completion of the following modules:

   VOLUME 1
   Assessment
   Charting
   Medical Asepsis

   VOLUME 2
   Sterile Technique
   Administering Oral Medications
   Giving Injections
   Preparing and Maintaining Intravenous Infusions

2. Satisfactory completion of the self-test on mathematics of dosages and solutions on pages 276–277. If you cannot meet this level of proficiency, you need additional practice in the mathematics of dosages and solutions. There are many programmed texts available for independent study.
3. A review of the anatomy and physiology of the vascular system.

SPECIFIC LEARNING OBJECTIVES

Specific Learning Objectives	Know Facts and Principles	Apply Facts and Principles	Demonstrate Ability	Evaluate Performance
1. *Equipment*	List various types of equipment available and purpose of each	Given a specific situation, identify equipment needed	In the clinical situation, choose correct equipment	Validate choice with instructor
2. *Intravenous medication administration*				
a. *Preparing the medication*	Know where to find information on preparation of IV medication. Explain compatibility of IV fluids.		Read directions on package. In the clinical area, prepare IV medication correctly.	Double-check preparation and recheck with instructor
b. *Adding medications to IV fluid container*	State reason for injecting only at injection ports	Identify entry port on fluid container into which medication should be injected	Add medication to IV fluid container maintaining sterility	Evaluate own performance using Performance Checklist
c. *Using a controlled-volume administration set*	Identify purpose of controlled-volume set. State amount of fluid to be used for diluting medication when using controlled-volume set.	Identify situations in which controlled-volume set is necessary	Give medication using controlled-volume administration set	Evaluate own performance using Performance Checklist
d. *Using a minibottle and secondary administration set*	Identify purpose of minibottle	Identify situations in which minibottle and secondary administration set could be used	Give medications correctly using minibottle and secondary administration set	Evaluate own performance using Performance Checklist

e. IV push	Explain reasons for difference in rate of injection. Explain how to decrease discomfort of IV push medications.	Identify entry port on IV tubing to be used for injection	Maintain sterile technique while injecting medication at correct rate	Evaluate own performance using Performance Checklist
f. Using a heparin lock (intermittent infusion set)	List reasons for use of heparin lock. Explain purpose of heparin solution in lock.	Identify situations in which heparin lock would be useful	Give medication into heparin lock. Add heparin solution to lock to maintain patency of heparin lock.	Evaluate own performance using Performance Checklist
3. Hazards	State objective signs that can indicate adverse reaction to IV medication		In the clinical area, evaluate patient's response to IV medication	Verify own evaluation with instructor

LEARNING ACTIVITIES

1. Review the Specific Learning Objectives.
2. Read the section on intravenous infusions in Ellis and Nowlis, *Nursing: A Human Needs Approach,* or comparable material in another textbook.
3. Look up the module vocabulary terms in the glossary.
4. Read through the module.
5. In the practice setting:
   a. Draw up medication as you would for an IM injection, using a 21- or 22-gauge needle.
      (1) Inject the medication into an IV fluid container through the correct port, using sterile technique.
      (2) Invert the bottle, observe, and withdraw the needle.
   b. Draw up a second dose of medication.
      (1) Inject this into the air vent of the IV bottle.
      (2) Withdraw the needle, invert the bottle, and observe the result.
   c. Draw up medication.
      (1) Set up a controlled-volume administration set (Peditrol, Soluset, Volutrol).
      (2) Fill the controlled-volume reservoir with 100 ml fluid.
      (3) Add the medication.
      (4) Start the flow rate.
      (5) Close both the airway and inlet to the reservoir. Observe the effect.
      (6) Close the airway and open the inlet to the reservoir. Observe the effect.
      (7) Close the exit to the reservoir, and open the airway and inlet. Observe the effect.
      (8) Regulate the flow to administer medication in 30 minutes. (Figure the correct rate.)
   d. Draw up the medication using a small-gauge needle (25 or 26 guage). On an existing IV line, choose an entry port.
      (1) Inject the medication directly into the IV line.
      (2) Watch for air bubbles forced into the line.
      (3) Consider the speed with which the medication can be given.
   e. Draw up the medication using a large-gauge needle. On an existing IV line, choose an entry port. Repeat (1)–(3) in step d, above. Note the difference in effect of the large- and small-gauge needles.
   f. Draw up medication and heparin solution. Inject into the heparin lock.
   g. Set up a minibottle, adding medication in the same way you added medication to the fluid container.
      (1) Attach the secondary set to an ongoing IV, and regulate the rate.

VOCABULARY

anticoagulant
compatible
diluent
intermittent infusion set
laminar airflow hood
venipuncture

ADMINISTERING INTRAVENOUS MEDICATIONS

Equipment

The basic equipment is the same you would use for an intramuscular injection. To begin, select the appropriate size of *syringe* for the quantity of medication. A small-gauge *needle* (one with a high gauge number, 25 or 26) gives medication slowly; a large-gauge needle (one with a low gauge number, 19 or 20) injects medication rapidly. The size you select depends on how fast the medication must be given.

The *fluid container* has a special entry port for adding medications. In some facilities, medications are added to IV fluids in the pharmacy, where an area of minimal contamination from microorganisms is maintained through the use of a laminar airflow hood. If IV additives are added on the nursing unit, it is your responsibility to do so in an area as free from potential contamination as possible.

Minibottles, or partial-fill bottles, are small IV fluid containers that hold 50 to 100 ml solution. These are used to administer a small volume of medication that must be diluted. The medication is added to the minibottle, which is then hung as a secondary administration set.

Controlled-volume administration sets (Peditrol, Soluset, Volutrol) are attached to a regular, large IV fluid container. These allow a measured volume of fluid to be withdrawn from the large container. The medication can then be added to the controlled-volume reservoir and given at the appropriate rate.

Intermittent infusion sets, which are also called *heparin locks* or *heparin traps,* are designed to provide ready access to a vein without having an IV infusing continuously. A needle is placed in the vein. Attached to the needle hub is a very short tubing with an IV entry port at the end. A dilute heparin solution (an anticoagulant) is injected into the needle and tubing to fill them. This prevents blood from coagulating and block-

ing the needle. Because the solution is diluted, and only a small quantity is used, the person does not receive enough heparin for systemic effects. Whenever the trap is used, it must be refilled with fresh dilute heparin solution. Most facilities establish a routine for the strength of heparin solution and the amount needed to fill the particular intermittent infusion set in use. Often, 1 ml containing 100 units heparin is used. (A prefilled Tubex syringe is available in this strength and quantity for this purpose.)

You need an *alcohol swab* for cleaning whenever a surface is punctured by a needle, as well as tape, which may be needed to reinforce the point of attachment.

SELECTING THE EQUIPMENT

Often, the physician's orders will specify the method of IV administration.

IV push means the medication should be given directly into the vein, usually through an existing IV line or a heparin trap. If an access to the vein is not present, the medication must be given by a nurse skilled in doing venipuncture. When multiple IV push medications are needed, the nurse may request an order for a heparin trap from the physician.

Add to the IV indicates that the medication should be placed in the large-volume container, and will be administered over the time period designated for the fluid. Medications given this way must be stable in solution for the length of time the infusion is to run.

Medications that are not stable over time or that must be diluted and given more slowly than is practical with IV push are often added to minibottles or controlled-volume administration sets. The minibottles have the advantage of one-time use. They are hung piggyback, using a secondary administration set attached to an injection port of the primary IV. The controlled-volume sets can be used several times within 24 hours and usually cost less. They should be used only for a single medication or for medications that are compatible.

If the physician has not designated a method of administration, select one on the basis of the recommendations of the drug manufacturer and the existing equipment procedures in your hospital.

Preparing the Medication

Each IV medication has specific properties. The literature accompanying the medication is the best source of information for such things as appropriate diluent, amount of diluent, and how slow or how fast to give the medication. The speed of injection is related to the desired effect of the medication. If no speed is designated, use a slow rate, which is less irritating to the vein. (A rate of 1 ml per minute is considered slow.)

You must know the medication's expected actions and potential adverse reactions when you administer IV medication. Because the system is affected so rapidly, the patient must be observed very closely for side effects or reactions while the medication is being given and in the period immediately after it is given. Be prepared to act swiftly should an emergency occur.

Patient Education

As with all procedures, you should explain to the patient what you are doing. In particular, focus on what the patient will experience.

Adding Medication to a Fluid Container

NEW CONTAINER

1. Check the physician's orders.
2. Verify the compatibility of all medications and fluids being mixed. The pharmacist is a good resource for this information.
3. Wash your hands.
4. Prepare the medication using sterile technique. Remember the three checks and the five rights.
5. Label the new fluid container with the name and amount of additive, the date and time, and your initials.

6. Open the top of the new fluid container and identify the injection port. This may be designated by the word *Add,* or by a triangle on the rubber top. On a plastic bag, the injection port usually appears as a conventional, soft-rubber injection port, which is self-sealing. If you inserted a needle through the plastic, you would cause a leak.
7. Clean the port with an alcohol swab.
8. Inject the medication. If there is an air vent, be sure you do not inadvertently inject into it.
9. Hang as a conventional IV.
10. Dispose of the equipment.
11. Wash your hands.
12. Chart.

CONTAINER ALREADY ATTACHED TO AN IV

1. Check the physician's orders.
2. Verify the compatibility of all additives.
3. Wash your hands.
4. Prepare the medication.
5. Check the patient's identity.
6. Turn off the flow.
7. Invert the fluid container.
8. Clean the injection port with an alcohol swab.
9. Inject the medication.
10. Hang the container.
11. Start the flow.
12. Label the container.
13. Dispose of the equipment.
14. Wash your hands.
15. Chart.

Using a Controlled-Volume Administration Set

1. Check the physician's orders.
2. Verify the compatibility of all additives.
3. Wash your hands.
4. Prepare the medication.
5. Identify the patient.
6. Label the chamber with the name and amount of medication, the date, time, and your initials.
7. Open the inlet to the controlled-volume

chamber. Fill with 50 to 100 ml, depending on the dilution suggested by the drug manufacturer. (Usually 100 ml is used unless there is a fluid restriction.)

8. Tightly close the inlet to the chamber.
9. Check the chamber. If it is hard plastic, make sure that the air vent is open.
10. Turn on the drip from the chamber to check that the system is functioning correctly *before* adding medication.
    a. If the system does not work, the filters may be clogged, and you will have to replace the set.
    b. If the system is functioning, turn off the drip again.
11. Clean the entry port of the fluid chamber with an alcohol swab.
12. Insert the needle through the entry port and inject the medication.
13. Calculate the drip rate and regulate the flow. Remember that the controlled-volume set usually has a microdrip orifice. In all sets that deliver 60 gtt per ml, the drip rate will be the same as the number of milliliters per hour.
14. Dispose of the equipment.
15. Wash your hands.
16. Chart the medication and your observations.

Using a Minibottle

1. Check the physician's orders.
2. Verify the compatibility of all medications and fluids being mixed.
3. Wash your hands.
4. Prepare the medication.
5. Inject the medication into the minibottle, following the procedure for injection into any fluid container.
6. Label the minibottle with the name and amount of medication, the date and time, and your initials.
7. Attach a short secondary administration set, with a needle on the end, to the minibottle, using sterile technique.
8. Identify the patient.
9. Hang the minibottle on the IV standard.

10. Open the regulator to fill the tubing and eliminate air.
11. Close the regulator.
12. Locate the highest injection port.
13. Clean the injection port with an alcohol swab.
14. Remove the needle guard and insert the needle fully into the injection port.
15. Turn the regular IV line to a very slow rate. This prevents losing the IV when the minibottle is all given.
16. Calculate the drip rate and regulate the flow of the minibottle.
17. Place the needle guard alongside the port and needle hub, and tape around the connection, to hold the needle in place and to keep the needle guard there. This preserves the needle guard for use later when you discontinue the minibottle. (Keeping needles covered is a safety precaution for the staff.)
18. When the minibottle is empty, turn off its fluid line.
19. Regulate the regular tubing to the correct rate.
20. Withdraw the needle.
21. Dispose of the used equipment correctly.
22. Wash your hands.
23. Chart the medication, the route of administration, the dosage time, and any pertinent observations, and sign the entry.

Giving Medication by IV Push into an Existing IV

1. Check the physician's orders.
2. Wash your hands.
3. Prepare the medication.
4. Identify the patient.
5. Check to see that the existing IV is functioning properly.
6. Identify the injection port closest to the patient. (An injection port must be used because it is self-sealing. Puncturing the plastic tubing will create a leak.)
7. Clean the port with an alcohol swab.
8. Insert the needle firmly into the port.
9. Pinch off the IV line between the port

and the end of the bottle to close it off. This prevents the medication from going up into the bottle.
10. Inject the medication at the correct rate.
11. Observe the patient.
12. Release the tubing when the injection is completed.
13. Withdraw the needle.
14. Dispose of the equipment.
15. Wash your hands.
16. Chart.

Giving Medication into a Heparin Lock

This is a variation of giving an IV push medication.

1. Check the physician's orders.
2. Wash your hands.
3. Prepare the medication and the dilute heparin solution in separate syringes.
4. Identify the patient.
5. Locate the heparin lock. It is usually on the forearm or the back of the hand.
6. Inspect the site. Look for signs of phlebitis and check that the needle has not dislodged.
7. Clean the port of the heparin lock with an alcohol swab.
8. Insert the needle of the syringe with medication firmly through the soft rubber.
9. Aspirate *gently* to see if blood returns. This verifies the lock's position in the vein.
10. If blood returns, inject the medication at the recommended rate.
11. If blood does not return, the needle may be against the wall of the vein or it may be dislodged. Inject a very small amount of medication while feeling the tissue over the site with your fingertips.
    a. If the fluid is being injected into the tissue, you can feel a small swelling. Also, ask the patient whether he or she feels discomfort; the dilute heparin solution usually produces burning when injected into the subcutaneous tissue. If evidence indicates that the medication is going into the subcutaneous tissue, remove the heparin lock and replace it.
    b. If there is no evidence that fluid is moving into the tissue, inject a bit more medication, continuing to check for burning and swelling. Continue to give the medication in this manner.
12. Withdraw the needle after all medication is given.
13. Clean the injection port again.
14. Insert the needle of the heparin-filled syringe.
15. Inject the heparin solution slowly.
16. Remove the syringe and needle from the port.
17. Dispose of the equipment.
18. Wash your hands.
19. Chart the information regarding the medication and your observations.

Hazards of Administering IV Medication

Because an IV medication is immediately available to body tissue, any severe reactions to a medication happen quickly. The major danger is from reactions that interfere with respiratory, circulatory, or neurological function. Whenever a medication is given intravenously, watch for noisy respirations, changes in pulse rate, chills, nausea, or headache. These can be early signs of severe reaction. If these occur, discontinue the medication and carefully assess the patient. Then notify the physician.

In addition to these general symptoms, you must also be aware of the possible adverse reactions specific to medication being given. To detect reactions early, you must plan to make the appropriate observations.

PERFORMANCE CHECKLIST

Adding medication to a new fluid container	Unsatisfactory	Needs more practice	Satisfactory	Comments
1. Check physician's orders.				
2. Verify compatibility of all additives.				
3. Wash your hands.				
4. Prepare medication.				
5. Label container correctly.				
6. Open new fluid container and identify point for injecting medication.				
7. Clean entry point with swab.				
8. Inject medication into container.				
9. Hang bottle according to correct procedure.				
10. Dispose of equipment.				
11. Wash your hands.				
12. Chart.				

Adding medication to an attached fluid container				
1. Check physician's orders.				
2. Verify compatibility of all additives.				
3. Wash your hands.				
4. Prepare medication.				
5. Identify patient.				
6. Turn off IV flow.				
7. Invert fluid container.				
8. Clean additive site with swab.				
9. Inject medication.				
10. Hang up IV container.				
11. Start up flow.				
12. Label container correctly.				
13. Dispose of equipment.				
14. Wash your hands.				
15. Chart.				

Using a controlled-volume administration set	Unsatisfactory	Needs more practice	Satisfactory	Comments
1. Check physician's orders.				
2. Verify compatibility of additives.				
3. Wash your hands.				
4. Prepare medication.				
5. Identify patient.				
6. Label container correctly.				
7. Open inlet and fill.				
8. Close inlet.				
9. Check chamber.				
10. Check system for functioning.				
11. Clean entry port.				
12. Insert needle and inject medication.				
13. Calculate rate and regulate flow.				
14. Dispose of equipment.				
15. Wash your hands.				
16. Chart.				
Using a minibottle				
1. Check physician's orders.				
2. Verify compatibility of additives.				
3. Wash your hands.				
4. Prepare medication.				
5. Inject medication into minibottle.				
6. Label minibottle correctly.				
7. Attach secondary administration set.				
8. Identify patient.				
9. Hang minibottle.				
10. Open regulator to fill tubing with fluid.				
11. Close regulator.				
12. Locate injection port.				
13. Clean port with swab.				
14. Insert needle.				
15. Slow regular IV line.				

	Unsatisfactory	Needs more practice	Satisfactory	Comments
16. Calculate and regulate minibottle drip.				
17. Tape connection with needle cover.				
18. When empty, turn off minibottle.				
19. Regulate regular line.				
20. Withdraw needle.				
21. Dispose of used equipment.				
22. Wash your hands.				
23. Chart.				
Giving medication into a heparin lock				
1. Check physician's orders.				
2. Wash your hands.				
3. Prepare medication and dilute heparin.				
4. Identify patient.				
5. Locate heparin lock.				
6. Observe site.				
7. Clean port with swab.				
8. Insert needle of medication syringe.				
9. Aspirate.				
10. If blood returns, give at appropriate rate.				
11. If blood does not return, give small amount while checking for swelling and discomfort.				
12. Withdraw needle.				
13. Clean site again.				
14. Insert needle of heparin-filled syringe.				
15. Inject heparin into lock, slowly.				
16. Remove needle.				
17. Dispose of equipment.				
18. Wash your hands.				
19. Chart.				

Giving medication by IV push	Unsatisfactory	Needs more practice	Satisfactory	Comments
1. Check physician's orders.				
2. Wash your hands.				
3. Prepare medication.				
4. Identify patient.				
5. Check IV functioning.				
6. Select injection port.				
7. Clean port with swab.				
8. Insert needle through rubber.				
9. Pinch off tubing above port.				
10. Inject medication at appropriate speed.				
11. Observe patient.				
12. When all is injected, release tubing.				
13. Withdraw needle.				
14. Dispose of equipment.				
15. Wash your hands.				
16. Chart.				

QUIZ

Short-Answer Questions

1. Why is a needle inserted into an IV line only at an injection port?

   _____

2. If there is no designated speed of injection for an IV push medication,
   how fast should it be injected and why? _____

   _____

3. What is the purpose of an intermittent infusion set? _____

   _____

4. Why is a heparin solution left in the heparin lock? _____

   _____

5. How many milliliters of fluid are used to dilute the medication in a
   controlled-volume administration set? _____

Module 48 Starting Intravenous Infusions

MAIN OBJECTIVE

To start intravenous infusions safely and comfortably for patients using the equipment correctly.

RATIONALE

Depending on the facility's procedure, unit nurses may or may not start intravenous infusions. If it is the unit nurse's responsibility to start intravenous infusions, the nurse must follow the five rights and three checks, as well as manipulate the required equipment skillfully, keeping the patient comfortable and safe. If house staff or specially trained IV nurses are responsible for starting intravenous infusions, the unit nurse must still be sufficiently familiar with the equipment and the procedure to be of assistance.

PREREQUISITES

1. Successful completion of the following modules:

   VOLUME 1
   Assessment
   Charting
   Medical Asepsis

   VOLUME 2
   Sterile Technique
   Administering Oral Medications
   Giving Injections
   Preparing and Maintaining Intravenous Infusions

2. A review of the anatomy and physiology of the vascular system

SPECIFIC LEARNING OBJECTIVES

	Know Facts and Principles	Apply Facts and Principles	Demonstrate Ability	Evaluate Performance
1. *Psychological implications*	State three reasons why patients become anxious about IV infusions	Given a patient situation, assess and plan appropriate nursing intervention to decrease patient's anxiety about receiving IV infusion	Prepare patient psychologically for IV therapy immediately before initiating. Bring equipment into room at time IV is to be started.	Evaluate own performance with instructor
2. *Indications for intravenous fluids*	State four indications for intravenous fluids	Given a patient situation, state why patient is receiving IV fluids	In the clinical facility, discuss reason(s) for IV therapy for assigned patient(s)	Evaluate own performance with instructor
3. *Equipment*	List four kinds of equipment generally available for starting IV infusions	Correctly identify equipment for starting IVs	Choose correct equipment for particular clinical situation	Evaluate own performance with instructor
4. *Locating a vein*	State usual sites for adult and infant IVs, and give rationale for their use. State four methods that can be used to distend veins.	Given a patient situation, state potential IV site. Given a patient situation, discuss which method of distending veins might be used.	In the practice area and/or clinical facility, locate potential IV sites on peers and/or patients. In the practice area and/or clinical facility, demonstrate how to cause vein to distend using peer and/or actual patient.	Evaluate own performance with instructor

5. *Procedure for starting an intravenous infusion*	Describe steps in procedure	Given a patient situation, describe how procedure might be adapted	Start IV in practice area and/or clinical facility	Evaluate with instructor using Performance Checklist
6. *Charting*	State items of information to be included when charting insertion of IV infusion	Given a patient situation, do sample charting for insertion of IV infusion	In the clinical setting, correctly chart insertion of IV infusion	Evaluate with instructor

LEARNING ACTIVITIES

1. Review the Specific Learning Objectives.
2. Read the section on administering fluids intravenously (in the chapter on nutrition and fluids) in Ellis and Nowlis, *Nursing: A Human Needs Approach,* or a comparable chapter in another textbook.
3. Look up the module vocabulary terms in the glossary.
4. Read through the module.
5. In the practice setting:
   a. Examine the various pieces of equipment available for starting an IV. Identify each of the following:
      (1) 18-, 19-, or 20-gauge, short-beveled needles. (Compare a short-beveled needle with a regular needle.)
      (2) A butterfly
      (3) An IV catheter inside a needle (Intracath, Venocath)
      (4) An IV catheter over a needle, or catheter-threaded needle (Abbocath)
      (5) Any other available devices
   b. Read the package instructions accompanying each of the above devices. Handle the equipment and attempt to follow the instructions.
   c. Using a mannequin or IV "arm," start an IV with a 20-gauge, short-beveled needle. Do the complete procedure, including the explanation to the "patient," and taping and dressing. If time permits, review Module 46, Preparing and Maintaining Intravenous Infusions, and set up the IV as well. When you feel you have had sufficient practice, ask your instructor to evaluate your performance.
   d. If sterile equipment is available and school policy permits, practice starting an IV on another student. Perform the entire procedure and have the student evaluate your performance.
   e. Practice charting, using the form used in the facility to which you are assigned, as well as a narrative note.
6. In the clinical setting:
   a. Ask your instructor to arrange for you to observe an IV being started.
   b. Ask your instructor to arrange for you to start an IV under supervision in your clinical facility, if the facility's policies permit. For your first experience, a patient with "good" veins (for example, a young male) is preferable.
   c. If your facility employs an IV nurse, ask your instructor if arrangements can be made for you to accompany him or her as an observation experience. If time permits, ask if you can practice locating a suitable vein, and have the nurse evaluate your choice. If policy permits, ask if you can start an IV on a patient with good veins.

VOCABULARY

antecubital space
armboard
bevel
bifurcation
butterfly
cutdown
laminar air flow hood
N.P.O.
Penrose drain
tortuous
tourniquet

STARTING INTRAVENOUS INFUSIONS

Psychological Implications

To some patients, the knowledge that they are about to receive intravenous fluids is threatening. Certain patients feel the procedure implies serious illness; others are frightened by the threat of pain, discomfort, and immobility. Previous experience can help make the patient less apprehensive, assuming the experience was a good one; for other patients, however, the memories of problems related to the IV make the impending experience truly frightening.

Explain the procedure just a few minutes before the IV is to be started; this prepares the patient without giving him or her a long time to worry. In addition, keep the equipment out of the room until you are actually going to begin ("out of sight, out of mind"). Lastly, in some facilities, it is the policy to use ½ to 1 ml local anesthetic intradermally before starting an IV, to numb the skin and the vein. This makes it easier for the patient to cooperate and removes most of the pain and discomfort associated with the insertion.

Indications for Intravenous Fluids

Intravenous fluids are ordered for a variety of reasons. They maintain the daily requirements for fluid (in the patient who is NPO or who is nauseated and vomiting); they replace lost fluid (in the postoperative patient); they provide large amounts of fluid rapidly (for a patient who has taken a drug overdose); and they serve as a vehicle for medications, most commonly antibiotics.

The fluid is ordered by the physician specifically to meet the needs of the individual patient. A seemingly endless variety of solutions are available, including simple dextrose in water or sodium chloride solution, sophisticated electrolyte solutions, plasma volume expanders, and concentrated dextrose and protein solutions, to mention only a few. Each fluid has a specific purpose, and they cannot be interchanged. Carefully check the order and the label to be certain that you have the correct solution. Also check the expiration date. And finally, check the clarity; any cloudiness or particulate matter could indicate that the solution is not suitable for use and should be returned to its source.

Equipment

No single type of equipment is ideal: all have advantages and disadvantages. When choosing equipment, you must consider the age and mobility of the patient, the length of time the equipment will be in place, and the individual patient's vein structure. Then, compare these factors to the characteristics of the equipment, and make your choice.

Most facilities select a single manufacturer of intravenous solutions and equipment as their supplier. It is this equipment with which you will become familiar over time. The varieties of fluid containers and administration sets were discussed in Module 46, Preparing and Maintaining Intravenous Infusions. A similar variety of equipment is available for starting infusions.

A *straight sterile needle* (usually 18, 19, or 20 gauge) with a short bevel can be used for short-term IVs (Figure 48.1). The short bevel prevents puncturing the posterior wall of the vein as the needle enters. A metal needle tends not to irritate the vein but may damage or puncture the vein if the patient moves about, which would cause an infiltration.

A *butterfly* (or scalp vein infusion set)

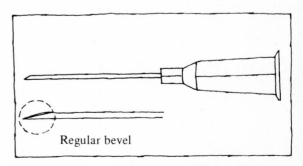

Regular bevel

FIGURE 48.1 STRAIGHT NEEDLE WITH A SHORT BEVEL

comes with plastic "wings" that are attached to the needle's hub for easier manipulation during insertion (Figure 48.2). After the vein has been entered, the wings lie flat against the skin and provide a means for securing the needle and tubing. Available from 16 gauge to 25 gauge, the butterfly can be used in a variety of situations. The smaller sizes (25 and 23) are particularly useful for infant scalp veins and for those patients with small, fragile, or rolling veins. A butterfly is also available for intermittent use (Figure 48.3), for example, on a heparin trap.

An *intravenous catheter inside a needle* (Figure 48.4) (Intracath, Venocath) is "threaded" into the vein and is used when the intravenous is expected to remain in place for several days. After the needle is pulled back out of the skin, leaving the approximately 11-inch-long catheter in place, a guard is secured over the needle, covering it completely. This device is usually quite stable, and affords the patient maximum mobility. It is available in several sizes. The plastic is less likely to puncture or injure the vein, but may be a source of irritation leading to phlebitis.

Still another device consists of an *intravenous catheter* about 2 inches long *over a needle* (Figure 48.5). The needle and catheter are inserted. When blood returns, the needle is removed, leaving the catheter in place. This device is used when veins are tortuous and will not receive a long catheter. The over-the-needle catheter is more likely to be damaged by the needle's sharp edge, which can result in the plastic catheter breaking off in the vein and becoming an embolus.

Selecting a Vein

For the adult patient, intravenous infusions are usually started in an arm or a hand. Legs

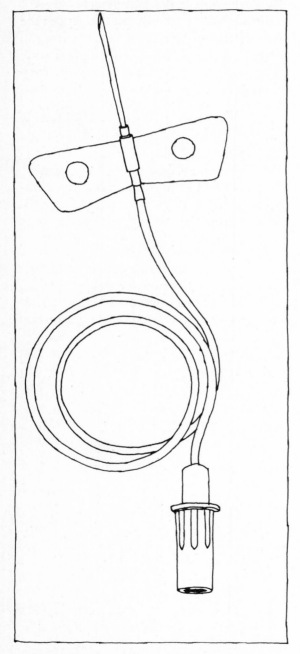

FIGURE 48.2   BUTTERFLY INFUSION SET

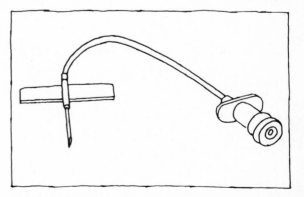

FIGURE 48.3   BUTTERFLY FOR INTERMITTENT USE

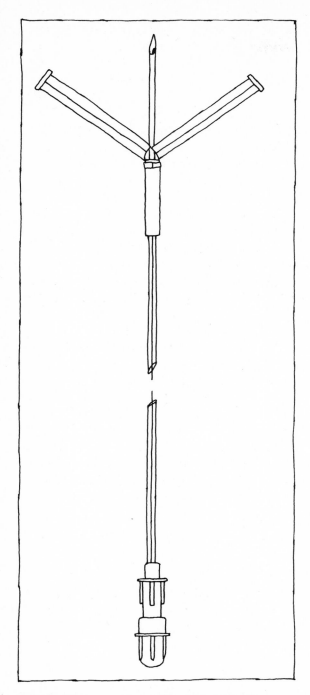

FIGURE 48.4   INTRAVENOUS CATHETER
INSIDE A NEEDLE

are avoided because of the danger of thrombus formation and subsequent pulmonary
emboli. Selection depends on a number of
factors, including the reason for the IV, the
length of time it is expected to be needed,
the condition of the patient's veins, and the
comfort and safety of the patient.

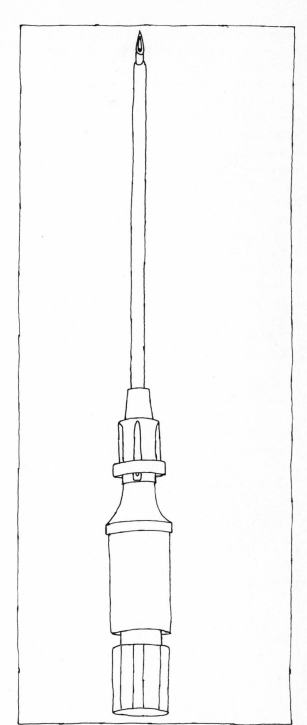

FIGURE 48.5   INTRAVENOUS CATHETER
OVER A NEEDLE

Although it is usually easy to start an IV
in the branches of either the cephalic or the
basilic vein located near the antecubital
space (inner aspect of the elbow), these veins

are often *not* a good choice. Insertion there limits the patient's mobility in that arm, and laboratory technicians often rely on these veins for their blood samples. They should be used as a last resort and in emergency situations.

Better sites in the adult patient are the lower branches of the basilic and cephalic veins (see Figure 48.6); the scalp veins are used in the infant because there is less movement there and hence less chance of dislocation.

It is best to start low in the vein (in the hand or forearm). Then, if you are unsuccessful or if the IV comes out at a later time, you can choose a vein proximal to, or higher than, the first one. A site where there is bifurcation may be easier to enter if you can enter from below. Compare the length of the device you plan to use with the available vein. Given that you have a choice, it is preferable not to use the dominant hand or arm and also better to change sides with subsequent IVs. Your choices are often limited by the diagnosis, the condition of the patient's veins, the presence of additional equipment, and so forth.

Select the vein by looking, palpating, and attempting to distend any veins in the area.

You want a clearly visible vein that can be palpated and that has a straight section for entry. If one is not visible, look for the faint outline of a blue vein under the skin to determine where to begin. When even an outline is not visible; you must begin to distend the veins, to make them visible or palpable. To distend the veins, place a tourniquet (using a length of Penrose drain) a few inches above the area where you want to start the IV, and ask the patient to "pump," opening and closing his or her fist. Generally, these maneuvers distend the vein, making it easier to locate and enter. If you are still unable to locate a vein, place the limb in a dependent position for a period of time, or apply warm wet packs to the area. (See Figure 48.7.) Veins that are not visible but are palpable can be used.

Some veins can be entered without using a tourniquet, a procedure that is advisable when a patient's veins are particularly fragile or rolling. The extra distention produced by a tourniquet can cause a vein to burst or roll even more.

If you have tried two times and have been unable to enter a vein, it is best to get assistance. The procedure is uncomfortable for the patient, and you do not want to use

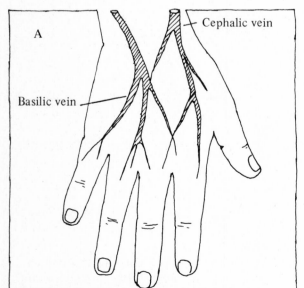
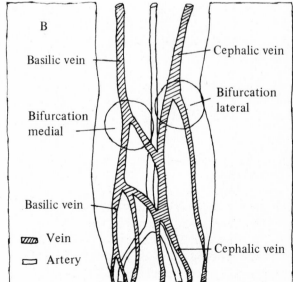

FIGURE 48.6 SUITABLE VEINS FOR STARTING IVs *A:* Hand; *B:* forearm.

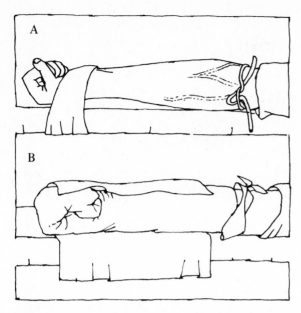

FIGURE 48.7   WAYS TO DISTEND A VEIN
A: Tourniquet; *B:* moist heat.

up all the available veins. If no member of
the nursing staff can start the IV, it may be
necessary to ask the anesthesia department
for help (depending on the policies in your
facility) or the physician to do a cutdown
(surgical opening of a vein to start an IV).

Starting an Intravenous Infusion

1. Check the physician's orders. The
   orders include the type and amount
   of solution, as well as the length of
   time over which the solution should
   run. The physician may also order
   additional medications to be added to
   the solution. Depending on the policies
   of the facility in which you work, you
   may add them yourself or they may be
   added in the pharmacy under a laminar
   airflow hood. (See Module 47, Administering Intravenous Medications.)
2. Select the equipment. You will need to
   choose equipment both to set up the IV
   (as discussed in Module 46) and to start
   the IV. This last includes the following:
   a. A tourniquet
   b. An antiseptic swab
   c. A means of entry into the vein

d. Tape. (Tear four 6-inch strips and
   place them conveniently.)
e. Ointment
f. Dressing materials
Keep this equipment together in a box
or on a cart. This is a convenient practice because you often will not know
which device you'll want to use until
you have examined the patient.
3. Identify the patient. Starting an intravenous infusion should be handled with
   all the same careful checking as the
   administration of any medication.
4. Prepare the patient psychologically.
   Just a few minutes before you plan to
   start the IV, tell the patient that he or
   she is to have one and for what reason.
   Do not take the equipment to the bedside until you are actually ready to
   start. (See Psychological Implications,
   page 373, and refer to Module 46.)
5. Adjust the lighting. Make sure you have
   adequate lighting, a factor that is extremely important and is often over-
   looked. If the room lights are not
   adequate, locate a portable lamp for
   temporary use.
6. Prepare the patient physically. First
   provide for the patient's privacy. Look
   at the gown or pajamas the patient is
   wearing, and help him or her to change
   if necessary. A pajama top with narrow
   sleeves or a long nightgown may be
   difficult if not impossible to remove
   once the IV is in place. A regular hospital gown is often the easiest and best
   "clothing" for the patient to wear. Then
   position the patient as comfortably as
   possible. Place a towel under the arm to
   protect the bed. And, you may have to
   remove the patient's watch or change
   the position of the nameband if either
   is in the way.
7. Wash your hands. Starting an IV is a
   sterile procedure, for which your hands
   must be clean.
8. Position yourself. In order to start an
   IV, you'll find that it is equally important for you to be comfortable as it
   is the patient. The position you choose

must be comfortable for you, and may
not be so orthodox as a chair at the bedside. Some nurses put the bed in high
position and stand; others put the bed
in low position and kneel on a towel;
still others sit on the bed. Of course, the
policy in your facility may somewhat
limit your range of choices.

9. Locate a vein in which to start the IV.
Examine both forearms and select a
site to begin. Place a tourniquet a few
inches above the area where you want
to start, and ask the patient to open and
close his or her fist. If the vein does not
distend, you may have to place the limb
in a dependent position or apply warm
moist packs to the area. Remember not
to use a tourniquet if the veins are
extremely fragile or rolling.

10. Clean the area thoroughly. Start from
the point at which you want to enter
and move with a circular motion away
from it, cleaning the skin thoroughly at
and around the vein you have selected.
If the area is especially hairy, shave it
before you attempt to start the IV,
both for aseptic reasons and to prevent
the tape from pulling. Clean the area
after it has been shaved. The antiseptic
agent used for cleaning is usually indicated by unit or facility procedure. Try
not to touch the area after it has been
cleaned.

11. Anesthetize the area if policy allows.
Use a local anesthetic to decrease the
sensitivity of the skin and vein. Be sure
to check whether the patient is allergic
to local anesthetics.

12. Insert the needle. Using the thumb of
your nondominant hand, gently retract
the skin away from the site. Holding
the needle at about a 45-degree angle,
with the bevel up, pierce the skin immediately beside the vein you have
selected (Figure 48.8). When the needle
is through the skin, decrease the angle
until it is almost parallel with the skin,
and enter the vein (Figure 48.9). When
blood comes back into the tubing or
syringe (depending on the device you

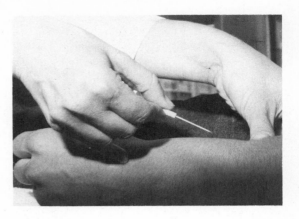

FIGURE 48.8 SKIN RETRACTED AND NEEDLE
AT ANGLE TO PIERCE SKIN
Courtesy Ivan Ellis

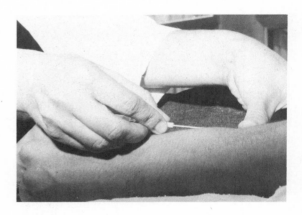

FIGURE 48.9 NEEDLE AT ANGLE TO ENTER
VEIN
Courtesy Ivan Ellis

are using), insert the needle almost the
full 1½ inches. Follow the package instructions for the use of any other device.

13. Release the tourniquet. Holding the
needle or other device steady with your
dominant hand, release the tourniquet
with your other hand.

14. Connect the tubing and initiate the
flow. Remove the protective cap from
the IV tubing (maintaining sterile technique), connect it securely to the
needle, and open the regulator to initiate the flow. This should be done
quickly to prevent the patient's blood
from clotting and clogging the needle.

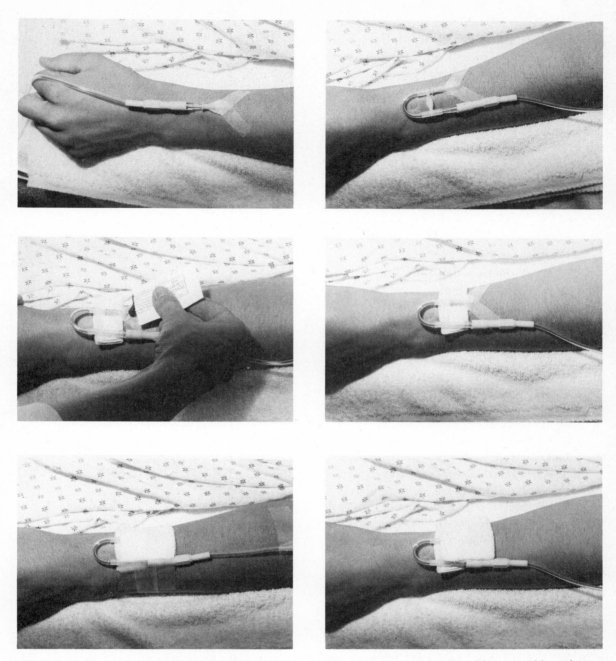

FIGURE 48.10 TAPING AND DRESSING THE IV *A:* Chevron tape in place; *B:* tubing curved by using a U-shaped connector; *C:* gauze square under hub to support position; *D:* applying antiseptic ointment on needle entry site; *E:* 3 × 3 dressing; *F:* dressing and tubing taped in place.
Courtesy Ivan Ellis

15. Tape the needle securely and dress the site. (See Figure 48.10.) This should be done according to unit or facility procedure. If you have no procedure, use the following:
   a. Place a sterile folded 3 × 3 or 2 × 2 gauze square under the needle (folded side toward the needle).
   b. Place a small amount of antiseptic ointment (Betadine is commonly used) at the needle site.
   c. With ¼-inch adhesive tape (check for

patient allergy), tape the needle in place, using a chevron configuration.

d. Place a sterile 3 × 3 or 2 × 2 gauze square open over the IV site.

e. Tape the needle and tubing in place, using paper tape (if available—it is usually less traumatic to the patient's skin), and make a loop near the point of entry. This helps prevent the weight of the tubing from pulling the needle out of place. A commercially produced firm plastic insert is available for this purpose.

f. Tape the armboard in place if necessary.

g. Write the date and time and your initials on the tape.

16. Adjust the flow rate. The physician will have ordered a specific amount of fluid to be administered over a certain period of time. In some facilities, you will figure the rate of flow yourself, based on the number of drops per milliliter administered by the equipment you are using. In others, the rate will be figured by pharmacy personnel, but you still must be able to check that rate and to figure it again in the event the IV gets "ahead" or "behind." Many facilities stock narrow strips of paper calibrated according to the number of hours the IV is to run (Figure 48.11); the nurse adds the specific times appropriate for the individual IV. These forms make it easier for the nursing staff to assess the progress of the infusion.

17. Dispose of the equipment.

18. Wash your hands.

19. Chart the IV. Usually a special form is used for this purpose (see Module 46, Figure 46.15). Include the time the IV was started, the type of fluid, any additives, where the IV was started, and by whom. When an IV is discontinued, include the time and the amount of fluid absorbed. A patient receiving an IV is usually on intake and output as well.

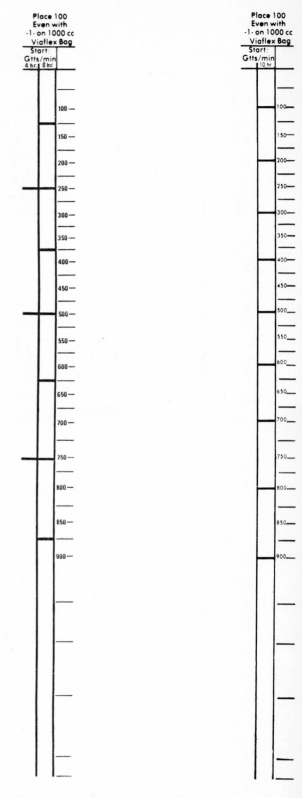

FIGURE 48.11   CALIBRATION LABELS   *A:* 4- or 8-hour label; *B:* 10-hour label.

PERFORMANCE CHECKLIST

	Unsatisfactory	Needs more practice	Satisfactory	Comments
1. Check physician's orders.				
2. Select equipment.				
3. Identify patient.				
4. Prepare patient psychologically.				
5. Adjust lighting.				
6. Prepare patient physically.				
7. Wash your hands.				
8. Select position of comfort for yourself.				
9. Locate vein. Apply tourniquet.				
10. Clean area thoroughly.				
11. Anesthetize area if allowed.				
12. Introduce needle.				
13. Release tourniquet.				
14. Connect tubing and initiate flow.				
15. Tape needle and dress site.				
16. Adjust flow rate.				
17. Dispose of equipment.				
18. Wash your hands.				
19. Chart.				

QUIZ

Short-Answer Questions

1. List three reasons why patients often fear intravenous infusions.

    a. _____

    b. _____

    c. _____

2. List two reasons why a patient might be receiving IV fluids.

    a. _____

    b. _____

3. List the four pieces of equipment discussed in this module that can be used to start an IV.

    a. _____

    b. _____

    c. _____

    d. _____

4. a. Where is an IV usually started in an infant? _____

    b. Why? _____

5. List four methods that can be used to distend a vein.

    a. _____

    b. _____

    c. _____

    d. _____

6. What term is used to describe the surgical opening of a vein to start an IV? _____

Glossary

abdominal breathing Respirations in which the abdominal muscles and diaphragm are active; the abdomen moves out on inspiration and in on expiration; also called *diaphragmatic breathing.*

accommodation The adaptation or adjustment of the lens of the eye to permit the retina to focus on images or objects at different distances.

acetone A colorless volatile solvent; commonly used as a synonym for ketone body; see *ketone body.*

acid A substance that ionizes in solution to free the hydrogen ion; turns litmus paper pink.

adhesive A substance that causes two surfaces to stick to one another.

adventitious sounds Abnormal sounds, as in the lungs.

alkaline Having characteristics of a base; neutralizes an acid.

alveoli Air sacs of the lungs, at the termination of a bronchiole.

amoeba Any of various protozoans of the genus *Amoeba* and related genera, occurring in water, soil, and as internal animal parasites, characteristically having an indefinite, changeable form and moving by means of pseudopodia.

ampule A small, sterile glass container that usually holds a parenteral medication.

anesthesia (1) The total or partial loss of sensation. (2) The agents that are used to induce a loss of sensation.

Selected definitions in this glossary are from *The American Heritage Dictionary of the English Language,* © 1976 by Houghton Mifflin Company. Reprinted by permission from *The American Heritage Dictionary of the English Language.*

anesthesiologist A physician with special training in the science and skill of administering anesthetic agents.

anesthetic Any agent that causes unconsciousness or insensitivity to pain.

anesthetist A nonphysician who is skilled in administering anesthetic agents.

anoxia A pathological deficiency of oxygen.

antecubital space A depression in the contour of the inner aspect of the elbow; also called *antecubital fossa.*

anticoagulant Any substance that suppresses or counteracts coagulation, especially of the blood.

antiembolic stockings Stockings that are designed to aid the venous flow of immobilized persons or persons with circulatory impairment, or to decrease peripheral venous disorders; also called *support hose* or *TEDs.*

antimicrobial Capable of destroying or suppressing the growth of microorganisms.

antiseptic Any substance that halts the growth of microorganisms, not necessarily by killing them.

anus The excretory opening of the alimentary canal.

apex The narrow or cone-shaped portion of an organ. In the heart, the point located in the area of the midclavicular line near the fifth left intercostal space; in the lung, the narrower, more pointed, upper end.

apical pulse A term used to denote the hearing of the heartbeat through a stethoscope held over the apex of the heart.

apnea The absence of respiration.

appliance Any device worn by a person to facilitate the meeting of basic needs; for example, any device worn to contain drainage from an ostomy.

armboard A firm, flat padded device that is used to straighten the arm and/or hand, to keep an intravenous infusion in place.

ascitic fluid An abnormal accumulation of serous fluid in the abdominal cavity; also called *ascites*.

aseptic Preventing contamination by microorganisms; also see *surgical asepsis*.

asepto syringe A medical instrument that is used to aspirate and instill a fluid. The tip is graduated in size so that it fits into tubings of various sizes; the rounded bulb is used to create suction to fill the barrel and pressure to expel the fluid.

asphyxiation Suffocation.

aspirate To remove gases or fluids by suction.

aspiration pneumonia An acute disease, marked by inflammation of the lungs, that is caused by inhaling substances (vomitus, mucus) into the lungs.

atelectasis The collapse of a group of alveoli due to blockage of the bronchiole passage by secretions.

auricle The external part of the ear; the pinna.

auscultation Listening with a stethoscope to the sounds produced by the body.

autoclave A device that establishes special conditions for sterilization by steam under high pressure.

barrel In a syringe, the cylinder that holds the fluid.

base The broad or wide end of an organ. In the heart, the area located at the second left and right intercostal spaces at the sternal borders; in the lungs, the wide lower end.

bell On the stethoscope, the cone-shaped head that is most often used for listening to heart sounds.

bevel On a needle, the slanting end that contains the opening.

bifurcation The point at which a blood vessel divides or separates into two parts or branches.

bilirubin A yellowish pigment that is derived from the normal or pathological destruction of hemoglobin.

bronchi The branches of the trachea that lead directly to the lungs.

bronchial Pertaining to or affecting one or more bronchi; see *bronchi*.

bronchiole The fine, thin-walled, tubular branches of a bronchus.

burette (1) A plastic, baglike container with tubing that is used to instill a tube-feeding formula. (2) Any glass or plastic tube with graduated levels.

butterfly (1) A type of tape that is used to secure two wound edges together. (2) A device that is used to start intravenous infusions; named for its plastic "wings," which are used to secure the device in place.

button A small, round, plastic device that is used to plug a tracheostomy opening.

cannula A tube that is inserted into a bodily cavity to drain fluid or to insert medication.

canthus The corner at either side of the eye that is formed by the meeting of the upper and lower eyelids. The *inner canthus* is the corner next to the nose; the *outer canthus* is the corner to the outside of the face.

capsule A soluble gelatinous sheath that encloses a dose of oral medication.

catheter A slender flexible tube, of metal, rubber, or plastic, that is inserted into a body channel or cavity to distend or maintain an opening; often used to drain or to instill fluids.

catheterization   The process of inserting a catheter; most commonly used to refer to inserting a catheter into the bladder.

caustic   Able to burn, corrode, dissolve, or otherwise eat away by chemical action.

cecostomy   A surgically devised opening directly from the cecum to the abdominal wall.

cerumen   A yellowish waxy secretion of the external ear; earwax.

claustrophobia   A pathological fear of confined places.

clockwise   In the same direction as the rotating hands of a clock.

colostomy   A surgically devised opening directly from the large intestine to the abdominal wall.

comatose   Unconscious.

combustion   Burning.

compatible   In agreement, harmony, or congenial combination.

complete blood count (CBC)   A measurement that establishes the values of a variety of components of the blood, usually including red blood count, white blood count, hemoglobin, and hematocrit.

concentration of solution   The amount of a specified substance in a unit amount of another substance; may be expressed as a percentage (20% solution), or as a ratio (1:1,000), or as a weight in a fluid amount (100 mg per liter).

conjunctival sac   The saclike inner fold of membrane on the lower eyelid.

constriction   A feeling of pressure or tightness.

contaminated   Having been in contact with microorganisms.

cough   To expel air from the lungs suddenly and noisily.

cough reflex   An involuntary nerve response that causes a cough.

counterclockwise   In a direction opposite that of the movement of the hands of a clock.

culture   The growing of microorganisms in a nutrient medium.

cutdown   A small surgical incision into a vein that is used to establish an intravenous line.

cyanotic   The presence of a bluish discoloration of the skin due to oxygen deficiency.

dead air space   The portion of the airway in which gas exchange does not take place.

dehiscence   The splitting or bursting open of a wound, usually of the abdomen.

dependent edema   See *edema*.

depilatory   A substance or device that is used to remove hair.

dermatological   Pertaining to the skin.

diaphragm   (1) A muscular membranous partition that separates the abdominal and thoracic cavities and that functions in respiration. (2) On a stethoscope, the flat, drumlike head that is used most often for listening to blood pressure, and lung and bowel sounds.

diastole   The normal rhythmic relaxation and dilatation of the heart cavities, during which the cavities are filled with blood.

dilatation   The condition of being abnormally enlarged or stretched.

diluent   A substance that is used to dilute or dissolve.

disinfect   To clean or rid of pathogenic organisms.

disinfectant   An agent that disinfects by destroying, neutralizing, or inhibiting the growth of pathogenic microorganisms.

displacement   The act whereby a substance is replaced by another either in weight or in volume.

distention   Bloat and turgidity from pressure from within; usually referring to the stomach, bowel, or bladder.

diuretic A drug that increases the production of urine.

dorsal recumbent position Person lies on back with knees bent.

dose A specified quantity of a therapeutic agent, prescribed to be taken at one time or at stated intervals.

double-barreled colostomy A colostomy in which there are two openings; one that leads to the proximal colon and one that leads to the distal colon.

douche A stream of water that is applied to a part or cavity of the body for cleaning or medicinal purposes; most frequently, in relationship to the vagina.

droplet nuclei Microscopic particles that, when surrounded by moisture, become airborne.

dullness In percussion, not sharp or intense.

dyspnea Difficulty in breathing.

edema An excessive accumulation of serous fluid in the tissues. *Dependent edema* is fluid that has accumulated in the lower areas of the body due to gravity; *periorbital edema* is a fluid that has accumulated in the soft tissue around the eyes; and *pretibial edema* is fluid that has accumulated over the tibia.

embolus A moving particle in the blood stream.

emulsify To combine two solutions that do not normally mix into one liquid, resulting in a suspension of globules.

endotracheal tube A rubber or plastic tube that is placed in the trachea for purposes of ventilation.

epithelial Related to the cellular surface of the skin or mucous membrane.

ethmoid sinus The open cavity in the ethmoid bone that lies between the eyes and forms part of the nasal cavity.

evisceration To protrude through an incision of a part after an operation.

expectorate To eject from the mouth; spit.

expiration Breathing out.

explosive Pertaining to a sudden, rapid, violent release of energy.

exudate Fluid drainage from cells.

febrile Having an elevated body temperature.

feces Waste excreted from the bowels.

first-intention healing Uncomplicated wound healing that occurs when tissue is constructed between two wound surfaces that touch; also called *primary-intention healing*.

five rights A safety measure that is used to ensure the correct drug administration process. (1) The right drug is given (2) in the right dosage, (3) by the right route, (4) to the right patient, (5) at the right time.

flatness A short, high-pitched sound without resonance or vibration.

flowmeter A mechanical device that monitors the flow of oxygen or other gases or liquids.

fluid overload A situation in which there is more fluid in the circulatory system than it can handle; also called *circulatory overload*.

Foley catheter A rubber catheter with an inflatable balloon at its end. When inflated the balloon holds the catheter in place.

foreskin The loose fold of skin that covers the glans of the penis; the prepuce.

gag reflex A sudden involuntary spasm of the pharynx.

gastric gavage Introducing a feeding by tube into the stomach.

gastrostomy A surgical opening into the stomach; usually for feeding by tube.

gatched bed   A hospital bed that can be bent and raised at the knee area.

gauge   A measurement of the diameter of a needle; a large number indicates a smaller diameter.

gavage   Feeding by means of a tube.

glucose   A dextrose sugar.

glycogen   A carbohydrate that is stored in the tissues.

guaiac   A natural resin that is used as a reagent to test for blood in specimens.

hemoglobin   The oxygen-bearing component of red blood cells.

hemorrhage   Bleeding; especially copious discharge of blood from the vessels.

Homan's sign   Pain in the dorsal calf when the foot is forcibly flexed; indicative of thrombophlebitis.

hub   On a needle, the portion that attaches to a syringe or tubing.

humidifier   An apparatus that increases the humidity of an enclosure.

hydrogen peroxide   A colorless, strongly oxidizing liquid made of hydrogen and oxygen.

hydrometer   An instrument that is used to determine specific gravity.

hyperventilation   Abnormally fast or deep respiration in which excessive quantities of air are taken in and excessive carbon dioxide is expelled, which causes buzzing in the ears, tingling of the extremities, and sometimes fainting.

hypoventilation   Abnormally slow or shallow respirations that result in inadequate air movement and, thus, inadequate oxygenation.

hypoxemia   Inadequate oxygenation of the blood.

hypoxia   An oxygen deficiency of body tissues.

ileoconduit   A surgically constructed pathway for urinary drainage in which a segment of ileum is detached from the rest of the bowel, the ureters are attached to this ileal segment, and one end of the segment is closed while the other opens onto the abdomen in a single stoma; also called *ileobladder* and *ileoloop.*

ileostomy   A surgically devised opening from the ileum to the abdominal wall, the drainage of which is liquid and contains some digestive enzymes.

impaction   Compressed material in a confined space; for example, hardened feces in the bowel.

incubate   To provide conditions for growth.

infiltration   Leaking of fluid from an intravenous line into the tissue surrounding the vein.

inflammation   Localized heat, redness, swelling, and pain as a result of irritation, injury, or infection.

inflatable cuff   A plastic balloon-like device, such as the one around a tracheostomy tube, that, when filled with air, expands, producing pressure on surrounding tissues.

infusion   The introduction of a solution into a vessel; commonly, the introduction of a solution into a vein.

inspection   A careful, critical visual examination.

inspiration   The act of breathing in; inhalation.

instill   To pour in drop by drop; commonly used to indicate very slow fluid introduction.

instillation   The process of pouring in drop by drop; commonly used to indicate a slow process of introducing fluid.

intensive care unit (ICU)   An area of a hospital set aside for the care of the critically ill.

intermittent   Stopping and starting at intervals.

intermittent infusion set   A set that delivers intravenous solutions into a vein at intermittent time periods; also called *Heparinlock* and *Heparin trap*.

intradermal   Injected into the skin layers.

intramuscular (IM)   Injected into the muscle tissue.

intravenous   Placed into a vein; often used to refer to the fluid being given directly into a vein.

intubation   The placement of a tube into an organ or passage; often used to refer to placing an endotracheal tube into the trachea.

irrigate   To wash out with water or a medicated solution.

karaya   A vegetable gum that is produced from the species *sterculia;* commonly used as a sealing material for ostomy appliances because of its nonirritating and protective properties.

ketone body   A chemical compound that is produced as an abnormal end product of fat metabolism, and is excreted in the urine and through the lungs.

laminar airflow hood   A device that provides a controlled flow of microorganism-free air layers within a hood; used to create an environment for the sterile preparation of medications.

laparotomy   A surgical incision into any part of the abdominal wall.

lateral   Toward the side; away from the midline of the body.

lather   A light foam that is formed by soap or detergent agitated in water.

lavage   Washing, especially of a hollow organ (stomach or lower bowel) by repeated injections of water.

Levin tube   A slender rubber or plastic tube that is usually used for decompres-

sion or nasogastric feedings; also called *nasogastric tube*.

liniment   A medicinal fluid that is applied to the skin by rubbing.

liter   The metric equivalent of 1.0567 quarts.

lithotomy position   Person lies on back with legs flexed and spread apart.

litmus paper   White paper that is impregnated with litmus and is used as an acid-base indicator.

lobe   A subdivision of the lung that is bounded by fissures and connective tissue.

local   Of or affecting a limited part of the body; not systemic.

lotion   A medicated liquid, especially one containing a substance in suspension for external application.

Luer-Lok   A brand name that is commonly used to refer to a type of syringe tip that fastens securely to the needle by a twisting action.

lumbar puncture (LP)   The insertion of a needle into the spinal canal for purposes of withdrawing spinal fluid or instilling contrast-dye materials; also called *spinal tap*.

lumen   The inner, open space of a needle, tube, or vessel.

lung   A spongy, saclike respiratory organ; also see *lobe* and *segment*.

maceration   An area of skin that has softened and deteriorated following prolonged contact with moisture.

meatus   The opening of the urethra onto the surface of the body.

medial   Toward the midline of the body.

meniscus   The curved, upward surface of a liquid in a container.

microorganism   An animal or plant of microscopic size, especially a bacterium or protozoan.

mucousPertaining to mucus.

mucusThe viscous suspension of mucin, water, cells, and inorganic salts that is secreted as a protective lubricant coating by glands in the mucous membranes.

nasal mucosa The mucous-membrane lining of the nose.

nasogastric tubeA long slender rubber or plastic tube that is introduced through the nose and esophagus into the stomach, for purposes of feeding or aspiration.

nebulizerA device that converts a liquid into a fine spray.

necrosisThe death of living tissue.

needleA hollow pointed device that is used to deliver medication into the tissue or to aspirate from the tissue.

normal flora Those microorganisms that are usually found at a site and that do not cause disease by their presence there.

NPONothing by mouth.

objectiveBased on observable phenomena.

obturatorAny device that closes the opening in a channel such as a tracheostomy tube.

occultHidden.

ocularOf or pertaining to the eye.

ointmentOne of the numerous, highly viscous or semisolid substances that are used on the skin as a cosmetic, an emolient, or a medicament; an unguent; a salve.

ophthalmicOf or pertaining to the eye or eyes; ocular.

ostomateA person who has an ostomy.

ostomyA surgically constructed opening from a body organ to the exterior of the body.

oticOf or pertaining to the ear.

oxygenationTreating, combining, or infusing with oxygen.

palpationExamining or exploring by touch.

paracentesisThe insertion of a trocar into the abdominal cavity for the removal of excess fluid.

paralytic ileus Immobilization of the intestinal wall caused by acute obstruction and distention.

parenteral fluid Fluid given directly into tissues or blood vessels.

patentOpen.

pathogenAny agent, especially a microorganism such as a bacterium or fungus, that causes disease.

pectoralis muscles Four muscles of the chest.

pedal pulseA pulse wave that can be felt over the arteries of the feet.

penisThe male organ of copulation and urinary excretion.

Penrose drainA very flat, soft-latex tubing; short lengths are often used to provide drainage from a surgical wound, while longer lengths are sometimes used as tourniquets.

percussion(1) A process of striking a finger held against the body surface with a fingertip of the opposite hand and listening to the resulting sound as an assessment tool. (2) The striking of a hand on the chest wall to produce a vibration or shock that loosens secretions retained in the lungs.

perinealPertaining to the perineum.

perineumThe portion of the body in the pelvic area that is occupied by urogenital passages and the rectum.

pHA measure of the acidity or alkalinity of a solution; 7.0 is neutral, and numbers below that are acidic and numbers above it are alkaline, in a range of 1 to 14.

pharynxThe section of the digestive tract that extends from the nasal cavities to the larynx, there becoming continuous with the esophagus; functions as a passageway for both food and air.

phlebitis   Inflammation of a vein.

plunger   In a syringe, the pistonlike rod that expels the fluid from the barrel.

pneumonitis   Acute inflammation of the lung.

point   On a needle, the sharpened end.

postural hypotension   A sudden drop in blood pressure that is caused by a change in position, from lying to sitting or standing; may cause dizziness, fainting, and falling; also called *orthostatic hypotension.*

prongs   (1) Sharp or pointed projections. (2) A device that delivers oxygen at the nares.

prophylactic   Acting to defend against or to prevent something, especially disease.

protein   An organic compound of living matter that contains amino acids as its basic structural unit.

pulmonary embolus   Obstruction of the pulmonary artery or one of its branches by an embolus.

purulent   Containing or secreting pus.

rales   Abnormal or pathological respiratory sounds heard on auscultation.

reagent   A substance that is used in a chemical reaction to detect, measure, examine, or produce other substances.

rebound tenderness   The pain or discomfort that is experienced when pressure is quickly withdrawn from an area.

recovery room (RR)   An area of a hospital set aside for the care of the immediate post-operative patient; also called the post-anesthesia room (PAR).

rectal   Pertaining to the rectum.

recumbent   Lying down; reclining.

regurgitation   Flowing backward, as in vomiting; also as blood flows backward through incompetent valves in the heart.

resonance   In percussion, a vibrating sound that is produced in the normal chest.

respirator   A mechanical apparatus that administers artificial respiration; a ventilator.

retraction   An abnormal pulling in of soft tissue of the chest on inspiration; commonly seen in the supraclavicular, intercostal, and substernal areas.

rhonchi   Coarse rattling sounds that are produced by secretions in the bronchial tubes; a type of rale.

route   In medication, a path of administration.

saliva   The secretion of the salivary gland, which contains mucus and digestive enzymes.

sanguinous   Pertaining to or involving blood; containing blood.

second-intention healing.   Healing that occurs through granulation beginning at the base of the wound; also called *secondary-intention healing.*

secretions   Substances that are exuded from cells or blood.

segment   A subdivision of a lobe of the lung.

semi-Fowler's position   A supine position with the head raised 12 to 18 inches.

serosanguinous   Containing both serum and blood.

serous   Containing, secreting, or resembling serum.

shaft   On a needle, the long narrow stem.

shock   A syndrome characterized by insufficient blood and oxygen supply to the tissues; may be caused by hemorrhage, infection, trauma, and the like.

sigmoidostomy   A surgically constructed opening from the sigmoid colon to the abdominal wall.

Sim's position   A side-lying position with the top leg flexed forward.

singultus   Hiccup.

sphenoid sinus   The open area in the center of the sphenoid bone that lies at the base of the brain.

spore   (1) An asexual, usually single celled reproductive organism that is characteristic of nonflowering plants, such as fungi, mosses, and ferns. (2) A microorganism in a dormant or resting state that is especially resistant to destruction.

sputum   Expectorated matter that contains secretions from the lower respiratory tract.

sterile   Free from bacteria or other microorganisms.

sterile technique   A method of functioning that is designed to maintain the sterility of sterile objects.

sterilize   To render sterile; also see *sterile.*

sternum   A long flat bone that forms the midventral support of most of the ribs; the breastbone.

stethoscope   An instrument that is used for listening to sounds produced in the body; also see *bell* and *diaphragm.*

stock drugs   Medications kept in a general supply, to be dispensed to individual patients.

stoma   The opening on the skin of any surgically constructed passage from a body organ to the exterior of the body.

straight catheter   A plain catheter without a bulb or balloon on its end.

subcutaneous (SC)   Pertaining to tissue beneath the layers of the skin; sometimes called *hypodermic (H),* a term that can also mean "injection," and is, therefore, not good usage.

subjective   Personal; in assessment, refers to information from the patient's viewpoint.

suction   Withdrawing (gas or fluids) through the use of negative pressure.

suppository   A solid medication that is designed to melt in a body cavity other than the mouth.

suppuration   The formation or discharge of pus.

surgical asepsis   The techniques that are designed to maintain the sterility of previously sterilized items and to prevent the introduction of any microorganisms into the body.

suspension   A relatively coarse, noncolloidal dispersion of solid particles in a liquid.

symmetry   The equal configuration of opposite sides.

symphysis pubis   The area at the front center of the pelvis, where the pubic bones from either side fuse into one bone.

syringe   A medical instrument that is used to aspirate and expel fluids.

systemic   Of, pertaining to, or affecting the entire body.

systole   The rhythmic contraction of the heart, especially of the ventricles, by which blood is driven through the aorta and pulmonary artery after each dilation, or diastole.

tablet   A small flat pellet of medication that is taken orally.

TEDs   A brand name that is commonly used as a synonym for antiembolic stockings; see *antiembolic stockings.*

thoracotomy   A surgical incision of the chest wall.

three checks   A safety measure that is used to ensure procuring the correct drug. The label is checked (1) before picking up the medication, (2) while holding it in the hand, and (3) after returning the container to its storage place.

thrombophlebitis   Inflammation of a vein resulting from the presence of a thrombus.

thrombus A clot occluding a blood vessel or formed in a heart cavity, produced by coagulation of the blood.

thyroid gland A two-lobed endocrine gland that is located in front of and on either side of the trachea.

tolerance In activity, the capacity to endure.

Toomey syringe A large-barreled syringe with a graduated tip that fits into a tubing.

topical Applied or pertaining to a local part of the body.

tortuous Having or marked by repeated turns or bends; winding; twisting.

tourniquet Any device that is used to stop temporarily the flow of blood through a large artery in a limb.

trachea A thin-walled tube of cartilaginous and membranous tissue that descends from the larynx to the bronchi, carrying air to the lungs.

tracheal ring The proximal, cartilaginous ringlike structure that surrounds the trachea.

tracheostomy A surgically devised opening into the trachea from the surface of the neck.

transfer forceps A sterile instrument with pincer or pronglike tips that is used to move sterile items from one sterile area to another.

Trendelenburg position A position in which the head is down from the horizontal.

tympanic membrane The thin, semitransparent, oval-shaped membrane that separates the middle ear from the inner ear; also called *eardrum.*

tympany In percussion, a low-pitched, drumlike sound.

umbilicus The navel; the site on the abdomen where the umbilical cord was attached during gestation.

unit dose A system of dispensing drugs in which each dose is packaged and labeled individually.

ureterostomy A surgically devised opening in which a ureter is brought out to drain directly through a stoma onto the abdomen.

urethra The tubular structure leading from the bladder to the surface of the body.

urinometer An instrument that is used for determining the specific gravity of urine.

uvula The small, conical fleshy mass of tissue that is suspended from the center of the soft palate above the back of the tongue.

vagina The passage leading from the external genital orifice to the uterus in female mammals.

vaginal Pertaining to the vagina.

venipuncture The puncture of a vein; for example, in drawing blood or administering intravenous fluids and medication.

venous pressure The pressure of blood in the veins; often measured in the superior vena cava. This measurement, called *central venous pressure* (CVP) is normally between 4 and 10 cm water.

vial A small glass container that is sealed with a rubber stopper; may be used for single or multiple doses.

vibration A rapid, rhythmic to-and-fro motion

viscosity Having relatively high resistance to flow; thickness.

void The emptying of urine from the bladder through the urethra; to urinate.

vulva The external female genitalia, including the labia majora, the labia minora, the clitoris, and the vestibule of the vagina.

wheal A small acute swelling on the skin; may be caused by intradermal injections or by insect bites and allergies.

wheezes Hoarse whistling sounds, produced by breathing, that are considered abnormal.

xiphoid process The lower tip of the sternum.

Z-track A method for injecting medications that are particularly irritating or which stain the tissues; does not allow medication to track out through the needle hole.

Answers to Quizzes

Module 27

1. Urinometer
2. A measurement of the concentration of a liquid
3. The measurement of hydrogen ions
4. Far fewer drugs interfere with testing.
5. Percentages of glucose
6. Testape
7. If the patient has eaten red meat within the last three days
8. Because the material may dry out or change in character if left standing
9. b
10. d
11. b

Module 28

1. Any three of the following: feeding; instilling medications; irrigating the stomach; gastric suction
2. So as not to damage the mucosa on insertion
3. c
4. b
5. c
6. a
7. d
8. b

Module 29

1. a
2. c
3. b
4. b
5. a
6. c
7. a

Module 30

1. An opening from the ileum (small intestine)
2. The drainage is liquid and contains digestive enzymes, which increases the potential for skin breakdown.
3. An ileoloop drains urine; it serves as a drainage path from the ureters. An ileostomy drains fecal material.
4. a. To protect the skin
   b. To prevent occlusion of the stoma
5. Seated on a toilet or commode
6. Approximately 1,000 ml
7. 240 ml in each syringe, for a total of 720 ml
8. 3 to 5 inches
9. Approximately 15 minutes
10. Approximately 30 minutes after the patient gets up from the toilet
11. Because of the potential for urinary-tract infection

Module 31

1. a. Oxygen tent
   b. Nasal catheter
   c. Nasal cannula
   d. Oxygen mask
2. c
3. b
4. d
5. a
6. b
7. b
8. d

Module 32

1. Any five of the following: color, odor, size, shape, symmetry, movement

2. a. Size
   b. Shape
   c. Equality of pupils
3. In a position above 45 degrees
4. 4 and 10 centimeters
5. a. What is being done
   b. Why it is being done
   c. What the patient can do to make it easier for himself or herself and the nurse
6. Around the eyes
7. Because the breasts may be particularly sensitive at the time of menstruation
8. Because palpation and percussion can change the bowel sounds that might be heard
9. Fifth intercostal space near the nipple line (the apex)
10. Any one of the following: bronchial obstruction; chronic lung disease; shallow breathing

Module 33

1. Because persons who are immobile tend to breath shallowly, leaving areas of the lungs unused, which may collapse or accumulate secretions. Deep breathing opens and expands these areas, and encourages secretions to move.
2. 1:2
3. To use gravity to facilitate the movement of secretions from the lungs to an area where they can be coughed up and expectorated
4. a. Sitting upright
   b. Leaning 45 degrees to right
   c. Leaning 45 degrees to left
   d. Leaning 45 degrees forward
   e. Leaning 30 to 45 degrees backward
5. All positions are lying head down at a 30- to 45-degree angle:
   a. Lying on right side, shoulders at a 90-degree angle to bed
   b. Lying on right side, shoulders at a 45-degree angle to bed
   c. Lying flat on back
   d. Lying on abdomen

6. To loosen secretions so that they will drain
7. To encourage deep breathing by giving immediate feedback on performance

Module 34

1. Elective surgery is planned; emergency surgery is urgent.
2. Your care must fit the specific time frame; but will include the essentials of care.
3. a. Deep breathing and coughing
   b. Moving in bed and getting in and out of bed
   c. Leg exercises
4. To empty the contents of the stomach, thereby preventing vomiting and possible aspiration
5. a. To remove dirt, oil, and microorganisms from the skin
   b. To prevent the growth of remaining microorganisms
   c. To leave the skin undamaged and unirritated
6. Because studies have shown a reduced infection rate over earlier preoperative shaves
7. a. It is more comfortable for the patient.
   b. There is less chance of nicks and cuts.
8. a. To establish a baseline
   b. To detect whether the patient is febrile, which might indicate the presence of infection
9. a. Removing colored nail polish
   b. Removing makeup
   c. Removing dentures
10. a. To notify them in case of emergency
    b. To tell them when the surgery is completed

Module 35

1. a. Tissues
   b. Emesis basin
   c. Equipment for taking vital signs

(thermometer, stethoscope, sphyg-
momanometer, blood pressure cuff)
   d. IV stand
2. Any six of the following: time of arrival on unit; responsiveness; vital signs;
   skin condition; dressing; presence of IV;
   presence of bladder catheter; presence
   of other drainage tubes; safety and comfort
3. a. Is the catheter unclamped?
   b. Is the catheter connected to the
      appropriate drainage container?
   c. Is the catheter freely draining?
   d. What are the amount and character-
      istics of the urine?
4. 2:30 p.m. Received from RR. Drowsy,
   but answers to name call. T = 97°; P =
   78; R = 20, deep and easy; and BP =
   128/88. Skin warm and dry. Dressing
   clean, dry, and intact. P. Johnson, RN
5. Any seven of the following: operation
   performed; postoperative diagnosis;
   anesthetic agents used; estimated blood
   loss; blood and/or fluid replacement in
   surgery and RR; type and location of
   drains; vital signs when patient left RR;
   medications administered in RR; output; physician's orders
6. Any two of the following: encourage
   early ambulation; encourage patient's
   participation; keep patient and unit
   tidy; listen; do patient teaching

Module 36

1. d
2. d
3. d
4. b
5. c
6. c
7. a
8. d
9. T
10. F
11. T
12. F
13. F

14. Any two of the following: heat sensitive
    tape on outside of package; glass-tubing
    indicator inside pack; vacuum seal on
    bottle; intact seal on commercial pack-
    age

Module 37

1. a. To remove microorganisms
   b. To remove dirt and oil
   c. To leave an antibacterial residue on
      the skin
2. Wood is too difficult to sterilize.
3. Fingernails and knuckles (or areas with
   folds and crevices)
4. It continues to inhibit the growth of
   microorganisms.
5. So that the water containing dirt, oil,
   and microorganisms drains off the
   elbows, keeping the hands the cleanest
   part
6. It lessens the possibility of contaminating the gloves while putting them on.
7. a. When serving as a scrub nurse in the
      operating room
   b. When serving as a scrub nurse in the
      delivery room
   c. When assisting with certain invasive
      diagnostic procedures

Module 38

1. a. Cleaning
   b. Instilling medications
2. To instill medication
3. One of the following: eye; wound;
   bladder; catheter
4. One of the following: ear; nasogastric
   tube; vagina
5. a. Too high temperature
   b. Too great pressure
   c. Incorrect solution concentration
6. That the drainage or outflow tubing
   not be blocked or clamped while fluid
   is being introduced
7. When the tympanic membrane is not
   intact

8. The fluid will tend to drain out too quickly and not come in contact with all vaginal surfaces.

Module 39

1. Any three of the following: fear of pain; anxiety over intrusion into body; embarrassment over loss of modesty; anxiety over relationship to reproductive system
2. There was no opportunity for the patient to express concerns or ask questions.
3. b
4. c
5. c
6. c
7. d
8. a
9. c

Module 40

1. a. Protection
   b. Absorption
   c. Application of pressure
2. a. To maintain sterile technique
   b. To observe and describe the wound
   c. To use appropriate dressing materials
3. a. Amount
   b. Color
   c. Consistency
   d. Odor
4. Any three of the following: edges approximated; smooth contour; minimal inflammation; minimal edema
5. Nonadherent
6. Paper tape

Module 41

1. a. To allay fears
   b. To elicit cooperation
2. Because pathogens can travel down the moist, continuous respiratory tract
3. To remove amniotic fluid and mucus

that accumulates in the back of the throat and interferes with breathing
4. To obtain adequate suction or pull
5. 15 seconds
6. Three times

Module 42

1. b
2. a
3. d
4. c
5. b
6. c
7. c
8. a
9. d

Module 43

1. a. Stock supply
   b. Individual patient supply
2. a. As it is taken off the shelf
   b. Before opening
   c. Before it is replaced
3. a. Right drug
   b. Right dose
   c. Right route
   d. Right patient
   e. Right time
4. a. Identification band
   b. Ask to state name
5. gr 1/60
6. 30 ml
7. 15 or 16 min
8. 1 ʒ
9. 300 mg
10. 2 teaspoons
11. d
12. c
13. b

Module 44

1. a
2. c

3. b
4. Because of the danger of aspiration pneumonia with oil-based solutions
5. Ethmoid and sphenoid sinuses
6. Any three of the following: to protect; to soften; to soothe; to provide relief from itching
7. a. Dorsal recumbent position with knees elevated
   b. Sim's position
8. 20 minutes
9. Beyond the internal sphincter
10. To help the patient relax

Module 45

1. a. Glass or Luer-Lok
   b. Disposable plastic
   c. Prefilled
   d. Insulin
   e. Tuberculin
2. U-100
3. length, gauge
4. a. Vials
   b. Ampules
5. Vial
6. Any three of the following: almost complete absorption; more rapid absorption; gastric disturbances do not affect the medication; patient does not have to be conscious or rational
7. 25-gauge, 5/8-inch needle
8. a. Upper arms
   b. Anterior aspect of thighs
   c. Lower abdominal wall
9. Intramuscular route
10. 22-gauge, 1½-inch needle
11. a. Upper iliac crest
    b. Inner crease of the buttocks
    c. Outer lateral edge of the body
    d. Lower (inferior) gluteal fold
12. Any three of the following: no large nerves or blood vessels; cleaner; less fatty; several positions can be used; better for small children because gluteal muscle is not well developed until after a child walks
13. a. Smaller muscle, so not capable of absorbing larger amounts of medication
    b. Danger of injury to the radial nerve.
14. The plunger is pulled back (aspiration).
15. To see whether the needle has penetrated a blood vessel
16. a
17. b

Module 46

1. a. Sterile solution
   b. Administration set
   c. IV stand
   d. Means of entry into the vein
   e. Tape and cleaning and dressing materials
   f. Ointment as indicated
2. No contaminated air can enter the container and come in contact with the sterile fluid.
3. Obtain another container and return the cloudy one to the source.
4. a. Hang it so the fluid level is higher.
   b. Put the second container on an extension hanger to make it lower than the first.
5. a. 32 gtt/min
   b. 24 gtt/min
   c. 33 gtt/min
   d. 33 gtt/min
6. Container every 24 hours, tubing every 48 hours
7. Too much fluid over a short period of time will simply be excreted *or* will cause fluid overload; too little fluid may not meet the body's needs for fluid.
8. a. Direct pressure on the site
   b. Raising the patient's arm above the head
9. a. Clot over the needle lumen
   b. Clogged filter
   c. Lumen of the needle against the vein wall
   d. Kinking or pressure on the tubing
   e. Arm position
10. a. Pain
    b. Redness

c. Swelling
d. Warmth
11. a. Pallor
    b. Swelling
    c. Coolness
    d. Pain
    e. Diminished IV flow
12. a. Review entire system.
    b. Check bottle.
    c. Check drip chamber.
    d. Check tubing.
    e. Check IV site.
    f. Check extremity if armboard is in use.

Module 47

1. Because they are made of a self-sealing rubber; if a needle were inserted in the plastic, the system would leak.
2. Slowly (approximately 1 ml per minute), because it will be less irritating
3. To provide access to the circulatory system without having to do repeated venipuncture
4. To keep blood from coagulating in the lock
5. 50–100, depending on the drug manufacturer's directions

Module 48

1. a. May imply serious illness
    b. Pain
    c. Immobility
2. Any two of the following: to maintain daily fluid requirements; to replace past losses; to provide large amount of fluid rapidly; to provide medication
3. a. Short-beveled needle
    b. Butterfly
    c. Intravenous catheter inside a needle
    d. Intravenous catheter over a needle
4. a. Scalp
    b. Less chance of dislocation because of less movement in that area
5. a. Applying a tourniquet
    b. Hand pumping
    c. Keeping limb in dependent position
    d. Applying warm moist heat
6. Cutdown